Introduction to
Evidence-Based Practice
A Practical Guide for Nursing

SECOND EDITION

Lisa Hopp, PhD, RN, FAAN
Dean and Professor
College of Nursing
Director, Indiana Center for Evidence Based Nursing Practice: A JBI
    Affiliate Center
Purdue University Northwest
Hammond, Indiana

Leslie Rittenmeyer, PsyD, RN, CNE
Professor Emerita
College of Nursing
Purdue University Northwest
Hammond, Indiana

F.A. DAVIS
Philadelphia

Printed in the United States of America

Last digit indicates print number: 10 9 8 7 6 5 4 3 2

Acquisitions Editor: Jacalyn Sharp

Manager of Project and eProject Management: Catherine H. Carroll

Senior Content Project Manager: Christine M. Abshire

Art and Design Manager: Carolyn O'Brien

As new scientific information becomes available through basic and clinical research, recommended treatments and drug therapies undergo changes. The author(s) and publisher have done everything possible to make this book accurate, up to date, and in accord with accepted standards at the time of publication. The author(s), editors, and publisher are not responsible for errors or omissions or for consequences from application of the book, and make no warranty, expressed or implied, in regard to the contents of the book. Any practice described in this book should be applied by the reader in accordance with professional standards of care used in regard to the unique circumstances that may apply in each situation. The reader is advised always to check product information (package inserts) for changes and new information regarding dose and contraindications before administering any drug. Caution is especially urged when using new or infrequently ordered drugs.

ISBN 978-0-8036-6663-4

Library of Congress Cataloging-in-Publication Data

Names: Hopp, Lisa, 1956- author. | Rittenmeyer, Leslie, author.
Title: Introduction to evidence-based practice : a practical guide for nursing / Lisa Hopp, Leslie Rittenmeyer.
Description: Second edition. | Philadelphia : F.A. Davis, [2021] | Includes bibliographical references and index.
Identifiers: LCCN 2020045424 (print) | LCCN 2020045425 (ebook) | ISBN 9780803666634 (paperback) | ISBN 9781719645553 (ebook)
Subjects: MESH: Evidence-Based Nursing | Nursing Process | Models, Nursing
Classification: LCC RT41 (print) | LCC RT41 (ebook) | NLM WY 100.7 | DDC 610.73–dc23
LC record available at https://lccn.loc.gov/2020045424
LC ebook record available at https://lccn.loc.gov/2020045425

For my mate, Eric, who inspires me to think big;
for my parents, who taught me to work hard;
for my girls, who are my reason to be;
and for patients, who are the reason we nurse.

-LH

This book is dedicated to my husband Dennis,
who worries that I spend too much time on my computer;
our family, who sustains me;
and to nurses at the bedside,
who are heroic in their everyday work.

-LR

Foreword

Pressure ulcers, catheter-acquired urinary tract infections, falls, safe medication administration, and many other health problems are universal. As I interact with nurses, physicians, physiotherapists, and other health-care providers across the world, I am struck by the commonness of our problems and our desire to improve outcomes. Our cultures, contexts, and worldviews certainly vary; remarkably, we can share the same body of evidence. The way we use the evidence and how patients respond and experience their health are unique.

In this book, you will learn how to use the evidence-based practice process to provide the best nursing care possible in your local context. You will find that evidence-based practice is not merely an interesting academic exercise that you just "get through" whether you are in your undergraduate or graduate studies. Rather, you will learn how evidence informs the practical, everyday actions that you take on behalf of your patients.

Drs. Hopp and Rittenmeyer have written the book in any easy-to-read and pragmatic way. You will quickly understand how to begin using evidence to make the best decisions for your nursing practice. The authors intend that any nurse or student can use the book to get started with evidence. I particularly like that each chapter begins with a clinical story that you will likely connect to your own practice. These stories illustrate how practical and fundamental it is to have the right knowledge for the right patient at the right time.

You are busy clinicians, thinking on your feet. This book is meant to help you think in action but use the best available evidence with your clinical expertise to make decisions incorporating your patients' preferences and values. The time has come for a book that allows clinicians and students to learn about evidence-based practice in a straightforward, clear, and uncluttered manner.

ALAN PEARSON AM, RN, ONC, DIPNED, MSc, PHD, FRCNA, FCN, FAAG, FRCN
Founding Executive Director and Professor Emeritus
of Evidence-Based Health Care
Founding Executive Director, JBI
University of Adelaide

Preface

We conceptualized this text around the belief that nurses want what is best for their patients. Through our work in the evidence-based practice movement, we have come to learn that this is not always a simple endeavor. The rapid explosion of information and its sources has contributed to the complexity of practicing in a way that yields desirable outcomes. In order to access, appraise, and utilize the available information, students and practicing nurses alike need to learn first about evidence-based practice. In this book, we present the elemental principles that demystify the process in a way that is easily accessible and excites passion for patient care. We are keenly aware that there is significant need for nurses to gain a global perspective in order to truly find and implement the best available evidence. We believe this book provides that perspective as well.

We intend that clinicians and undergraduate and graduate students will find the book useful. Its aim is to present a comprehensive survey of evidence-based nursing practice that faculty can use throughout an undergraduate and graduate curricula and clinical educators can use throughout a staff development program. Our goal is to provide information that is thorough yet concise and practical for clinicians, students, and faculty. Each chapter begins with a clinical story that serves as a real-world illustration of evidence-based practice in action.

We have designed the material to be flexible. Educators may use the book across a curriculum or program as learning about evidence-based practice unfolds. Alternatively, they may use it as the primary text for a course focused on evidence-based practice. Faculty in graduate programs will find it particularly useful as a scaffold for upper division courses. We also believe this book could be valuable for any practicing nurses who want to learn the basic principles of evidence-based nursing practice.

In Unit I, we set the stage by addressing the basic questions of what evidence-based nursing practice is, how it makes a difference, and where evidence comes from. We present a global perspective in terms of both the history of evidence-based practice and appropriate sources of evidence. In Unit II, we address a sample of pragmatic models and framework of evidence-based practice. We emphasize that models help structure the process of making changes in practice. We have picked models that help individual nurses or systems transfer evidence into everyday nursing practice. Unit III deconstructs the evidence-based process from asking a question through evaluation. Using Hayes's 5 As structure, we align evidence-based practice and the nursing process. Finally, in Unit IV, we put it all together in examples of the entire evidence-based practice process in nursing specialty areas. Each chapter is structured in a parallel fashion to illustrate how evidence-based practice can address a nurse-sensitive outcome. These chapters integrate the evidence-based practice process from problem recognition to outcome evaluation and quality improvement.

Though the stages of the evidence-based practice process have remained stable since the first edition, our updates in the second edition reflect the most important advances how evidence-based practice improves health and health care. In addition to new references and knowledge that underpin all chapters, we have updated the clinical stories to match changes in the evidence base and priorities of practice. Readers will find substantial updates to the chapters related to models and frameworks (Chapter 5 and 6), evidence sources and searching (Chapter 9), advances in patient preferences (Chapter 12), progress in implementation science and interventions to move evidence into practice (Chapter 13), the intersections of evidence-based quality improvement and local policy development (Chapter 14) and national and international policy (Chapter 15) and assessment of outcomes (Chapter 16). In Unit IV, readers will find updates to the application of the evidence-based practice process to clinical exemplars and a completely revised chapter for pediatric nursing.

It is our hope that we have constructed a book that has utility in the beginning, middle, and end of an undergraduate curriculum or staff development program. We intend that it will remain not on bookshelves but in the hands of students and nurses as a useful resource for basic information about evidence-based practice.

Contributors

Manisa Baker, DNP, RN, APRN, CCNS, CCRN-k
Assistant Professor
Purdue University Northwest
Hammond, Indiana

Janet Davis, PhD, MSN, MBA, RN, CNE
Assistant Professor, Nursing
Purdue University Northwest
Hammond, Indiana

Amanda L. Kratovil-Mailhiot, PhD, RN
Assistant Professor, Nursing
Purdue University Northwest
Hammond, Indiana

Patti Ludwig-Beymer, PhD, RN, CTN-A, NEA-BC, CPPS, FAAN
Associate Professor
Purdue University Northwest
Hammond, Indiana

Ellen Moore, DNP, RN, FNP-BC
Associate Professor Emeritus, Nursing
Purdue University Northwest
Hammond, Indiana

Cheryl Moredich, DNP, RN, WHNP-BC
Associate Professor and Director of Online Programs, Nursing
Purdue University Northwest
Hammond, Indiana

Alan Pearson, RN, ONC, DipNED, MSc, PhD, FRCNA, FCN, FAAG, FRCN
Professor Emeritus of Evidence-Based Health Care
University of Adelaide
Founding Executive Director
JBI
Adelaide, South Australia

Beth Vottero, PhD, RN, CNE
Associate Professor, Nursing
Purdue University Northwest
Hammond, Indiana

Jane Walker, PhD, RN
Associate Professor Emeritus, Nursing
Purdue University Northwest
Hammond, Indiana

Kim Whalen, MLIS
Associate Professor of Library Services
Valparaiso University
Valparaiso, Indiana

Reviewers

Vera Dauffenbach, MSN, EdD, RN
Associate Professor
Bellin College
Green Bay, Wisconsin

Paula M. Davis-Huffman, DNP, APRN,
  PPCNP-BC
Assistant Professor
Florida Gulf Coast University
Fort Myers, Florida

Jenny D. Erkfitz, RN, MSN
Academic Coach, Nursing
Instructional Connections, Inc.
Noblesville, Indiana

Maria Kraft, MSN, RN
Adjunct Faculty
Concordia University
Portland, Oregon

Lori Rhudy, RN, PhD, CNRN, ACNS-BC
Nurse Scientist
Mayo Clinic
Rochester, Minnesota

Joy Whitlatch, EdD, MSN, RN
Associate Professor
Chamberlain University
Downers Grove, Illinois

Roseann M. Zahara-Such, DNP, APRN,
  PCNS-BC
Assistant Clinical Professor of Nursing
Purdue University-Northwest
Hammond, Indiana

Acknowledgments

Many people have supported us throughout the writing of this book. We have the good fortune to work with colleagues whom we look forward to seeing every day and who make our days at the university seem like working from home.

If we spend a bit too much time at work, it is because of the commitment and friendships we share with our fellow faculty at Purdue University Northwest. We are particularly thankful for Dean Emerita Peggy Gerard's support, whose leadership earned our college a legacy of respect upon which our careers in nursing and evidence based practice was founded.

To our contributors, Drs. Manisa Baker, Janet Davis, Amanda Kratovil-Mailhiot, Patti Ludwig-Beymer, Ellen Moore, Cheryl Moredich, Jane Walker, Beth Vottero, and Ms. Kim Whalen, we thank you for your willingness to contribute your stories, scholarly work, and collegiality. Your individual perspectives and unique talents added dimension and depth to the book. We wish to particularly acknowledge Dr. Alan Pearson, the founding executive director who had the "big idea" to launch JBI that has had such profound impact on our careers as well as evidence-based health care worldwide. Finally, we wish to acknowledge the work of Dr. Michelle Block who contributed to the first edition. We lost our dear friend and colleague between editions. We miss her intellect, friendship, and optimism every day.

At F. A. Davis, we would like to thank editors Jacalyn Sharp and Christine Abshire, who have kept us moving forward with the persistent kindness and nudging of gentlewomen.

Finally, we acknowledge our global colleagues within the Joanna Briggs Collaboration and Institute for their commitment to improve the health of people in every nation through evidence-based practice.

Contents

Background and Context

What Is Evidence-Based Practice and Who Cares?

This unit sets the stage for learning about evidence-based practice. In Chapter 1 you will learn the history of evidence-based practice worldwide and its progress in the United States. In Chapter 2, you will learn how to carefully define evidence-based practice by understanding each of its key elements and how it makes a difference in everyday clinical nursing practice. In Chapter 3, a global leader in evidence-based practice discusses the importance of global thinking and use of international evidence. These chapters are fundamental to understanding how evidence-based practice fits into your clinical practice as well as nurses' practice worldwide. Each chapter begins with a clinical story, and the story unfolds throughout each chapter. This will help you connect new concepts with clinical practice.

CHAPTER 1

Professional Nursing and Evidence-Based Practice

Lisa Hopp

- Define *evidence-based practice* in the context professional nursing.

- Defend the importance of using evidence to make professional nursing decisions.

- Differentiate clinical decisions based on nursing traditions from those based on evidence.

- Describe how evidence-based practice evolved from research utilization.

Agency for Healthcare
  Research and Quality
  (AHRQ)
Bibliographic databases
Centers for Medicare and
  Medicaid Services (CMS)
Cochrane Collaboration
Conduct and Utilization of
  Research in Nursing (CURN)
  Project

Cumulative Index to Nursing
  and Allied Health Literature
  (CINAHL)
Evidence-based practice
JBI
Medical Literature Analysis and
  Retrieval System (MEDLINE)
National Academy of Medicine
  (formerly Institute of Medicine
  [IOM])

KEY TERMS (continued)

National Guideline
  Clearinghouse (NGC)
Nursing traditions
Randomized controlled trial (RCT)

Research utilization
Western Interstate Commission
  for Higher Education (WICHE)
  Project

Clinical Story

It is 10:00 p.m. Maria is caring for a 50-year-old female patient who had abdominal surgery about 8 hours ago. Maria also has four other postsurgical patients assigned to her. She enters the room to assess the patient's vital signs and comfort level and to check her abdominal wound dressing. She sees that the patient has an IV catheter for fluid and medications, and the patient says that she has not been able to urinate since she returned from surgery. The patient tells Maria that her pain level is 5/10 and that she is reluctant to move around because "it hurts too much."

Maria knows that the patient's pain control is a priority and that abdominal surgery patients typically receive IV fluids until they are ready to drink fluids by mouth. She is concerned that despite receiving nearly 750 milliliters of fluid since surgery, the patient has not urinated. Maria understands that urinary catheters are not routinely used during general surgery to prevent urinary tract infections, but she wonders whether the patient is retaining urine or whether she is dehydrated. She decides to ask a more senior nurse about whether or not she should catheterize the patient to determine whether she has retained urine or whether there is another, less invasive way to find the answer.

The senior nurse assesses the patient with Maria. She tells Maria that, in her experience, patients can retain urine in the first hours after this type of surgery and that they will work together to assess the patient. First, the senior nurse asks the patient whether she feels pressure in her lower abdomen, but the patient could not sort out the discomfort of her surgery from bladder fullness. The senior nurse demonstrates how to palpate and percuss for a distended bladder but that is inconclusive. She decides to assess the patient using a bladder scanner. This takes just five minutes to reveal that indeed the patient has retained about 1 liter of urine. They ask the patient whether she would like to try get up to the toilet if they can improve her pain first. They accompany the patient to the toilet and, after a moment, she is able to void. The senior nurse takes a moment after they settle the patient to discuss the evidence that she used in her decision making.

Think Before You Read

- What did Maria need to know to help her decide what to do to help the patient urinate?
- Where might Maria have sought information to help her make her clinical decision?

Introduction

When nurses begin their day, they face many decisions. They decide when and how to assess their patients. They use what they learn from their assessment and the patient's desires to plan mutually determined goals. As expert nurses plan, they choose which interventions will most likely help them meet these goals. In other words, they use the nursing process to do what is best for their patients. Evidence-based practice is concerned with how to make these everyday decisions using the best available evidence from research, professional nursing expertise, and the patient's preferences.

What Is Evidence-Based Practice?

Evidence-based practice is about doing what works and doing it the right way to achieve the best possible patient outcomes (Muir-Gray, 1997, p. 18). More formally, it is "the conscientious, explicit, and judicious use of current best evidence in making decisions about the care of individual patients. . . . [It] means integrating individual clinical expertise with the best available external clinical evidence from systematic research" (Sackett, Rosenberg, Muir-Gray, et al, 1996, p. 71). These classic definitions persist today, as nursing leaders in evidence-based practice have adapted this definition to include four components that influence decisions: (1) the best available research evidence, (2) clinical expertise, (3) resources, and (4) patient preferences (DiCenso, Cullum, & Ciliska, 1998; Muir-Gray, 1997).

Each part of this definition is important. First, "conscientious, explicit, and judicious" means that nurses think carefully, weigh their use of information, and are able to tell others why they use the information. "Current best evidence" implies that someone must first thoroughly search and then judge the quality of the information to determine whether the evidence is indeed the best that is available. In other words, the definition indicates that nurses do not use any evidence that happens to be handy. Rather, they find and choose the highest quality information. When professional nurses make evidence-based decisions about individual patients, they also incorporate what they know from their clinical experience and past practices. However, clinical expertise means something different from **nursing traditions,** or, more simply, doing what you always do for no other reason than habit. Clinical expertise requires being able to tell others what you know, thinking about what you know, talking about what you know, and asking others to critique what you know; clinical expertise is practical know-how that someone else validates (Rycroft-Malone, Seers, Titchen, et al, 2004). Professional nurses incorporate patient preferences to morally and ethically provide care. Although much remains to be learned about how best to incorporate patient desires into clinical decisions, patient preferences include both what individuals prefer, and what groups within a community prefer (Rycroft-Malone et al, 2004). Finally, the component "available resources" refers to the reality of limited health-care dollars, human resource challenges such as adequate nurse–patient ratios, and the availability of technology. Perhaps the most complex aspect of evidence-based decision making is how to weigh the benefit, harms, and costs of providing the best care.

In this chapter's clinical story, Maria did what many nurses do first—she asked someone whose opinion she valued. The senior nurse used both her experience of caring for patients with abdominal surgery and the evidence she knew related to risk and assessment of postoperative urinary retention. The experienced senior nurse had worked with many postoperative patients. She could have advised Maria based on only her practical know-how or previous traditions such as simply catheterizing the patient without further assessment or more conservative approaches. Instead, she used recent evidence to support her decision to use the bladder scanner, manage the patient's pain, and then assist her in trying to void. Maria's colleagues could justify her approach not as "that's the way she has always done it." Rather, she could support her decisions with recent summaries of evidence regarding postoperative urinary retention (Porritt, 2019). In addition, she included the patient in the decision, having discussed the option of a voiding trial.

As you learn more about evidence-based practice, remember that it is like a three-legged stool, where the best available evidence from research, clinical expertise, and patient preferences support the best patient outcomes within a context of limited resources.

Why Is Evidence-Based Practice Important?

Rycroft-Malone, Buchnall, and Melnyk (2004) boldly stated, "One of the most prominent themes ever to characterize international health care is evidence-based practice" (p. 1). In the United States, many organizations, governments, regulators, and patients are calling for health-care providers to practice using evidence. Logic would indicate that the best, most current, information should inform nursing decisions. However, published studies about the effectiveness of using research in practice shows only modest improvements in patient outcomes. One study showed an overall 28% improvement in patient outcomes when nurses used research rather than standard interventions (Cheater, Becker, & Olson, 1988). But this evidence is not current, and the authors conducted the study before the evidence-based practice movement began. Nonetheless, it is very clear that evidence-based practice is here to stay, and most experts believe that when nurses use evidence to inform their decisions, patient outcomes will be the best they can be (Box 1■1).

Nurse scientists have been producing research since nursing's earliest days. Although the number of research studies continues to grow, there are still relatively few studies about how best to use this research. The general public may believe that as soon as scientists discover something that improves patient outcomes, health-care providers quickly adopt this new information. Unfortunately, new knowledge does not transfer quickly or easily, and a great deal of geographic variation exists in the United States (Institute of Medicine of the National Academies [IOM], 2008). Furthermore, treatments that evidence shows are effective are still not consistently used. For example, the Dartmouth Atlas Project showed that, even among highly rated hospitals, only 40% to 83% of patients had beta blockers (a highly effective

---

BOX 1■1 **Significance of Evidence-Based Practice**

- International importance
- Large, regional variations in use of evidence-based practices
- Rapid development of research but slow adoption of evidence-based practices
- Only about half of all patients in the United States receive recommended care
- There is a 28% improvement rate in patient outcomes when nurses use interventions based on research versus standard care
- "Pay-for-performance" requires that evidence-based practices are used
- "Know-do gap" keeps patients from receiving the best care

---

medicine that helps protect the heart from another heart attack and decreases sudden death and other causes of mortality) prescribed at discharge after having a heart attack (Wennberg, 2002). Evidence-based practice aims to speed up the transfer of new knowledge into everyday practice, but the best approach to help clinicians take up the evidence remains complex and no single answer exists.

A Brief History of Evidence-Based Practice

In some ways, evidence-based practice is nothing new. But since the 1990s, evidence-based practice has become a major movement in how nurses and all health professionals think about making clinical decisions. Florence Nightingale was one of the first nurses to advocate for health-care workers to create, interpret, and use research findings to give the best care. She understood the scientific method, statistics, and epidemiology, and she tried to influence health ministers to make better use of data they collected to improve health (McDonald, 2001). However, it was not until nurses were adequately educated and could fund research that findings were available to use.

In the 1970s, nursing leaders focused on a process called **research utilization.** Estabrooks (1999) defined *research utilization* as a "complex process in which knowledge, in this case in the form of research, is transformed from the findings of one or more studies into possible nursing interventions, the ultimate goal of which is use in practice" (p. 204). Today we consider evidence-based practice as an umbrella term that includes research utilization. Two big national projects in the United States were the **Conduct and Utilization of Research in Nursing (CURN) Project** and the **Western Interstate Commission for Higher Education (WICHE) Project.** Their goal was to increase the use of research by improving how nurses evaluated research. These projects helped nurses improve their appraisal skills and appropriate use of individual pieces of research. But these efforts predated our understanding that single studies rarely provide an adequate answer and the syntheses of many studies provide stronger evidence. The importance of patient preferences and clinical expertise is now stressed as part of the equation of best practice.

Some 80 years after Nightingale's frustration with how decision makers ignored the evidence, British epidemiologist and physician Archie Cochrane shocked the medical community when he publicly complained that physicians did not pay attention to evidence when they made clinical decisions (Cochrane Collaboration, n.d.). Like Nightingale, he saw that many infant deaths could have been prevented if only physicians made decisions based on many large, rigorous studies. Although he died before his idea became a reality, in 1992 the **Cochrane Collaboration** established its first collection of research trials on the health of mothers and babies. Cochrane emphasized that a particular type of study, the **randomized controlled trial (RCT),** was the best way to test whether an intervention works. An RCT is an experiment using human beings in which the investigator randomly assigns participants in the trial to either a treatment or control (no treatment) group. It is now considered the gold standard of effectiveness in research because it balances other confounding influences between groups and allows the researcher to link cause (treatment or control) with the effect (clinical outcome). This idea still guides the work of the Cochrane Collaboration, and its library of reviews of international evidence is regarded as one of the premier primary sources of evidence about the effectiveness of interventions, particularly for medicine (Cochrane Collaboration, n.d.).

Although the Cochrane Library contains some evidence that is directly related to the effects of nursing interventions, another organization is aimed at evidence more directly related to nursing and nurse midwifery. In 1996, Alan Pearson and colleagues founded the **JBI** in Adelaide, South Australia (Jordan, Donnelly, & Pittman, 2006). Like that of the Cochrane Collaboration, JBI's purpose is to develop a worldwide collaboration to address global health priorities through synthesis and dissemination of systematic reviews of evidence. The founders took a broader view of what constitutes legitimate evidence, including findings from many kinds of rigorous research, experience, and expertise. In addition, JBI focuses on all aspects of evidence-based practice, not only the summary of evidence. The collaboration now includes centers and members distributed throughout the world, representing diverse populations. The work of the institute and collaborating centers continues its strong focus on nursing and nurse midwifery but also embraces multiple health-care disciplines (Jordan et al, 2006).

In the United States, evidence-based practice efforts at the federal level have come from the **Agency for Healthcare Research and Quality (AHRQ),** which is considered the nerve center of evidence-based practice activity in the United States. In 1997, the AHRQ began awarding 5-year contracts to evidence-based practice centers in the United States and Canada for the production of technology assessment, health reports, and systematic reviews that have particular clinical, social, or economic importance. The agency also managed the **National Guideline Clearinghouse (NGC),** which was an online collection of guidelines for clinical practice. Many nurses relied on this resource for evidence-based guidelines, and it was particularly important when searching for practice guidelines. However, many organizations may develop guidelines about the same health problem; therefore, you may find many guidelines about certain topics and no guidelines about others. Another important organization that has had a deep impact on evidence-based practice in the United States is the **National Academy of Medicine (NAM)** (formerly known as the **Institute of Medicine [IOM]).** The NAM is a nongovernmental organization within the National Academies of Sciences, Engineering, and Medicine; its job is to study and advise about all scientific matters, including health. It is highly regarded because of the way it studies problems and holds open, public meetings during deliberations.

When it was known as the IOM, the organization published a series of reports about the safety of patients and the quality of health care in the United States. These reports caused many in the United States to take notice of the imbalance between what it spent on health care compared with the outcomes. In one report, authors estimated that only about 55% of Americans receive recommended care, that inadequate care resulted in 18,000 unnecessary deaths annually from heart attacks, and, on average, that 17 years pass before a new discovery becomes routine practice (IOM, 2003). Because of these reports, the NAM and other organizations have called for significant changes to accelerate the integration of evidence into practice.

Are U.S. Nurses Ready for Evidence-Based Practice?

Many agencies and groups are requiring nurses and other health-care professionals to use evidence to support their decisions. Accrediting groups, such as The Joint Commission, and payers such as the **Centers for Medicare and Medicaid Services (CMS),** the federal agency that administers Medicare and monitors Medicaid programs offered by states, require hospitals to demonstrate that evidence informs their policies. The focus on patient safety has shone a spotlight on evidence-based practice. In 2008, CMS denied payment for certain hospital-acquired conditions that could have been prevented if the health-care team had used evidence-based practices (Centers for Medicare and Medicaid Services [CMS], 2009). Many of these conditions are highly sensitive to nursing care. For example, in the clinical story, Maria could have inserted an indwelling catheter to solve the patient's urinary retention. If a Medicare patient in a hospital acquires a urinary tract infection after the catheter is inserted, then the hospital will not receive any reimbursement related to the infection. Researchers have estimated the cost of this type of infection could range from $4,694 to more than $27,000 depending on how severe the infection becomes (AHRQ, 2017). More patients can die, and lengths of stay can be longer, adding to cost (Chant, Smith, Marshall, et al, 2011). This "Pay-for-performance" incentive and other pressures have motivated hospitals to increase capacity and to use evidence-based practice. Ultimately, these incentives may stimulate support for nurses to enable them to use evidence in their everyday practice.

The call for evidence-based practice is strong, but are nurses in the United States ready to respond? Schools of nursing are working hard to prepare their

BOX 1■2 **Interdisciplinary Rounds**

Evidence-based practice is not unique to nursing. All health-related fields—medicine, physiotherapy, pharmacy, dentistry—are becoming evidence based. Evidence-based practice can provide a common language and path to pursue best practices with other disciplines.

Example

When designing an evidence-based protocol to discontinue urinary catheters as soon as possible after surgery, nurses would consider evidence from the Centers for Disease Control and Prevention and international practice guidelines. They would need to collaborate with infectious disease specialists, urologists, surgeons, and other physicians to develop a policy that is acceptable to the local providers yet consistent with the best available evidence.

To negotiate the process successfully, the lead nurses would need to be able to find, evaluate, and interpret the best available evidence and to advocate for the integration of patient preferences.

graduates to use evidence to make clinical decisions (Box 1■2). Prior to the 1990s, graduates of baccalaureate programs may have been somewhat prepared to use individual reports of research. More commonly, students learned practices steeped in traditions, learning the profession while in their clinical courses or through what they read in textbooks. In 2005, Pravikoff, Tanner, and Pierce found that nurses in the United States lacked many of the fundamental skills and resources needed for evidence-based practice (Pravikoff et al, 2005). For example, when nurses search for evidence, they need to know how to use **bibliographic databases** in which the health-care literature is indexed. Nearly 75% of respondents had never searched the **Cumulative Index to Nursing and Allied Health Literature (CINAHL),** the primary bibliographic database for nursing research, and nearly as many (58%) had never searched the **Medical Literature Analysis and Retrieval System (MEDLINE),** the primary bibliographic database for medicine and other health professions. In addition, most did not seek the help of a librarian (83%) or the hospital's library (82%). Even if they did know how to use the databases, only about half of the respondents thought they had access to the Internet. The investigators also asked about barriers (other than time) that prevented them from using evidence. Many of the top individual barriers related to knowledge and skills in finding, understanding, and analyzing research, and some respondents lacked access to a computer or library. Top institutional barriers included higher priorities, staffing, budget, and training challenges, and the feeling that evidence-based practice was not possible "in the real world." In 2012, Melnyk et al again surveyed American nurses about their perceptions of evidence-based practice. They found that nurses increasingly value evidence-based practice but that similar barriers remain, including lack of time and resistance from peers and managers. However, nurses reported that they

BOX 1■3 **Tools for Learning and Practice**

- Search the Internet for the Cochrane Collaboration and JBI. Explore the sites and bookmark for future use.
- Search the Internet for the Agency for Healthcare Research and Quality (AHRQ); explore and bookmark. Search the site for the "future of nursing," register for updates, and bookmark for future use.
- Use Google or another search engine to search for the phrase "evidence-based practice." Explore the sites and bookmark for later evaluation of their usefulness and genuineness.

need more knowledge and skills and an organizational culture that supports using evidence in clinical practice.

These challenges may seem overwhelming, but the emphasis on evidence-based practice in all disciplines will surely help us to improve skills, provide resources, and bridge the "know-do" gap (Box 1■3). The rest of this book is aimed at demystifying evidence-based practice so that students and practicing nurses can do what works and what is right for patients.

■ Summary

Evidence-based practice is more than using research. Maria, the new nurse in the clinical story, looked to a colleague to help her solve the patient's problem; together with the senior nurse, they used evidence from research and the patient's preferences. In her conversation with the senior nurse, Maria discovered that her colleague used her expertise gained through several years of experience and current evidence to decide how to manage a common clinical problem. By using noninvasive interventions, they may have prevented possible complications related to inserting a urinary catheter, avoiding costs that the hospital may not have recovered if the patient developed an infection because of the catheter. This scenario illustrates that the best practice can and should be a combination of the best available evidence (the evidence-based policy), the patient's desires, and thoughtful use of clinical expertise. The definition of evidence-based practice as a three-legged stool points to using particular types of information to guide practice and acknowledges that expert knowledge gained from experience and from patients is important to making good clinical decisions.

The Cochrane Collaboration and JBI have led international efforts to develop libraries of the best available evidence and tools for evidence implementation. Even though nurses in the United States may report that they do not possess some of the basic skills needed for using evidence in their practice, many governmental and nongovernmental agencies are calling for better safety and quality outcomes through the use of best available research evidence. Schools of nursing, students, and practicing nurses need to work together to meet the challenge of informing all aspects of patient care with evidence, not habit and tradition.

CHAPTER QUESTIONS

1. Define *evidence-based practice.*

2. What factors have contributed to making evidence-based practice a prominent theme in the United States and abroad?

3. What are the Cochrane Collaboration and JBI?

4. What is the difference between using evidence to inform practice and using traditions to inform clinical decisions? Do nursing traditions have a place in clinical decisions?

5. How do research utilization and evidence-based practice compare?

6. Explain what is meant by the "know-do" gap. Provide an example.

7. Think about a common nursing practice such as bathing. How might evidence-based practice guide how we bathe patients in different situations? Is there a place for evidence-based practice in simple skills such as bathing patients? Why or why not?

References

Centers for Medicare and Medicaid Services. (2009, April 15). Hospital acquired infections (present on admission indicator). Retrieved from http://www.cms.hhs.gov/HospitalAcqCond/

Agency for Healthcare Research and Quality (AHRQ) (2017). Estimating the additional hospital inpatient cost and mortality associated with selected hospital acquired conditions. Retrieved from https://www.ahrq.gov/hai/pfp/haccost2017-results.html

Chant, C., Smith, O. M., Marshall, J. C., et al. (2011). Relationship of catheter-associated urinary tract infection to mortality and length of stay in critically ill patients: A systematic review and meta-analysis of observational studies. *Critical Care Medicine, 39*, 1167–1173. doi:10.1097/CCM.0b013e31820a8581

Cheater, B. S., Becker, A. M., & Olson, R. K. (1988). Nursing interventions and patient outcomes: A meta-analysis of studies. *Nursing Research, 37*, 303–307.

Cochrane Collaboration. (n.d.). Chronology of Cochrane Collaboration. Retrieved from http://www.cochrane.org/docs/cchronol.htm

DiCenso, A., Cullum, N., & Ciliska, D. (1998). Implementing evidence-based nursing: Some misconceptions. *Evidence-Based Nursing, 1*, 38–39.

Estabrooks, C. A. (1999). The conceptual structure of research utilization. *Research in Nursing and Health, 22*, 203–216.

Institute of Medicine of the National Academies. (2003). *Priority areas for national priority: Transforming health care quality.* Washington, DC: National Academies Press.

Institute of Medicine of the National Academies. (2008). *Knowing what works in health care: A roadmap for the nation.* Washington, DC: National Academies Press.

Jordan, Z., Donnelly, P., & Pittman, E. (2006). *A short history of a big idea: The Joanna Briggs Institute 1996–2006.* Melbourne, Australia: Ausmed Publications.

McDonald, L. (2001). Florence Nightingale and the early origins of evidence-based nursing. *Evidence-Based Nursing, 4*, 68–69.

Melnyk, B. M., Fineout-Overholt, E., Gallagher-Ford, L., et al. (2012). The state of evidence-based practice in US nurses: Critical implications for nurse leaders and educators. *Journal of Nursing Administration, 42*, 410–417.

Muir-Gray, J. A. (1997). *Evidence-based health care: How to make health policy and management decisions.* New York, NY: Churchill Livingstone.

Porritt, K. (2019). Post-operative urinary retention: Assessment and diagnosis. Evidence summary in the Joanna Briggs Institute EBP Database, JBI@Ovid, JBI21696.

Pravikoff, D. S., Tanner, A. B., & Pierce, S. T. (2005). Readiness of U.S. nurses for evidence-based practice. *American Journal of Nursing, 105*(9), 40–51.

Rycroft-Malone, J., Buchnall, T., & Melnyk, B. (2004). [Editorial.] *Worldviews on Evidence-Based Nursing, 1,* 1–2.

Rycroft-Malone, J., Seers, K., Titchen, A., et al. (2004). What counts as evidence in evidence-based practice? *Journal of Advanced Nursing, 47,* 81–90.

Sackett, D. L., Rosenberg, W. M. C., Muir-Gray, J. A., et al. (1996). Evidence-based medicine: What it is and what it isn't. *British Medical Journal, 312,* 71–72.

Wennberg, J. E. (2002). Unwarranted variations in healthcare delivery: Implications for academic medical centres. *British Medical Journal, 32,* 961–964.

CHAPTER 2

Elements of Evidence-Based Practice

Leslie Rittenmeyer

Clinical Story

To fulfill the requirements of their capstone course, senior nursing students Jeni, Maggie, and Henrik have teamed up to work on an evidence-based practice project. Even though they have been learning about *evidence-based practice* throughout their curriculum, they feel their knowledge is somewhat fragmented. Because their project is comprehensive, they realize that they need to meld all the different components of evidence-based practice (EBP) into a cohesive whole that they understand and can then apply. They decide as a group that in order to better understand the core elements they should first begin by deconstructing the definition. In doing this, they begin to better understand the importance of taking a *pluralistic approach* while searching for the *best available research evidence* and, additionally, how clinical decision making is influenced by *clinical expertise* and the *preferences* and values of the patient within the context of *available resources*. They are now able to begin the process of identifying the desired outcomes for their project. The group is very excited about this assignment and realize that by going through this process, they are preparing themselves to implement the core principles of evidence-based practice when they venture into the workforce.

Think Before You Read

- What types of questions are important for you to answer for clinical decision making?
- What types of questions are important for understanding how patients experience health and health care?
- What do you think of when you hear "evidence-based practice" in the context of learning about nursing?

Introduction

At first glance, the definition of evidence-based practice (discussed in Chapter 1) does not appear complicated. However, when all of the elements are separated and the words and meaning are pulled apart, one begins to see the complexity. Sometimes, to understand things in their entirety, you have to deconstruct the whole into smaller pieces and then put the pieces back together again, much like a jigsaw puzzle. In doing so, you develop a better understanding of the big picture. When you understand the big picture, it then becomes easier to apply that knowledge to a variety of situations.

Components of Evidence-Based Practice

Recall the definition of evidence-based practice from Chapter 1: "the conscientious, explicit, and judicious use of current best evidence in making decisions about the care of individualized patients. . . . [It] means integrating individual clinical expertise with the best available external clinical evidence from systematic research" (Sackett, Rosenberg, Muir-Gray, et al, 1996, p. 71). It is important to realize that the nursing discipline has adapted this definition to include the components of best available research evidence, clinical expertise, resources, and patient preferences (DiCenso, Cullum, & Ciliska, 1998; Muir-Gray, 1997).

Best available research evidence is a term that suggests clinicians use the best evidence available to them to make informed clinical decisions. This is, of course, opposed to making decisions that are *not* based on the best evidence. An example is basing a clinical decision on the notion that "we have always done it this way." The complexity of the workplace seldom allows nurses time to search for the latest synthesized evidence, and even if they could, there is such a large amount of information that doing so would not be a realistic activity. There are many barriers to using the best available evidence at the bedside, so clinicians may tend to practice using outdated or incomplete knowledge. Things are often done because people have always done them that way. There may be a noticeable gap between evidence and practice. Information becomes outdated quickly, and evidence-based practice attempts to place updated and synthesized information in the clinician's hand. Therefore, the emphasis of evidence-based practice is to bring a synthesis of the external available research evidence to the busy clinician to improve clinical decision making, thereby improving patient outcomes. Without question, clinical expertise, patient preference, and available resources influence how the evidence is used to make clinical decisions. Haynes, Devereaux, and Guyatt (2002) suggest that vital to evidence-based clinical decision making is the individualization of care to the context of the patient's situation. These ideas are discussed in more depth later in this chapter.

What Is Best Available Research Evidence?

As novice practitioners, the students in the opening clinical story ask themselves: "What constitutes best available research evidence?" Data and information that come from many different sources can become the evidence used to influence clinical decision making.

Randomized Controlled Trials

The gold standard for evidence related to the **effectiveness** of a treatment is a randomized controlled trial (RCT). RCTs, very simply put, are clinical trials that involve at least one test treatment and one control treatment randomly assigned to groups. This type of trial is most often used to test effectiveness or safety (Hariton & Locascio, 2018). For example, an RCT can determine how effective a particular drug is in reducing a particular symptom without causing dangerous side effects. The idea of the term *gold standard* has a long history and was not always attached to medicine but to the financial world. It was not until 1982 that the term was more commonplace, and by the 1990s there was a parallel between the rise of evidence-based medicine and the phrase (Jones & Podolsky, 2015).

RCTs are not without some constraints and are sometimes subject to bias and chance. In all of the quantitative methods, there is an emphasis on measurement and statistical analysis. On the one hand, if a rigorous research method is used to generate data, other quantitative methods such as cohort studies and case control studies can also be considered good sources of evidence. On the other hand, quantitative methods are not appropriate for answering all research questions. Pearson (1998) suggests that RCTs are good for cause and effect questions, but not for all questions that are of interest to clinicians. The criteria used to appraise the rigor and quality of these types of studies are discussed in later chapters of this book.

Pluralistic Approach: Quantitative Versus Qualitative Research

Ask yourself the following: What if I have a pressing clinical question and, after searching the research literature, I come to find that there is not any quantitative work, including RCTs, in my area of interest? As a clinician, do you just forget about it and say, "Oh well, there isn't any evidence, so I guess I'll just wing it"? That is why, when considering the best available evidence, nurses need to take a **pluralistic approach.** *Pluralism* is a philosophical term that posits that there is more than one way to look at something. Pearson (1999, 2004) contends that professionals and consumers alike have broad evidence interests, and therefore there is a need to be able to systematically synthesize both quantitative and qualitative works. He argues that each is of equal importance in influencing clinical decision making.

Maggie, introduced in the clinical story, has accepted a job on an oncology unit after she graduates, and she wonders what it might mean to a person to be told that he or she has a terminal illness. She has completed her research course and knows she can answer this question by searching the qualitative research. She conducts a review of the literature and is surprised to find that there are numerous qualitative research studies on this subject. Seeing these studies, she realizes the importance of accessible, synthesized qualitative research as well as quantitative research. Nursing is a human science, which means a great deal of research is framed within qualitative methodologies, and it is necessary to have a vehicle to synthesize and disseminate this evidence. Others in the nursing profession agree with this. Monti and Tingen (1999) believe having multiple paradigms in nursing reflects a robust scientific community that encourages creativity and debate. Jensen and Allen (1996), Sandelowski and Barroso (2003), and Walsh and Downe (2005) all advocate for the need to move beyond just meta-analysis of quantitative research and embrace meta-aggregation of qualitative work. **Meta-analysis** is a statistical method that allows for the combination of the results of many studies to aggregate the conclusions into data that are stronger than are those of just one study. **Meta-aggregation** (sometimes referred to as **meta-synthesis)** combines the findings of qualitative research and synthesizes them to create major themes that accurately depict the meaning of a particular experience.

Expert Opinion

Another source of evidence is expert opinion. **Expert opinion** is evidence that draws on the expert knowledge of individuals or groups; it is not research-based evidence. Although some clinicians believe this type of evidence is not credible, most maintain it is valuable when there is little or no other evidence available or as a supplement to synthesized research. There are times when the best available evidence will come from expert opinion because there is no other rigorously generated research. McCracken and Marsh (2008) make the argument that applying expert knowledge is not the mechanistic process that some accuse it of being but encourages reflection and critical thinking, which they believe is essential in clinical decision making.

Pearson (2003) advocates for a process that systematically examines expert opinion in various types of documents. These documents include books, conference proceedings, reports, and consensus clinical guidelines. Although not completely mainstream, the systematic review of text and opinion is gaining momentum.

Local Data

Knowledge from **local data** is gaining recognition as a legitimate source of valuable evidence. These data can come from a variety of sources and may be useful in improving clinical or organization outcomes. Rycroft-Malone et al (2004) identify the following sources for local data:

- Audit data
- Performance evaluations
- Feedback from a wide range of stakeholders
- Information from social and professional networks
- Knowledge about the culture of an organization
- Patient stories and narratives
- Local and national policy

Stetler (2003) labels this evidence as "internal evidence." She asserts that these data are obtained systematically from local sources and then framed in a way to make improvements in patient outcomes. Rycroft-Malone et al (2004) believes that locally obtained data will play a future role in evidence-based practice but believes more understanding is needed about how this type of data is systematically collected and appraised, how it will be integrated with other types of evidence, and what role it will have in informing clinical decision making.

Big Data and Data Analytics

Westra et al (2017) reviewed literature related to big data science and identified that nurse scientists are increasingly engaging in data science research. They identified a challenge in defining how nurse scientists partner with data science experts to transcend human intellectual limitations. Hansell (2017) described **big data** science as an interprofessional collaborative research methodology that uses large data sets to answer research questions that might be of interest to various disciplines. The purpose is to examine large amounts of information to find hidden patterns, new correlations, market trends, preferences, and relationships with patient care outcomes. She claimed that big data methodology is important because it allows us to examine data sets too large for normal computers to analyze but they may provide large amount of valuable information using larger computing power. According to Brennan and Bakken (2015), big data and data science show promise in informing our understanding of patient experiences and personalized interventions.

What Types of Questions Does the Best Available Evidence Answer?

Pearson et al (2005) contend that health practitioners seek evidence to address a wide range of issues, and thus the type(s) of evidence that a practitioner needs depends on the nature and purpose of the activity. They propose four types of questions that might be asked by health-care professionals that would require different types of evidence (Box 2■1).

Questions of feasibility ask for evidence that addresses to what extent a particular activity would be practical or practicable. A feasibility question asks whether an intervention or activity is physically, culturally, or financially feasible within a given context.

Questions of appropriateness ask for evidence that addresses how appropriate a given activity or intervention is related to the context in which the care is given. In other words, is the activity appropriate to the situation?

Questions of meaningfulness look for evidence that addresses how people experience a particular phenomenon. This evidence explores opinions, thoughts, feelings, beliefs, and subjective interpretations of events.

BOX 2■1 Interdisciplinary Rounds

Questions of feasibility, appropriateness, meaningfulness, and effectiveness often address clinical questions that are of interest to more than one discipline. The same evidence can be framed by different disciplines to make clinical decisions that are appropriate to that discipline.

Example

An interdisciplinary team consists of a nurse, social worker, psychiatrist, and case manager. Their collective job is to provide support services to persistently mentally ill patients who reside in independent apartments. All of them want to know the most effective interventions to help these clients take their medications effectively. The psychiatrist wants to know because it influences her clinical decision about what medications to order. The nurse wants to know because he is to provide patient education about medications and is responsible for intervening in drug-related problems. The social worker wants to know because she is designing a program for support services. The case manager wants to know because he is to provide the day-to-day support for activities of daily living. Each of these disciplines will benefit from the same evidence but for different reasons.

Questions of effectiveness seek evidence that addresses whether an intervention, when used appropriately, achieves the desired outcome.

An easy way to remember these questions is with the acronym FAME.

The Influence of Clinical Expertise, Patient Preference, and Available Resources

Jeni, Maggie, and Henrik can now articulate their understanding of what evidence-based practice is, what constitutes best available evidence, and what questions can be answered. However, they believe there is one piece of the picture they need to explore further. They remain curious about the role that clinical expertise, patient preference, and available resources play in clinical decision making.

Clinical Expertise

Professional nurses, like other health-care professionals, are assumed to bring a certain amount of theoretical and clinical knowledge to their practice. Professional knowledge is respected because nurses are considered to be credentialed experts. Titchen (2000) labels this as "professional craft knowledge." Rycroft-Malone et al (2004) acknowledge the importance of this knowledge in clinical decision making but also argue that for clinical experience or tacit knowledge to be credible, it must be made explicit so that it can be disseminated, critiqued, and developed. In other words, for tacit knowledge to be a source of evidence, it needs to be subjected to rigorous analysis and critique.

Haynes et al (2002) view **clinical expertise** as an overlay to all other components of evidence-based practice because it is expected that nurses will integrate tacit knowledge automatically when making clinical decisions. Nurses' knowledge and clinical skills help in (1) accurately assessing the needs of patients' families, groups, communities, and systems; (2) creating a better understanding of the context or the circumstance of a particular situation; (3) creating a climate in which patients' values and preferences are considered more important than those of the practitioners; and (4) discussing how available resources influence health-care delivery. Haynes et al state this model is prescriptive rather than descriptive. That is, it is a guide for "thinking about how decisions are made rather than a schema for how they are made" (2002, p. 36).

Patient Preference

The term **patient preference** refers to how involved a patient is in the clinical decision-making process. Some patients have definitive views about their health-care decisions, and others have less stringent views. Some want to receive a full disclosure of risk versus benefits, and others trust the clinicians to assess the risk of a given treatment. Haynes et al (2002) suggest these choices are influenced by personal values, patient condition, available resources, aversion to risk, and amount of accurate or inaccurate information at hand.

Empowering patients to have a choice in their treatment sounds like an easy enough goal, but the ways in which clinicians honor individual beliefs, values, past experiences, and knowledge and meld those into the other elements of evidence-based practice are less clear. There are times when patients make a decision that is contrary to the belief of the health-care provider. Some examples include a patient who decides to keep smoking after a heart attack, a patient who refuses lifesaving chemotherapy, or a patient who chooses to treat a condition with alternative methods. Patient choices can be culturally driven or based on religious beliefs or a value system. There is much to learn about what patient preference really means. More specific information about patient preference is addressed in later chapters.

Available Resources

There are clearly times and circumstances when the best available evidence points us in a direction that, when considering the circumstances, is not feasible or practical. For example, there might be evidence that recommends an intervention or activity that is very appropriate and feasible in one context, but because of a lack of **available resources** would not be appropriate in another. One of the goals of the evidence-based practice movement is to improve global health, and it is important to remember there are many health-care disparities caused by a scarcity of resources throughout the world. Residents of industrialized countries may not be familiar with the daily constraints faced by residents of less developed countries. What is important is that all informed health-care decisions be made within the context of available resources (Box 2■2).

■ Summary

Jeni, Maggie, and Henrik meet to review what they have learned through their exploration of the elemental components of evidence-based practice. They have

---

BOX 2■2 **Tools for Learning and Practice**

■ Go to Google Scholar (http://www.scholar.google.com) and search for the following article:

Jordan, Z., Lockwood, C., Munn, Z., et al. (2018). Redeveloping the JBI model of evidence-based healthcare. *International Journal of Evidence-Based Healthcare, 16,* 227–241. doi:10.1097/XEB000000000000139

■ After reading the Jordan et al article, search this chapter's Reference list and choose one other article that interests you.
■ Share what you have learned from that article with a classmate.

come to appreciate that evidence-based practice provides a framework for clinical decision making and that better clinical decisions lead to better patient outcomes. The type of evidence needed to inform a clinical problem is driven by the type of questions asked. The types of questions we usually ask are questions of effectiveness, meaningfulness, appropriateness, and feasibility. The group now feels comfortable discussing how research evidence, clinical expertise, and patient values and preferences along with available resources provide the framework for evidence-based practice. They have learned that best available evidence can be gathered from different sources, such as synthesized qualitative evidence, quantitative research evidence, local data, and expert opinion. They also feel they can discuss how patient preference and available resources influence clinical decision making. Now that they have put all of the pieces of the puzzle together, Jeni, Maggie, and Henrik are ready to move on and start applying what they have learned to the design of their project.

CHAPTER QUESTIONS

1. Discuss the relationship between evidence-based practice and clinical decision making.

2. Explain the meaning of *best available evidence*.

3. What type of evidence would a nurse look for in questions of feasibility, appropriateness, meaningfulness, and effectiveness?

4. Define *meta-analysis* and *meta-synthesis*.

5. Explain why the concept of clinical expertise overlays the clinical decision-making model.

6. Discuss how patient values and preferences and available resources influence clinical decision making.

References

Brennan, P. F., & Bakken, S. (2015). Nursing needs big data and big data needs nursing. *Journal of Nursing Scholarship, 47,* 477–484.

DiCenso, A., Cullum, N., & Ciliska, D. (1998). Implementing evidence-based nursing: Some misconceptions. *Evidence-Based Nursing, 1,* 38–39.

Hansell, P. (2017). Advances in nursing research methodology: Big data analytics the future. *International Journal of Nursing & Clinical Practices, 4,* 220. doi: https://doi.org/10.15344/2394-4978/2017/220

Hariton, E., & Locascio, J. (2018). Randomized controlled trials: The gold standard for effectiveness research. *BJOG: An International Journal of Obstetrics and Gynaecology, 125*(13), 1716. doi:10.1111/1471-0528.15199

Haynes, R. B., Devereaux, P. J., & Guyatt, G. H. (2002). Clinical expertise in the era of evidence-based medicine and patient choice. *ACP Journal Club, 136,* A11–A14.

Jensen, L., & Allen, M. (1996). Metasynthesis of qualitative findings. *Qualitative Health Research, 6*(4), 553–560.

Jones, D., & Podolsky, S. (2015). The history and fate of the gold standard. *The Lancet, 385*(9977), 1502–1503. https://doi.org/10.1016/S0140-6736(15)60742-5

Jordan, Z., Lockwood, C., Munn, Z., et al. (2018). Redeveloping the model JBI of evidence-based healthcare. *International Journal of Evidence-Based Healthcare, 16,* 227–241. doi:10.1097/XEB000000000000139

McCracken, G., & Marsh, J. (2008). Practitioner expertise in evidence-based practice decision making. *Research on Social Work and Practice, 18,* 301–310. doi:10.1177/10497311507308143

Muir-Gray, J. A. (1997). *Evidence-based health care: How to make health policy and management decisions.* New York, NY: Churchill Livingston.

Monti, E., & Tingen, M. (1999). Multiple paradigms of nursing science. *Advances in Nursing Science, 21*(4), 64–80.

Pearson, A. (1998). Excellence in care: Future dimensions in effective nursing. *Nursing Times, 3,* 25–27.

Pearson, A. (1999). Evidence based nursing: Quality through research. In R. Nay & S. Garnett (Eds.), *Nursing older people: Issues and innovations* (pp. 338–352). Sydney, Australia: Churchill Livingstone.

Pearson, A. (2003). Liberating our conceptualization of "evidence." *Journal of Advanced Nursing, 44,* 441–442.

Pearson, A. (2004). Balancing the evidence: Incorporating the synthesis of qualitative data into systematic reviews. *JBI Reports, 2,* 45–64.

Pearson, A., Wiechula, R., Lockwood, C., et al. (2005). The JBI model of evidence-based health care. *The International Journal of Evidence-Based Health Care, 3,* 207–215.

Rycroft-Malone, J., Seers, K., Titchen, A., et al. (2004). What counts as evidence in evidence-based practice? *Journal of Advanced Nursing, 47,* 81–90.

Sackett, D. L., Rosenberg, W. M. C., Muir-Gray, J. A., et al. (1996). Evidence-based medicine: What it is and what it isn't. *British Medical Journal, 312,* 71–72.

Sandelowski, M., & Barroso, J. (2003). Creating meta-summaries of qualitative findings. *Nursing Research, 52*(4), 226–233.

Stetler, C. (2003). The role of the organization in translating research into evidence-based practice. *Outcomes Management for Nursing Practice, 7*(3), 97–103.

Titchen, A. (2000). *Professional craft knowledge in patient-centered nursing and the facilitation of its development* (Doctoral dissertation, University of Oxford, 2000). Kidlington, United Kingdom: Ashdale Press.

Walsh, D., & Downe, S. (2005). Meta-synthesis method for qualitative research: A literature review. *Journal of Advanced Nursing, 50*(2), 204–211.

Westra, B. L., Sylvia, M., Weinfurter, E. F., et al. (2017). Big data science: A literature review of nursing research exemplars. *Nursing Outlook, 65*(5), 549–561. doi:10.2016/j.outlook.2016.11.021

CHAPTER 3

Global Perspectives and Borderless Knowledge

Alan Pearson

- Differentiate between local, national, and international sources of evidence for nursing.

- Describe and debate the role of international evidence in local clinical decision making.

- Develop a clinical question and source international evidence that addresses the question.

"Borderless" evidence/ knowledge	External evidence
Experience	Local evidence
Expertise	Tacit knowledge
	Tradition

Clinical Story

Mapani has been the head nurse on the cancer ward in the teaching wing of a large government hospital in sub-Saharan Africa for 11 years. She is becoming increasingly worried about the number of patients who develop a very sore and ulcerated mouth while receiving chemotherapy and radiotherapy. She knows that this has always been a problem, but as she begins her shift by looking through the care plans, she sees that of the 36 patients in the ward, 31 have moderate to severe mucositis. She knows the staff nurses and nurses' aides are meticulous in trying to ensure that every patient has regular oral care with chlorhexidine, but the hospital budget is very small, and the staff is able to do this only once a day. This cannot, however, be the reason for this increase in sore mouths—Mapani and the ward nurses are practicing according to how things have always been done per hospital procedure—so she decides to press on with her work and hope for the best.

At the same time Mapani has these thoughts, Michael, the clinical nurse specialist (CNS) for the head and neck oncology unit in a prestigious academic health science center in the United States, is doing rounds at his hospital with the staff nurses on night duty. It is 2 a.m., and the unit is relatively quiet, so he and the two staff nurses sit at the nurse's station to review patients in the unit. They also notice the prevalence of mucositis in the current patient population and wonder about the change they have recently made from using chlorhexidine to using sunflower oil in their oral hygiene protocol. The change has increased the costs to the unit but occurred because the benchmarking exercise the hospital is involved in showed that the prevalence of mucositis in another, similar hospital in the same city runs at 5% less than their hospital. The only difference between the care delivered was found to be the substance used to clean the mouth.

For both of these nurses—living far apart from each other in very different cultures and systems—it is clear that their concerns and experiences are far more alike than they are different. What is also striking is their reliance on local evidence and their apparent indifference to the external, global evidence. In Mapani's case, her source of evidence is her own peers and the practices they have engaged in for years. Michael and his team compare their performance against that of another local team, without any thought that the hospitals they benchmark against may have much poorer outcomes than units across the rest of the world. Were both to explore the best available global evidence, they would find that evidence varies in strength and nine different treatments showed some effect. However, some were weak, and no single treatment is clearly supportable; frequent, gentle oral care with potable (drinkable) water and crushed ice may be as effective as any other intervention to prevent mucositis in patients undergoing radio- or chemotherapy (Worthington, Clarkson, Bryan, et al, 2010).

- Is it reasonable to consider evidence from across the world in your clinical decision making?
- What factors might influence how you consider evidence from another country?

Introduction

Chapters 1 and 2 indicated that evidence-based nursing occurs when nurses make clinical decisions (with patients and the health-care team), taking into account the patient's values and preferences, the social and cultural context, their own judgment, and the best available global evidence.

The evidence-based practice movement had its genesis in the United Kingdom, Europe, Canada, and Australia—all countries that are closely aligned and where evidence sharing has been well established for centuries (Donaldson, 2007; Normand & Vaughan, 1993). Nurses in these countries are aware of international developments and either read journals from outside their country or search for information through PubMed (a free search engine, primarily for the MEDLINE database, in the United States). This, to a large extent, explains why the concept of searching for and evaluating international literature and then developing appropriate local applications is now well understood in these countries.

The United States has an enormous population. U.S. health professionals publish frequently in a large number of U.S.-based journals, and the process of using local activity data from across the United States to establish benchmarks is more dominant in some regions of the United States than is the evidence-based approach. However, the escalating cost of health care is one of the greatest challenges in the United States. Spending per capita remains the highest worldwide, even though the rate of growth slowed after the 2008 great recession and changes related to the Affordable Care Act of 2010; more people are insured. Nonetheless, the United States still spends the most per person and 17% of its gross domestic product, more than 28% higher than the next country, Switzerland, which spends 12% of its gross domestic product (Sawyer & Cox, 2018). Compared with other, similar countries, the United States spends similar public funds on health but a much higher amount of private funds (Sawyer & Cox, 2018). In 2008, $2.38 trillion was spent on health care in the United States, but 45.7 million citizens remained uninsured. Since the implementation of the Affordable Care Act, many more Americans are insured. In 2018, 91.5% of Americans were insured, with 28,566,000 remaining uninsured. However, this represents a decrease from 2017 due to changes in the Affordable Care Act (Berchick, Barnett, & Upton, 2019).

While spending has shifted somewhat toward private insurance, the high cost of health-care delivery, critical staff shortages, and patient demand for more and better services all contribute to an increasing sense of urgency to improve access to quality care while reducing costs. Given these challenges, nurses and other health-care professionals are beginning to recognize the need to learn from the experiences and research of others, both in the United States and around the globe (Kuehn, 2010).

Whereas all nations focus on local problems and local solutions, the broader concerns of assessing health needs, surveillance, evidence-based decision making, and the social dimensions of health are truly global. The widespread movement of people and diseases across boundaries and the universal influence of the Internet serve only to emphasize how small the world really is. As society becomes knowledge based, evidence is generated at ever-faster rates and exchanged in ever-larger networks. Evidence-based nursing is fundamentally embedded in these global developments. The process focuses on clinical decisions that are informed by the best available global evidence and is critically dependent on nurses' ability to access valid and reliable borderless evidence and apply it to the local context (Box 3■1).

What Is "Borderless Evidence"?

The concept of evidence is often misunderstood. The following is a broad dictionary definition of the term *evidence*: "the available facts, circumstances etc. supporting or otherwise a belief, proposition etc. or indicating whether a thing is true or valid" (Pearsall & Trumble, 1995, p. 487). Whenever nurses make clinical decisions with and for their patients, using local evidence is important. However, it is equally important to consider the external, global evidence that crosses borders of nations and disciplines. This is considered "**borderless" evidence** (or **knowledge**).

BOX 3■1 **Significance of Global, Borderless Evidence**

- Rapidly escalating costs of health care and calls for better, safer patient outcomes mean that the best evidence should inform clinical decisions.
- Research and evidence generation tend to coalesce in highly industrialized nations, but scientific principles guide research in all countries that produce knowledge.
- Clinical problems are remarkably similar across the world; some solutions are not specific to the setting, whereas others are very dependent on the context.
- Internet availability and e-publication of evidence have created unprecedented access to international evidence.
- Best available evidence knows no national boundaries; to live up to the definition of evidence-based practice, clinicians must consider the international evidence.

Local Evidence

Local evidence refers to the everyday knowledge nurses use within the local health system; this includes both **tacit knowledge** (implicit, unspoken) and more formally generated knowledge derived from local research studies. Tacit knowledge in nursing is largely associated with expertise, experience, and tradition. It represents the ideas, concepts, and understandings that are part of a knowledge-to-action continuum. This type of knowledge can be associated with the simple, everyday aspects of life such as eating and drinking; sleeping; mobilizing; and the experience of pain, suffering, and recovery. However, what appears simple on the surface actually hides the complexity and sophistication of expert nursing practice; it is hard to capture, evaluate, and report on in the formal research sense.

Local research is a more formal approach to evidence generation that involves the use of explicit methods of gathering and analyzing data. Increasingly, bedside nurses are engaging in local research efforts. These small-scale, locally generated studies play an important role in evidence-based nursing. However, if nurses base their practice solely on the findings of local research without accessing the global evidence, their practice will not reflect the intent of evidence-based health care and its interest in borderless knowledge.

Expertise

Expertise is highly regarded in nursing and is linked to the ability of a nurse to have relevant information in a given area of practice. Expertise is difficult to quantify and even more difficult to rank in terms of its reliability. Despite these difficulties, a large proportion of nursing practice relies on expertise. Furthermore, the opinions of experts often represent the best available evidence in areas in which research is limited or research on a specific question is difficult to conduct (Pearson, Wiechula, et al, 2007).

Experience

Experience is knowledge and skill acquired through being involved in or exposed to practice over time. It is largely know-how, or procedural knowledge, rather than propositional knowledge, but it plays a major role in nursing practice. When nurses make clinical decisions, they often weigh external evidence with their own experience. Thus, experience in itself is a source of evidence in health-care practice (Pearson, Wiechula, et al, 2007).

Tradition

Tradition plays a major role in nursing, largely because nurses are required to participate in an extended period of education and training to become familiar with the traditions of their profession and of the particular school they attended. **Tradition** is an inherited pattern of thought or action that leads to a specific, long-standing practice. Tradition may stem from logic and evidence from trial and error, but this is often not the case (Pearson, Field, et al, 2007).

In this chapter's clinical story, Mapani relies on the traditions of the unit. They have even been formalized into the plans of care. She begins to wonder whether the methods they are using are correct, but she has stopped short of pursuing the question further because severely limited resources complicate her situation. Michael, however, has relied on local benchmarking to inform practice. Despite being in different hemispheres, both need to find better evidence to inform their practices.

External Evidence

Expertise and experience can be legitimate, internal sources of evidence for practice, and tradition can be seen as being not so legitimate. However, when the results of rigorous research are available, it is appropriate to weigh the results of external research against those internal sources of expertise, experience, and tradition. To date, much of the focus of evidence-based practice has been on determining the best available **external evidence** from research, almost to the exclusion of any other source of evidence. This is because evidence from rigorous research (external evidence) is least prone to bias.

Globalization and "Borderless" Knowledge

The desire to deliver the best possible care is a central concern of nurses across the globe, and an increased interest in improving health care is now universal. In diverse urban, suburban, rural, and remote communities across the world, there is a growing desire for a knowledge-based health-care system that is focused on the individual and accessible to all.

Within nursing circles, Sigma (formerly known as Sigma Theta Tau International) and the International Council of Nursing (ICN) have developed mechanisms to support a global approach to evidence-based nursing practice. These include providing education, training, and resources to expand nursing's capacity for evidence-based practice in both developed and developing nations.

How can you, as a busy and time-poor nurse, ensure the knowledge you access and apply in local situations is the best available internationally and not limited to your state or your country—that it is, in effect, "borderless"? Fortunately, the evidence-based health-care movement has spawned accessible sources of information generated through global collaboration. The most notable collections are the Cochrane Library and the JBI EBP resources. These sources draw together all of the world's best available knowledge/evidence to answer a specific clinical question and summarize it in a format that will inform nurses whenever they make a clinical decision.

Searching for the Global Evidence

The assumption of evidence-based nursing is that there is information nurses need to know in order to practice professionally. There are, however, substantial gaps in available knowledge. Sackett, Rosenberg, Gray, et al (1996) classically argued that almost every time a practitioner encounters a patient, new information is required about some aspect of the diagnosis, prognosis, or management. They note that there will be times when the question will be self-evident or the information will be readily accessible. This is increasingly the case as sophisticated information technology moves closer to the bedside.

Even so, there will be many occasions when neither condition prevails and there will be a need to ask an answerable question that will require the best available external evidence. This requires considerably more time and effort than most health professionals have at their disposal, and the result is that most information needs go unmet.

Asking Answerable Questions

The first step is to pose a question that is answerable. Asking answerable questions is a skill that can be learned. At the onset of the evidence-based medicine movement, Sackett et al (1996) offered useful advice in the context of evidence-based medicine and the effectiveness of interventions. A broader perspective of evidence-based health care extends beyond questions of effectiveness to consider the appropriateness and feasibility of practices. The sources of a clinical question are the following:

- *Assessment*—how to properly gather and interpret findings from the history and physical examination and care
- *Etiology*—how to identify causes for problems
- *Differential diagnosis*—when considering the possible causes of a patient's clinical problems, how to rank them by likelihood, seriousness, and treatability
- *Diagnostic tests*—how to select and interpret diagnostic tests to confirm or exclude a diagnosis, based on considering, for example, their precision, accuracy, acceptability, expense, and safety
- *Prognosis*—how to gauge the patient's likely clinical course and anticipate likely problems associated with the particular disease and social context of the person
- *Therapy*—how to select therapies to offer patients that do more good than harm and that are worth the efforts and cost of using them
- *Prevention*—how to reduce the chance of ill health by identifying and modifying risk factors, and how to detect early problems by screening and patient education
- *Meaningfulness*—how to understand the experience of patients and the social context within which practice takes place
- *Feasibility*—how practical it is to implement a practice within a given clinical setting, culture, or country

- *Self-improvement*—how to keep your knowledge up to date, improve your clinical skills, and run a better, more efficient clinical service (adapted from Sackett et al, 1996)

Drawing on these factors, a clear, well-formulated question is developed to give focus to the search (see Chapter 8 for more detail on questioning). A clearly defined question should include specific details on the following:

- *The participants.* Participants should be clearly defined, including condition(s) (e.g., people with a confirmed diagnosis of emphysema), the population characteristics (e.g., females between 15 and 20 years), and the setting (e.g., in hospital medical wards).
- *The activities or interventions.* The question should specify the intervention or activity of interest (e.g., chest percussion or the administration of oxygen via a facemask).
- *The outcomes that are of interest.* The question should include the outcomes of interest to the review. The patient's satisfaction with care, peak flow, and oxygen saturation levels is an example of several outcomes one might include in a review of interventions aimed at improving outcomes in people with emphysema.
- *The types of studies relevant to answering the question.* The question itself indicates the study designs that are most appropriate. When the question focuses on experiences of people or communities, interpretive studies are usually indicated, whereas questions of feasibility may warrant economic evaluations and/or critical designs or evaluative designs. When the focus is on the effectiveness of a treatment, randomized controlled trials are considered to be the most appropriate, and questions relating to etiology or risk factors may be best addressed by case-controlled and cohort studies (see Chapter 11 for full explanations of these types of studies).

Generally speaking, although nurses often want to answer very broad questions, the narrower a question is, the easier it is to conduct the search. For example, if one is interested in determining the most effective, appropriate, and feasible way of improving the quality of life for people with emphysema, it is desirable to conduct a series of searches based on specific, focused questions. A well-formulated question will give direction to the search strategy.

Finding the Evidence: Global Evidence Sources

After you have identified the question, issue, or problem, the next step is to find the evidence. To do this requires knowledge about the techniques used to unearth the evidence and make it available. Systematic reviews and evidence-based practice guidelines are designed to save practitioners time by presenting condensed information, so they may be your the first preference in a search. Just as research—published or unpublished—varies in quality, so can a systematic review or guideline. Practitioners who want to base their practice on the best available knowledge need to learn new skills to access the resources available (Grimshaw, Eccles, Lavis, et al, 2012).

Be open to the idea that evidence is generated throughout the world. Therefore, approach to evidence must not be limited to one country. Language may pose a barrier to finding (or using) evidence that is published only in a non–English-language journal. Increasingly, organizations are trying to use international collaborations and multilingual translations to break down language barriers and make evidence available to more clinicians.

In subsequent chapters, you will learn more details about searching. Here, it is important to focus on how to capture the international evidence in your effort to find the best available evidence.

- *What databases/resources do you have available in your setting?* Not all databases are accessible to clinicians, and databases may or may not search across languages and nations. Some resources are simpler to search and easily available in the clinical setting, whereas others are more complex and housed away from the point of care.
- *Who will do the search?* You may need to consult an expert to help find answers across a broad spectrum of international sources. That expert may be a librarian in your facility or an advanced practice nurse. See Box 3■2 for recommendations.
- *How can you seek help from your librarian?* Although librarians may not be well versed in the substantive area of the clinical question, they are highly skilled in electronic searching and in the retrieval of papers. Be sure to communicate clearly what your question is and that you are interested in the global evidence.

Certain databases are large and most likely to yield international evidence. However, it may be difficult to find full descriptions of the national origins of the journals included in the index. These databases include (Box 3■3):

- *CINAHL.* The Cumulative Index to Nursing and Allied Health (CINAHL) database provides authoritative coverage of the literature related to nursing and allied health. In total, more than 4,000 journals are regularly indexed.

BOX 3■2 Interdisciplinary Rounds

- Borderless evidence means gathering evidence from any nation and any discipline that produces high-quality, relevant knowledge for nursing practice.
- Librarians can help find the international evidence and modify searches to accommodate different spellings and words for key terms of the search.
- World health organizations that promote access to international evidence have come from many disciplines.
- When you are considering treatments, traditions vary across nations as to whose role particular treatments belong; therefore, do not limit searches to a specific discipline when exploring the international literature.

BOX 3■3   **Tools for Learning and Practice**
___

Evidence-Based Practice Organizations With an International Focus:
- **JBI (http://www.joannabriggs.org):** An international collaboration of health-care providers representing 32 nations. EBP resources are found at **http://know.lww.com/JBI-resources/relevantevidence.html.**
- **Cochrane Nursing (https://nursing.cochrane.org):** An international group of nurses volunteering to support increased awareness and use of the Cochrane Library of international systematic reviews and other evidence sources.
- **Contact, Help, Advice and Information Network (CHAIN) (https://www.networks.nhs.uk/nhs-networks/chain):** An international community of more than 10,450 people working in health care and social care.
- **Guidelines International (http://www.g-i-n.net):** International members from 84 countries and 96 organizations with a mission to lead, strengthen, and support collaboration and work within the guideline development, adaptation, and implementation community.
- **Sigma (formerly Sigma Theta Tau International) (https://www.sigmanursing.org):** An invitation-only international membership. Sigma publishes *Worldviews on Evidence-Based Nursing* and sponsors books and meetings relevant to evidence-based nursing.
- **World Health Organization (http://www.who.int/en/):** Coordinating authority for health within the United Nations system. It provides leadership on global health matters, shapes the health research agenda, sets norms and standards, articulates evidence-based policy options, provides technical support to countries, and monitors and assesses health trends.
- **Virtual Health Library (http://regional.bvsalud.org/php/index.php?lang=en):** An open network of literature databases and other resources. It includes a collection of multiple non–English-language databases.

- *MEDLINE.* MEDLINE is widely recognized as the best source for bibliographic and abstract coverage of biomedical literature. It contains more than 25 million records from more than 5,600 journals.
- *The Cochrane Library.* The Cochrane Library is a collection of databases provided by the international Cochrane Collaboration (with over 20,000 contributors across the globe) and other organizations. At its core is the *Cochrane Database of Systematic Reviews,* a database of systematic reviews and meta-analyses that summarize and interpret the results of research. The Cochrane Library aims to make the results of well-conducted controlled trials readily available and is a key resource in evidence-based health care. There are a number of Cochrane entities, including Cochrane Nursing Care and the Cochrane Library of Systematic Reviews, both of which can be searched to

find nursing care–relevant reviews. Because of the Cochrane approach, reviews are more likely to include global evidence in the library.

▪ *JBI EBP Resources.* The JBI Evidence Synthesis and JBI Evidence Implementation of systematic reviews and implementation reports is a fully refereed library that publishes systematic reviews provided by JBI, with an emphasis on nursing, the allied health professions, and medicine. The JBI EBP Database (distributed by OVID) is an online, point-of-care evidence source that enables health-care practitioners to search for, critically appraise, summarize, embed, use, and evaluate evidence-based information. It is a service of the international JBI (with almost 70 collaborating centers around the globe), whose mission is to facilitate evidence-based health-care practice globally. Because of the underpinning international collaboration, these sources are likely to include international, multilingual evidence.

▪ *Embase.* Excerpta Medica Database (Embase) is a biomedical and pharmacological database that contains more than 23 million records from 1947 to the present. Embase covers more than 7,000 biomedical journals from 70 countries and is more likely to index European journals than other indexes.

▪ *Virtual Health Library.* The Latin America and Caribbean Center for Health Sciences Information developed this open network of literature databases and other resources. It includes a collection of multiple non-English databases that can be searched using English words. The search will return the original language abstract as well as a translated abstract. Databases include LILACS (Latin American and Caribbean Center on Health Sciences Information) and international agencies such as the Pan American Health Organization (Virtual Health Network, n.d.).

Conducting the Search: Implications for International Sources of Evidence

In later chapters, you will learn more about conducting careful searches of electronic databases and other sources. If you work with skilled librarians, they can help you obtain international evidence if you emphasize that you would like to find all sources of evidence. For example, differences in spelling conventions such as "randomised" versus "randomized" and "paediatric" versus "pediatric" require expertise in searching. Similarly, different countries use different terms for the same condition (e.g., "mucositis" and "stomatitis").

▪ Summary

It is remarkable how practitioners, as global citizens, are concerned with many of the same health problems. Thus, practitioners share a similar desire to have the right information for the right people at the right time. For example, a simple search on CINAHL for "pressure ulcer" OR "pressure injury" filtered to Middle East journals nets articles such as "Measuring the Quality of Pressure-Sore Prevention Cushions Through the Use of a Pressure Mapping System," published in the *Journal of the*

Israeli Physical Therapy Society. Using the same search term but limiting the journal set to Australia yields a similarly focused article in the Australian journal *Wound Practice and Research.*

Of course, some health problems are unique or more pronounced in certain regions of the world because of environment, sociopolitical conditions, or other factors that contribute to unique risks. For example, searching "malaria prevention" in the African subset of journals results in 36 hits for the period of 2005 to 2020, whereas the same search generates only 7 hits for the Mexico–South American subset. Certainly you need to determine whether you can apply the results from any study in a local context, regardless of whether it was conducted in your own country or another. Remain open to all sources of evidence to determine the best available.

In this chapter's clinical story, the international evidence applied both to fully industrialized nations and as less wealthy nations. The available resources influenced the questions and the balance of the costs and benefits of the solution, but the evidence was applicable to both.

CHAPTER QUESTIONS

1. What is meant by *evidence for nursing?*

2. What are the differences between local and global evidence?

3. In what situation would the use of local evidence be more desirable than external evidence?

4. What databases/electronic sources of information enable you to access international evidence?

5. Develop a clinical question and search a database first by limiting the search to just a few country journal subsets. Repeat the experiment but broaden your search to include all subsets of journals. How did your results compare? Is it important to include the international journals and databases in your search? Why or why not?

6. Think about a current issue or problem in your setting. Your search yields a systematic review that includes studies from India, Africa, the United Kingdom, and the United States. What will you consider to determine whether these results have relevance to your local setting?

7. Consider this statement: "Health is global." How does this statement relate to your way of thinking, or does it have any relevance to you?

References

Berchick, E. R., Barnett, J. C., & Upton, R. D. (2019*). Health insurance coverage in the United States: 2018* (U.S. Census Bureau Report No. P60-267 [RV]). Retrieved from https://www.census.gov/library/publications/2019/demo/p60-267.html

Donaldson, L. (2007). *Health is global: Proposals for a UK government-wide strategy.* London: Department of Health.

Grimshaw, J. M., Eccles, M. P., Lavis, J. N., et al. (2012). Knowledge translation of research findings. *Implementation Science, 7.* https://doi.org/10.1186/1748-5908-7-50

Kuehn, B. M. (2010). How the UK uses data on comparative effectiveness. *Journal of the American Medical Association, 304,* 1058–1059. doi:10.1001/jama.2010.1289

Normand, C. E. M., & Vaughan, J. P. (Eds.). (1993). *Europe without frontiers: The implications for health.* Chichester, United Kingdom: John Wiley.

Pearsall, J., & Trumble, B. (Eds.). (1995). *Oxford English reference dictionary.* Oxford, United Kingdom: Oxford University Press.

Pearson, A., Field, J., & Jordan, Z. (2007). *Evidence-based clinical practice in nursing and health care: Assimilating research, experience and expertise.* Oxford, United Kingdom: Blackwell.

Pearson, A. P., Wiechula, R., Court, A., et al. (2007). A re-consideration of what constitutes "evidence" in the healthcare professions. *Nursing Science Quarterly, 20,* 85–88.

Sackett, D. L., Rosenberg, W. M. C., Gray, J. A. M., et al. (1996). Evidence-based medicine: What it is and what it is not. *British Medical Journal, 312,* 71–72.

Sawyer, B., & Cox, C. (2018). How does health spending in the US compare to other countries? [Chart]. Peterson-Kaiser Health System Tracking. Retrieved from https://www.healthsystemtracker.org/chart-collection/health-spending-u-s-compare-countries/#item-start

Virtual Health Library. (n.d.). Information sources. Retrieved from http://regional.bvsalud.org/php/index.php?lang=en

Worthington, H. V., Clarkson, J. E., Bryan, G., et al. (2010). Interventions for preventing oral mucositis for patients with cancer receiving treatment. *Cochrane Database of Systematic Reviews, 2010*(12). doi:10.1002/14651858.CD000978.pub4

Models for Evidence-Based Practice

In this unit you will learn the different models of
evidence-based practice that help structure the process of
putting evidence into action. Some models are appropriate
for individual nurses whereas others help groups or
organizations transfer evidence into everyday practice. In
Chapter 4, you will discover some of the controversies that
surround evidence-based practice. Some nurse theorists have
criticized the evidence-based practice movement, claiming it
ignores nursing theory and regresses the profession toward
an era of thoughtless, antitheoretical practice. You will find
divergent points of view and then examine different
conceptual models and frameworks and how they can
increase the efficiency of integrating evidence into practice.
You will connect the frontline nurses' critical role in moving

(continues on page 38)

evidence into practice and the emerging concept of "knowledge translation." In Chapter 5, you will explore a sampler of the many models of evidence-based practice and see how the models can be used in the clinical story. You will find tools to help you compare each to help you choose which model fits a particular clinical situation. In Chapter 6, you will learn about the common principles among the models and find the key issues that emerge from the models.

Why Bother With Theory?

Leslie Rittenmeyer

- Explain the divergent points of view surrounding evidence-based practice.

- Describe the characteristics of a comprehensive model of evidence-based practice.

- Discuss how comprehensive models of evidence-based practice are congruent with the broader theoretical constructs important to nursing.

- Discuss the challenges and barriers that frontline nurses confront in moving evidence into practice.

Epistemology
Evidence-based practice
  movement
Evidence generation
Evidence/knowledge transfer

Evidence synthesis
Evidence utilization
Nursing theory
Systematic reviews
Theory-guided practice

Clinical Story

Arshay, Golda, Kyle, and Ruby are taking an introductory research course and are developing a presentation about certain aspects of evidence-based practice. In their presentation, they must address the divergent points of view and controversies surrounding the evidence-based practice movement. They also need to discuss the characteristics of comprehensive models of evidence-based practice and address whether those models are congruent with the broader theoretical constructs important to nursing. Finally, they must provide a broad overview of the challenges and barriers frontline nurses face when moving from best evidence to bedside practice. Even though the students have been learning about evidence-based practice since the beginning of their curriculum, they realize they need to deepen their knowledge to do this assignment well. Their first step is to search the literature and start reading.

Think Before You Read

- How do you go about organizing your thinking when you want to learn about a nursing intervention or a patient experience?
- What might very experienced nurses debate if they were to think about how they make decisions in their practice?
- Does it matter how you structure your thinking about the decisions you make in your clinical practice?

Introduction

As you have read in the previous chapters, evidence-based practice has been around many years and is far from a new notion. As far back as 1992, the Evidence-Based Medicine Working Group advocated for an approach to clinical decision making in medicine that used research evidence instead of pathophysiological rationales, intuition, previous clinical experience, and expert opinion to determine appropriate interventions for patient care. Early emphasis on randomized controlled trials (RCTs) as the gold standard of evidence set the tone for the initial **evidence-based practice movement.** Further, assigning a descending order of credibility to other forms of evidence spurred debate over what constitutes acceptable evidence.

Although some in nursing embraced the evidence-based practice movement early on, others feared it was atheoretical and was causing the profession to regress to an era of mindless, process-driven practice. The more narrow definitions of *evidence-based practice* fueled this perspective. However, expanded definitions of evidence-based practice and a wider understanding of what constitutes evidence in nursing have eased the discomfort with the evidence-based practice movement and have allowed for healthy academic debate. There is now a greater understanding of how the models of evidence-based practice are congruent with the broader theoretical constructs that are important to nursing.

Evidence-Based Practice: Historical Perspectives

Definitions

While beginning research for their presentation, Arshay, Golda, Ruby, and Kyle find that some of the earliest debates about the evidence-based practice movement in nursing began more than two decades ago. The team discovers that many of the concerns expressed about the evidence-based practice movement in nursing stemmed from the influences exerted by evidence-based medicine on evidence-based practice in general. One of the sources of conflict in the early debate was the presence of differing definitions of evidence-based practice in the literature. The definition proposed by the Evidence-Based Medicine Working Group (1992, p. 2420) stated that "evidence-based medicine de-emphasizes intuition, unsystematic clinical experience, and pathophysiologic rationale as grounds for clinical decision making and stresses the examination of evidence from clinical research." Sackett, Rosenberg, Gray, et al (1996) proposed a more expansive definition that did not restrict evidence to RCTs, and it allowed for clinical expertise also to be used as evidence. This was an important departure in the evidence-based medicine movement, and it continues to be influential today.

Stelter, Brunell, Guiuliano, et al (1998, pp. 48–49) proposed the following definition: "Evidence-based nursing de-emphasizes isolated, and unsystematic clinical experiences, ungrounded opinions, and tradition as a basis for nursing practices, and stresses instead, the use of research findings and, as appropriate, quality improvement data, other operational and evaluation data, the consensus of recognized experts and affirmed experience to substantiate practice." Gerrish and Clayton (1998, p. 58) stated that evidence-based practice "uses research findings derived from randomized controlled clinical trials or other experimental designs to evaluate specific interventions." Ingersoll (2000, p. 152) extended Sackett's (1996) definition as follows: "Evidence-based nursing practice is the conscientious, explicit and judicious use of theory-derived research-based information in making decisions about care delivery to individuals or groups of patients and in consideration of individuals' needs and preference." Ingersoll conceptualized evidence to include information from theory and research and, more important, a consideration of patient preferences; you can see that Ingersoll's definition moved us a little closer to where we are today. In a similar way, DiCenso, Guyatt, and Ciliska (2005, p. 4) defined evidence-based practice as "the integration of best research evidence with clinical expertise and patient values to facilitate clinical decision making."

A comprehensive definition of evidence-based practice and its relationship to nursing is provided by JBI, an interdisciplinary not-for-profit international research and development agency: "Simply defined, evidence-based practice is the melding of individual clinical judgment and expertise with the best available external evidence to generate the kind of practice that is most likely to lead to a positive outcome for a client or patient. Evidence-based nursing is nursing practice that is characterized by these attributes. Evidence-based clinical practice takes into account the context in which care takes place; the preference of the client; the clinical judgment of the health professional, as well as the best available evidence" (Joanna Briggs Institute, n.d.).

Controversies

The variability in the definitions of evidence-based practice, particularly early on, led to some criticism of the evidence-based movement by nursing theorists and scholars. With the emphasis on RCTs and a narrow definition of what constitutes evidence, some professionals failed to see how the evidence-based practice paradigm would benefit nursing. Some even argued that there was not enough empirical nursing research to embrace the model.

Some scholars questioned how well the evidence-based medical model fits with nursing's **epistemology** (foundations of knowledge). Carper (1978), in her classic article, and White (1995), in her expansion of Carper's work, provide an important framework for identifying the different forms of knowledge that reflect the ethos, or worldview, of nursing. They labeled these empirical, personal, ethical, aesthetic, and sociopolitical. In the earlier days of the evidence-based medicine movement, even though there was some room for clinical expertise to play a role in clinical decision making, emphasis was placed predominantly on the empirical way of knowing (e.g., RCTs). It was not that nurses devalued empirical knowledge but pointed to the value of other research paradigms to inform clinical decision making. Walker and Redmond (1999) suggest that medically dominated models, which value only empirical forms of evidence, present a threat to nursing's perspective of theory-guided practice. Mitchell (1999) recognizes the relevance of RCTs for providing directions for procedures, techniques, and protocols while also providing additional resources for clients and nurses about the latest developments in diagnosis and treatment, but she expresses several concerns about the evidence-based practice movement. She suggests that evidence-based practice constrains nurses from defining their own values to guide the nurse–person process and takes away from the humanness of that process. This creates a scenario that allows nurses to relinquish professional responsibility to patients and devalues nursing as a human science. She states strongly that nurses must choose a path that ensures a value-specific, theory-guided knowledge base, in which the client is considered the expert about his or her health and change. Her thoughts in 1999 provoked thoughtful reflection, and continue to do so today.

Fawcett, Watson, Neuman, et al (2001), although not opposed to evidence-based practice, expressed concern that the art of nursing might be subjugated to an emphasis on the science of nursing, threatening nursing's holistic roots. They clearly acknowledge the connections among theory, research, and practice; in fact, they believe that theories provide a lens through which critique and interpretation of various types of evidence may be viewed, which is essential for theory-guided, evidence-based holistic practice.

Upton (1999) suggests that, despite the honorable goals of evidence-based practice, the concept has exacerbated an already existing theory–practice gap because there are fundamental differences in contexts and beliefs among what she calls the four pillars of nursing: management, practice, research, and education. She states that "the present principles of evidence-based practice threaten to continue to exacerbate the theory-practice gap by the recognition that some of the principle beliefs underpinning the concept are in direct contrast to contemporary nursing's opinion and subsequently limit practitioner's creativity and autonomy" (p. 554). She believes these inconsistencies need to be resolved before the concept of evidence-based practice can be successfully implemented.

Ingersoll (2000) contends that ethical issues are raised if reimbursement in health care is connected solely to documented sources of evidence. Nolan and Bradley (2008) express skepticism about the evidence-based practice movement as well, concluding that although evidence-based practice can play a role in improving the treatment provided to patients, nurses should be aware of other kinds of evidence and appreciate that any single approach to determining care, no matter how popular, is likely to lead to a service that does not truly meet the complex individual needs of the patient.

Although the evolution of the evidence-based practice movement has been a little rocky and messy at times, the students preparing their presentation in this chapter's Clinical Story are fascinated by the progress that evidence-based practice has made in just two short decades. In following the historical progression of the movement, they are able to see how much of the debate and criticism came about, and how most of the criticisms have been addressed. The expanded definition that includes patient preferences, insight and clinical expertise, the consideration of context, the consideration of local data, and acceptance of a pluralistic approach about what constitutes evidence has made it possible to have rigorous academic dialogue. This is good both for health care, patients, and the discipline of nursing.

As the students prepare the next part of their presentation, they reflect on the key points they have just learned:

- It is in the interest of nursing as a discipline that practice be grounded in theory; some professionals in nursing fear that evidence-based practice is atheoretical and forces a "cookbook" approach to care that might cause nursing to lose its value of holism.
- The current definitions of evidence-based practice have expanded over the past two decades to include patient preferences, context of care, and clinical expertise.
- There is an expanded conceptualization of what constitutes evidence, moving beyond randomized clinical trials to a more pluralistic approach.

The students now feel they understand the issues, and they are ready to tackle the last part of their presentation. This means looking broadly at what constitutes a comprehensive model of evidence-based practice and addressing whether it is congruent with the broader theoretical constructs of the discipline.

Comprehensive Models of Evidence-Based Practice

There are several models of evidence-based practice, which are discussed in Chapter 5. In general, any comprehensive model views evidence-based practice as a process, with the goal of informing clinical decision making to improve global health. For instance, the JBI Model of Evidence-based Health Care (Pearson, Wiechula, Lockwood, et al, 2005) is organized to address evidence generation, evidence synthesis, evidence/knowledge transfer, and evidence utilization.

Evidence generation points to the best available evidence and indicates where there is a lack of primary evidence. It helps us to see where there are holes in the body of available research. **Evidence synthesis** is a pooling of available research findings through the process of systematic review. **Systematic reviews** include systematically searching international databases to identify and summarize the best evidence surrounding a clinical question. Because the JBI model is a pluralistic model, systematic reviews can focus on evidence from quantitative research, qualitative research, economic analysis, expert opinion, and text. **Evidence/knowledge transfer** is the part of the process that moves the evidence to where it needs to go. This may be accomplished through journals, clinical guidelines, electronic media, educational programs, other publications, and professional conferences. Knowledge transfer is also about targeting specific groups that should receive the information and packaging it so that it aids utilization and clinical decision making. The last part of the process, **evidence utilization,** is the use of evidence to bring about practice or system change. Evidence utilization is influenced by many outside factors such as the institutional culture, power structures, and available resources.

A decade or more later, the JBI model was reexamined to determine its relevancy in light of where the evidence-based movement is at the present time. The end result was the proposal of a revised model that further attempts to clarify the conceptual integration of evidence generation, synthesis, transfer, and implementation, linking these components with the challenging dynamics that influence whether translation of evidence into policy and practice is successful. This model provides a theory-rich, evidence-informed model that facilitates an organizational approach to best practices (Jordan, Lockwood, Munn, et al, 2018; Lockwood, 2017). The revision of this model will be discussed in more depth in Chapter 5.

In summary, evidence-based health care is a process that begins with clinical questions and concerns or interests of clinicians, patients, or consumers. The process attempts to answer these questions by generating knowledge and evidence through the process of systematic review. The knowledge/evidence is then transferred to target groups of professionals who utilize and evaluate its impact on health outcomes, health systems, and professional practice (Pearson, Field, & Jordan, 2007).

Congruency of Evidence-Based Practice With Theoretical Constructs of Nursing

In an attempt to answer the question of how current comprehensive models of evidence-based practice are congruent with the theoretical constructs important to nursing, the students decide to start out by examining the word *theory*. The word *theory* stems from the Greek word *theoreo,* which means to "look at, to observe, to contemplate."

Theories are sets of interrelated concepts with propositional statements that describe or link those concepts (Fawcett, 1999). Chinn and Kramer (2004) state that theories are a creative and rigorous structuring of ideas that project a systematic view of phenomena. **Nursing theory** aims to describe, predict, and explain the phenomena important to nursing. Theories help organize knowledge. Theories also guide the research process and the development of research questions that are pertinent to nursing. Most important, theories are meant to improve practice, not by dictating specific actions but by providing an overreaching guide for action. This is accomplished through the relationship between theory and research.

As long as one adheres to the broader definitions of evidence-based practice, it is hard to see the conflict between the aims and structures of **theory-guided practice** and evidence-based practice. Theory-guided practice is based on the assumption that practitioners can describe, explain, or predict why they do things. Evidence-based practice is a set of tools, procedures, and resources used to find the most current, best available evidence from research or other sources (if research is not available). It also involves applying that evidence to clinical decision making, taking into account the situation, culture, resources, and common sense. The overarching aim is to improve global health.

Challenges of Evidence-Based Practice

Arshay, Golda, Kyle, and Ruby now believe they have a good understanding of the controversies and critiques surrounding evidence-based practice. Although they believe evidence-based practice will help them provide better care, the students want to understand some of the challenges and barriers they will confront when attempting to implement it.

As they finish preparing this last part of their presentation, the students realize that implementation of a comprehensive model of evidence-based practice is sometimes messy and almost always complicated. They begin to realize it might be difficult for frontline nurses to implement an evidence-based practice on their own.

Hannes, Vandermissen, DeBlaeser, et al (2007) conducted a study of 53 Flemish nurses that attempted to identify the barriers to evidence-based nursing (Box 4■1). Melnyk and Fineout-Overholt (2005) also identified barriers to the implementation of evidence-based nursing practice (Box 4■2).

BOX 4■1 **Research Finding on Barriers to Evidence-Based Nursing**

- Known existing barriers to the use of evidence-based nursing include a lack of time, resources, evidence authority, and support.
- Known internal barriers include a lack of motivation and resistance to change.
- Nurses acknowledge a lack of responsibility in the uptake of evidence-based nursing.
- Elements of power are visible in nurses' relationships with physicians, managers, and patients, the latter being more outspoken with nurses providing home-based care who consider themselves "guests" in the patient's environment.
- Different education levels might lead to two-tier nursing practice.

BOX 4■2 **Barriers to Evidence-Based Practice in Nursing**

- Lack of knowledge in relation to evidence-based practice strategies
- Negative views and misperceptions about research and evidence-based practice
- Failure to believe that evidence-based practice will result in more positive outcomes than will traditional care
- Voluminous amounts of information in professional journals
- Lack of time to search for and appraise evidence
- Large patient loads
- Lack of administrative support
- Demands by patients for certain types of care
- Peer pressure to follow established conventions
- Inadequate content and skills regarding evidence-based practice in educational settings

As you can see, the evidence-based practice movement has come a long way in the past decade. Many of the controversies are being addressed and resolved through a process of scholarly discourse. Obviously, challenges and barriers still exist, but there is an increasing body of knowledge on how to address them.

■ Summary

As they prepare the final version of their presentation, this chapter's Clinical Story students have learned that the road to implementing evidence-based practice might be challenging. Despite that, they now have some insight into how to approach the process, and they are confident in their abilities to discuss the criticisms of the evidence-based practice movement (Box 4■3 and Box 4■4). They also embrace the

BOX 4∎3 **Interdisciplinary Rounds**

As stated in the work of Hannes et al (2007), one of the barriers to implementing evidence-based practice is the power inequalities in the health-care system that exist between physicians and frontline nurses.

Example
Nurses are often in a dependant position and contradicting physicians' opinions is hard for many of them. Some nurses reported that sometimes physicians would even do the opposite to reaffirm the dominant position. Many nurses feel that physicians will take advice from other professionals before they will do so from nurses. Some nurses in this study admitted that sometimes because they don't take the initiative, they automatically defer to physicians. How would you begin to address this in your practice?

BOX 4∎4 **Tools for Learning and Practice**

- Search the JBI Web site (https://jbi.global) and print out the revised Joanna Briggs Comprehensive Model of Evidence-based Health Care.
- Search Google Scholar (http://scholar.google.com) for the phrase "controversies in evidence-based nursing." Print out one article and read it in its entirety.
- Reflect on the definition of the word *theory* and give some examples of the way in which nursing theory can provide an overreaching guide for action.
- Explore the nursing theory Web site (http://healthsci.clayton.edu/ eichelberger/nursing.htm).

concept of both theory-guided practice and evidence-based practice and see nothing inconsistent between the goals of both systems. They understand there are barriers and challenges to the implementation of evidence-based practice but feel they are prepared to face them now that they know what to expect.

CHAPTER QUESTIONS

1. Discuss the belief by some that evidence-based practice is atheoretical.

2. Compare and contrast earlier definitions of evidence-based practice with a more current definition.

3. Answer the argument that the evidence-based practice movement is incongruent with the epistemologies of nursing.

(continues on page 48)

CHAPTER QUESTIONS (continued)

4. Compare and contrast the aims of theory-guided practice with the aims of evidence-based practice.

5. Explain ways in which evidence-based practice is congruent with the theoretical constructs of nursing.

6. Explain the process of knowledge transfer and how it is connected to knowledge utilization.

7. Explain how the barriers of lack of administrative support and unequal power structures might hinder a frontline nurse from implementing an evidence-based practice.

References

Carper, B. (1978). Fundamental patterns of knowing in nursing. *Advance in Nursing Science*, *1*(1), 13–23.

Chinn, P., & Kramer, M. (2004). *Integrated knowledge development in nursing* (6th ed.). St. Louis, MO: Mosby.

DiCenso, A., Guyatt, A., & Ciliska, D. (2005). *Evidence-based nursing: A guide to clinical practice*. St. Louis, MO: Mosby.

Evidence-Based Medicine Working Group. (1992). Evidence-based approach to teaching the practice of medicine. *Journal of the American Medical Association*, *268*(17), 2420–2425.

Fawcett, J. (1999). *The relationship of theory and research* (3rd ed.). Philadelphia, PA: F. A. Davis.

Fawcett, J., Watson, J., Neuman, B., et al. (2001). On nursing theories and evidence. *Journal of Nursing Scholarship*, *33*(2), 115–119.

Gerrish, K., & Clayton, J. (1998). Improving clinical effectiveness through an evidence-based approach: Meeting the challenge for nursing in the United Kingdom. *Nursing Administration Quarterly*, *22*(4), 55–65.

Hannes, K., Vandermissen, J., DeBlaeser, L., et al. (2007). Barriers to evidence-based nursing: A focus group study. *Journal of Advanced Nursing*, *60*(2), 162–171.

Ingersoll, G. L. (2000). Evidence-based nursing. What it is and what it isn't [Op-ed]. *Nursing Outlook*, *48*(4), 151–152.

Joanna Briggs Institute. (n.d.). Definition of evidence-based practice and nursing. Retrieved from http://www.joannabriggs.edu.au/

Jordan, Z., Lockwood, C., Munn, Z., et al. (2018). Redeveloping the model of evidence-based healthcare. *International Journal of Evidence-Based Healthcare*, *16*, 227–241. doi:10.1097/XEB000000000000139

Lockwood, C. (2017). Applying theory informed global trends in a collaborative model for organizational evidence-based healthcare. *Korean Academy of Nursing Administration*, *23*, 111–117. http://dx.doi.org/10.11111/jkana.2017.23.2.111

Melnyk, B. M., & Fineout-Overholt, E. (2005). Making the case for evidence-based practice. In B. M. Melnyk & E. Fineout-Overholt (Eds.), *Evidence-based practice in nursing & healthcare: A guide to best practice* (pp. 3–24). Philadelphia, PA: Lippincott Williams & Wilkins.

Mitchell, G. J. (1999). Evidence-based practice: Critique and alternative view. *Nursing Science Quarterly*, *12*, 30–35.

Nolan, P., & Bradley, E. (2008). Evidence-based practice implications and concerns. *Journal of Nursing Management*, *16*, 388–393.

Pearson, A., Field, J., & Jordan, Z. (2007). *Evidence-based clinical practice in nursing and health care: Assimilating research, experience and expertise*. Oxford, United Kingdom: Blackwell.

Pearson, A., Wiechula, R., Lockwood, C., et al. (2005). The JBI model of evidence-based health care. *International Journal of Evidence-Based Health Care*, *3*, 207–215.

Sackett, D. L., Rosenberg, W. M. C., Gray, J. A. M., et al. (1996). Evidence-based medicine: What it is and what it isn't. *British Medical Journal, 312*(7023), 71–72.

Stelter, C., Brunell, M., Giuliano, K. K., et al. (1998). Evidence-based practice and the role of nursing leadership. *Journal of Nursing Administration, 28*(7–8), 45–53.

Upton, D. J. (1999). How can we achieve evidence-based practice if we have a theory-practice gap in nursing today? *Journal of Advanced Nursing, 29*(3), 549–555.

Walker, P. H., & Redmond, R. (1999). Theory-guided, evidence-based reflective practice. *Nursing Science Quarterly, 12,* 298–303.

White, J. (1995). Patterns of knowing: Review, critique, and update. *Advances of Nursing Science, 17*(4), 73–86.

CHAPTER 5

A Sampler of Conceptual Frameworks and Models

Lisa Hopp

LEARNING OBJECTIVES

■ Differentiate evidence-based practice conceptual frameworks and models based on their focus, purpose, origins, and practical tools that help make the model operational.

■ Given a clinical situation, apply a specific model to a patient problem using the model's way of relating concepts.

■ Debate the practical usefulness of conceptual models to guide evidence-based nursing practice.

KEY TERMS

Conceptual framework
Context
Descriptive framework or model
Explanatory framework or model
Facilitation
Heuristic
Innovation
Iowa model

JBI model
Model
Ottawa Model of Research Use (OMRU)
PARIHS and i-PARIHS framework
Potential adopters
Practice environment
Predictive framework or model
Worldview

Clinical Story

Jaspar, Mina, Alfredo, and Grace often work the night shift together in a medical intensive care unit, and they have become good friends. They often tease one another about how they represent the "United Nations of Nursing." Jaspar was raised in a small town in southern England, moving to the city to attend school; Mina emigrated from Morocco when she was a teen; Alfredo started his career in Italy and moved to the United States when he married; and Grace is a native of this U.S. city, having recently graduated from a nearby school of nursing. They care for one to three patients each night, depending on the patients' acuity, yet they often talk with one another about the correct approach to patient care.

Tonight, the unit is at full capacity with 14 critically ill patients. Some of these patients are quite unstable, and others are physiologically stable but still require close nursing vigilance. The group members know that they cannot stop for a break, yet they consult with one another when they are unsure about the best way to assess or intervene with their patients and their families.

Jaspar's patient had a heart attack about 12 hours before he started caring for her. The patient, Mrs. B., is a 55-year-old woman whose husband and two grown children have not left the hospital since she was admitted. Jaspar is caring only for Mrs. B. because she has been very unstable, is on a ventilator, has several invasive catheters, and is on multiple intravenous medications. Her daughters and husband are at Mrs. B.'s bedside when her heart rhythm suddenly deteriorates to ventricular tachycardia. Jaspar and his colleagues begin resuscitation.

While the others continue to defibrillate and resuscitate Mrs. B., Mina attends to the family members. Mina gently draws them to the side, calmly tells them what they are seeing, and asks them if they want to stay by Mrs. B.'s side or if they wish to go to the waiting room. They decide that, for now, they want to stay. Mina stays by their side, explaining what they are seeing and how Mrs. B. is responding to the resuscitation efforts. Although the family members are clearly distressed that Mrs. B is so critically ill, they ask Mina questions and tell her that they are glad they are able to stay in the room. Mrs. B. improves and becomes more stable. Mina stays with the family until Jaspar is once again able to bring them closer to the bedside.

When the four nurses are finished with their shift, they have breakfast together and talk about their night. They realize the ways they were raised in households with different cultural backgrounds influence how they think about families being present during resuscitation. They talked about Mrs. B and her family's cultural backgrounds, their accompanying beliefs, values, and preferences. The nurses also have their own clinical strengths and preferences concerning the manner in which they make decisions about their nursing care. Nonetheless, even though they have unique approaches to the "how" of nursing, they share a common "what"—the evidence base of their decisions. If they use a framework, they can integrate their unique worldviews, hows, and common whats to develop a shared roadmap for using evidence to help them make decisions about supporting families during the resuscitation of a loved one.

Think Before You Read

- How do you organize your thinking when faced with a complex problem?
- Is a role for theories, frameworks, or models in your everyday nursing practice?
- If you are faced with a problem, what is the first question or thought that you have to begin to solve it?
- Think about what you do if you are in a new area and you need to find a specific place at a certain time. Do you simply start driving or walking or do you use some type of aid to help you get there? How might you think about theories, frameworks, and models like a roadmap for nursing practice?

Introduction

Sometimes students and clinicians find theory too abstract and impractical to help them in everyday nursing practice. Others claim that theory can stifle creativity and innovation when designing research about how to implement evidence into practice (Rycroft-Malone, 2007). Still others argue that if theory is neglected in the efforts to implement evidence, the theory–practice gap will expand, limit ingenuity, and lead us away from the essences of nursing as a discipline (Mitchell, 2013; Upton, 1999; Yancey, 2019). As you can see, these are nearly opposite opinions. As you read in the previous chapter, there is no need to approach evidence-based practice atheoretically. In fact, many would counter that theory is essential to advancing the evidence-based practice movement.

If you are new to using frameworks, theory, and models to shape how you use evidence in your practice, you need a good reason to pursue the challenge. In addition, you should remain open to different types before you select an approach. In fact, some models may be more applicable than others in different contexts and for different goals. We are not able to review all of the possible conceptual approaches to evidence-based practice in this chapter. Instead, we will offer you samples that we think are robust and practical. That means they should work in a variety of situations and guide you in sensible and functional ways.

Like the group of nurses in the clinical story, how one approaches nursing care, how one thinks about nursing, and, indeed, how patients experience health and health care are influenced by one's **worldview.** In other words, how you nurse is influenced by your frame of reference, your experiences, and how you think about and fit your experiences into your representation of the world. Patients and your beliefs and values that you share with your "group" influence your worldview. We use a system of symbols that "allows us to integrate everything we know about the world and ourselves into a global picture, one that illuminates reality as it is presented to us within a certain culture" (Aerts, Apostel, De Moor, et al, 2007; Wilson, Heaslip, & Jackson, 2018).

Why Bother Thinking Conceptually?

Before you read further, you may be asking, Why bother? Theory, conceptual frameworks, and models may simply seem like an academic exercise or an activity for people with extra time on their hands instead of a tool for busy clinicians. Consider the following analogy before you decide to stop reading: If you need to go somewhere but you do not know how to get there, you look at a map or use a device that provides the map. Depending on the purpose of your journey, you use a certain type and scale of map. You can also use a map to generate what-ifs. That is, if you go in a specific direction, you can find certain points of interest, hazards, or other places of note. Using theories, frameworks, and models is like using various types of maps to help you understand where you are going and how the places along the way relate to one another and to help you to generate hypotheses. They help you avoid getting lost in the process of moving evidence into practice (see Box 5■1).

In this chapter's clinical story, the four nurses come from very different cultural and family backgrounds and began their nursing careers in different contexts. These experiences shaped how they think about family members being present during resuscitation and how they view the evidence related to the practice. The patient and her family members also bring their own beliefs, values, and ways of thinking about their world. Nevertheless, the nurses all participated in helping Mrs. B.'s family through this very difficult experience by recognizing and responding to both their own and Mrs. B's family's worldviews.

Frameworks, Theories, and Models

Translating knowledge gained from evidence into action is complex. This complexity exists in the even more intricate context of nursing practice and the worldviews of

---

BOX 5■1 Significance of Frameworks, Theories, and Models

- Trying to use evidence in practice without a conceptual approach is like driving in a new area without a map or directions.
- Frameworks, theories, and models provide practical and creative guidance for implementing evidence in your practice.
- Using a conceptual approach can improve efficiency and speed the uptake of evidence.
- Frameworks, theories, and models provide research questions to advance nursing practice and health-care agendas.

those who do nursing. A variety of frameworks, theories, and models exists to help you navigate this complexity. They vary in their purpose, origin, how far along they are in their development, intended users, and scope. This chapter provides only a sample of frameworks and models that will be useful as you try to make evidence actionable. You may want to explore others that are beyond the scope of this book.

Definitions

Words and language are the building blocks of frameworks, theories, and models. Before exploring them, we need to be clear about the meanings of *conceptual framework, theory,* and *model* and how they relate to one another. Some people use these three expressions interchangeably, whereas others are very careful to differentiate each, even though they all represent some kind of "mental device" (Kitson, Rycroft-Malone, Harvey, et al, 2008).

Conceptual frameworks identify "a set of variables and relationships that should be examined in order to explain phenomena. They need not specify the direction of relationships or identify critical hypotheses. In contrast, a theory provides a denser and logically coherent set of relationships. Theories can offer views on the causal relationships and seek to explain the phenomena" (Kitson et al, 2008, p. 5). Several theories can be consistent with a single conceptual framework (Kitson et al, 2008).

Models are generally less ambitious than either theories or conceptual frameworks. They are still representations of a real phenomenon, but they are narrower, usually represent a specific situation, and are made of more precise assumptions (Nilsen, 2015; Rycroft-Malone & Bucknall, 2010b). Several models may fit a single theory.

Figure 5■1 may help you understand the relationship among conceptual frameworks, theories, and models and how worldview and context shape how they are

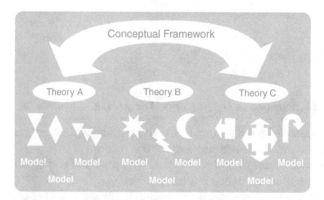

FIGURE 5■1 Relationship of conceptual frameworks, theories, and models. A conceptual framework describes, explains, or predicts a set of variables and relationships to further explain a phenomenon (shapes). Theories describe a denser, more logical, coherent set of relationships (set of ideas). Many theories may be consistent with a framework. Models are more narrowly focused but may be skeletal or precise; several models may fit one theory (schema sharing a theme such as triangles, arrows, or weather symbols).

used. Some people think of the relationship among conceptual frameworks, theories, and models in layers of specificity and scope.

In this chapter's clinical story, nurses in the critical care unit used a particular framework to guide how they approached developing their unit-specific policies as well as how individual nurses used evidence to make clinical decisions. Their unit practice council chose a conceptual framework because it was practical and clear and helped them structure the process of evidence utilization. It helped them choose appropriate tools to implement and evaluate evidence uptake.

Organizing Your Thinking About Frameworks, Theories, and Models

When you explore different conceptual frameworks and models, use a systematic approach to sort them. Much like organizing a closet, you will be able to select the right conceptual "clothes" for a particular situation if you understand their purpose, what situation they best fit into, what concepts they address, and how best to use them.

Rycroft-Malone and Bucknall (2010b) reviewed literature about theory use and developed a series of criteria to help organize your thinking and evaluate frameworks and models (see Table 5■1).

- Begin by determining the scope of the framework or model. Does it address a very broad, large range of abstract concepts, or is it more narrow and precise and perhaps more concrete in focus? Think about whether the framework or model aims to describe, explain, or predict.
- Consider how far along it is in its development by looking at how the authors designed the framework and model and if they provide evidence to support it. Have others used or tested the framework or model in a practice or a research setting?
- Think about the intended users. How should they use the model or framework? For what functions should they use it? For example, is it intended to help a certain discipline assess, intervene, or evaluate implementation of evidence?
- Consider if it is testable and how useful the model or framework is for you in the context that you intend to use it. In other words, think about the what, why, who, when, where, how, and how well of the framework or model.

Use these criteria to help you determine how well any particular model suits you, your setting, and need. We explore four models in more depth in this chapter and the next, but there are other models and frameworks that may interest you.

Specific Frameworks and Models for Evidence-Based Practice

Rycroft-Malone and Bucknall (2010a, 2010b) suggest the purposes of evidence implementation frameworks and models fall into one of three categories: descriptive,

TABLE 5■1   **Criteria for Organizing Frameworks and Models**

Criterion	Comments
Structure	▪ Frameworks vary in how extensive and abstract they are ▪ Models tend to be more precise and prescriptive
Purpose	▪ Descriptive—describes properties, characteristics, and qualities of a phenomenon ▪ Explanatory—explains causal relationships and mechanisms of a phenomenon and relates it to other concepts ▪ Predictive—predicts relationships through propositions or hypotheses
Development	▪ Inductive approaches—generated from gathering information and building the model or framework ▪ Deductive approaches—beginning with generalizations and gathering information to support the generalizations ▪ Support sources—evidence from research, systematically derived consensus, or analyses to support or refute the framework or model
Theoretical basis	▪ Theories provide a foundation for the framework or model ▪ One framework may borrow from several theories or be consistent with more than one theory ▪ These may be implied or clearly identified
Conceptual clarity	▪ Definition of terms and how they relate to each other ▪ Ability to identify differences and similarities among the theories that underpin the framework and model ▪ Ability to promote new theoretical understanding
Users and context	▪ Aimed at individuals, groups, or organizations ▪ Intended for certain disciplines (nurses, medicine, or multiple disciplines) or groups of disciplines (all health-care providers or groups that create policy) ▪ Real or simulated/hypothetical use
Functionality	▪ Tools related to using the framework, such as assessment tools, implementation strategies, and evaluation methods ▪ Ease of adoption or adaptation to clinical situations
Testability	▪ Ability to generate and test hypotheses using a variety of research methods ▪ Ability to use evidence to support or refute the framework or model

Adapted from Rycroft-Malone and Bucknall (2010a, 2010b).

explanatory, or predictive. **Descriptive frameworks** or **models** describe the nature of the elements of a phenomenon or process without making claims about relationships. **Explanatory frameworks** or **models** specify cause-and-effect relationships and mechanisms. **Predictive frameworks** or **models** forecast how phenomena will behave and how they relate to one another, and tend to generate propositions and hypotheses (Rycroft-Malone & Bucknall, 2010a, 2010b). The purpose statement of the framework or model tells you what to expect of it and may help you make a decision about whether to use it.

Another way to sort frameworks, theories, and models is to analyze their intended use and users. For example, some are meant to guide individuals in making specific clinical decisions. Others are meant to guide groups or organizations in developing policy. Still others are aimed at enhancing the context to improve the chance that individuals and groups will use evidence in some way.

In the next section, you can review brief descriptions of frameworks or models that are best suited to help frontline nurses make decisions in clinical settings. Other excellent frameworks and models exist (e.g., the Stetler model, the Knowledge to Action model, and Dobbin's Dissemination model), but they are more complex and beyond the scope of this book. You can review more about them thorough descriptions in texts and journal articles related to these and other frameworks and models (e.g., Rycroft-Malone & Bucknall, 2010a, or Nilsen, 2015). For each model discussed in this book, you will see how nurses can use each one to guide the policies related to family presence in the critical care unit, as illustrated in this chapter's clinical story.

Iowa Model

The **Iowa model** (Fig. 5■2) was developed at the University of Iowa hospital and was originally a guide to research utilization. The authors developed it further, based on feedback from staff nurses and nursing leaders and published the first version in 2001. After more than 3,900 requests to use the model, the authors again revisited and published their refined model in 2017 (Iowa Model Collaborative, 2017). They based their revisions on a systematic, multiphase process to revise and validate the model. The model is popular in part because it is very practical and avoids abstract concepts. It is aimed at individuals or groups who collaborate within a system to change practice.

The purpose of the model is to guide practitioners through a series of decision points as they move through the evidence implementation process. The schema looks like an algorithm or flowchart of decision points that provides a linear process of putting evidence into action (Iowa Model Collaborative, 2017; Titler, 2010).

The revised process begins with five types of triggers (clinical or patient identified issue; organization, state, or national initiative; data or new evidence; accrediting agency requirements/regulation; and philosophy of care) that motivates health-care providers to consider a change in practice. After stating the problem, the first decision the practitioner or group must make is whether the issue is a priority for the organization. If it is not, then the model recommends that the practitioner

The Iowa Model Revised: Evidence-Based Practice to Promote Excellence in Health Care

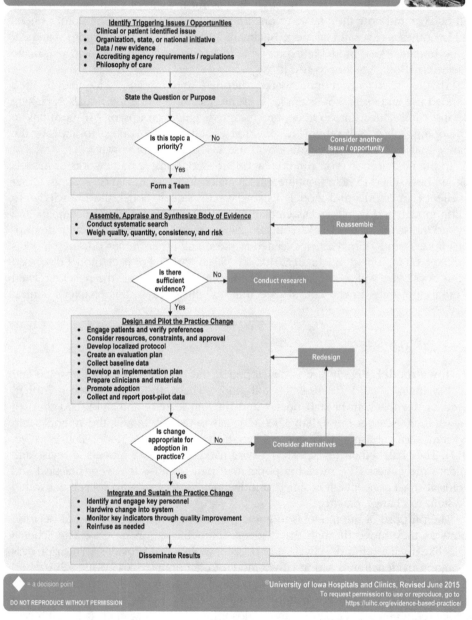

FIGURE 5■2 The Iowa Model Revised: Evidence-Based Practice to Promote Excellence in Health Care. (© 2015 University of Iowa Hospitals and Clinics, with permission.)

refocus on another issue. If it is a priority, a team forms and its members search, appraise, and synthesize research and other types of evidence. This requires members of the team to have skills in searching for evidence and weighing its quality, quantity, consistency, and potential risks. Next, the group decides whether there is a sufficient evidence base to guide practice. If the group determines that there is not a sufficient evidence base, then someone (the team may not feel they have adequate skills to conduct research but others may) must conduct further research and reassemble the new evidence and feed this knowledge back for appraisal and decision making about the adequacy of the evidence base. If they decide that the evidence base is adequate, they design and pilot the practice change that includes considering patient preferences and resources, developing a protocol and evaluation plan for the local context, collecting baseline data, implementing the plan, working with clinicians and developing any required materials, promoting the change, and measuring outcomes. Based on the outcome of the pilot phase, the group decides whether they should adopt the practice change. If they decide not to, the team redesigns the practice change and reruns the pilot phase. If the change is appropriate, then the team moves to integrate and sustain the practice by engaging key stakeholders, embedding the practice change in the monitoring of the practice change and reinforcing as needed. Finally, the team disseminates the results of their efforts (Iowa Model Collaborative, 2017; Titler, 2010). The Iowa Model Collaborative incorporated the feedback from more than 600 users in this last revision. You are encouraged to seek out the tools and further discussion of the model at the collaborative's Web site (https://uihc.org/evidence-based-practice).

In this chapter's clinical story, if the practice council used the Iowa model to develop a family presence initiative, Mina would begin with a trigger, such as reading a journal article about family presence and the organization's philosophy of patient-centered care. The article may have intrigued her because of her own view of the importance of supportive families in the critical care unit. In addition, close extended family relationships are at the center of her Moroccan heritage. She would then form a unit-based team if others validated that the initiative was aligned with the organization's goal of family-centered care. Once the unit leaders agreed that the initiative fit their strategic philosophy, Mina would seek the help of the unit practice council and information scientist to search and appraise, including weighing the quality, quantity, and potential risks associated with the evidence. Mina and the team would synthesize the evidence. After Mina presented her findings, the council would decide whether the evidence from research and other types of evidence was strong enough to proceed. Assuming it was, they may design goals such as the following: (1) families express satisfaction, comfort, and support during witnessed resuscitation; (2) families experience no ill effects of witnessed resuscitation; and (3) health-care providers are able to complete resuscitation smoothly. They would determine what tools they would need to evaluate if they met their goals. Then they would adapt existing evidence by melding somewhat older Emergency Nurses Association guidelines with subsequent research findings to create their own unit policy, and conduct pilot tests to carefully evaluate the impact of the new policy on families and health-care workers by interviewing or surveying both groups.

Finally, the team would analyze the findings from the evaluation to determine whether they should make changes and institute the policy more widely and permanently. They may also present their findings to local groups or even more broadly at conferences and via publication.

The Ottawa Model of Research Use

Researchers from the Canadian province of Ontario developed the **Ottawa Model of Research Use (OMRU)** (Fig. 5∎3) to help facilitators guide valid research implementation (Logan & Graham, 2010). It is descriptive and prescriptive, as well as practical. The model reflects Roger's Diffusion of Innovation Theory because it focuses on six key elements:

- Research-informed innovation
- Potential adopters
- Practice environment
- Implementation strategies for transferring the evidence into practice
- Adoption of the innovation
- Health-related and other outcomes

FIGURE 5∎3 The Ottawa Model of Research Use (OMRU). (Copyright © 2004 McGill University School of Nursing, with permission.)

Facilitators assess, monitor, and evaluate during a dynamic, interactive, multiple-feedback process (Logan & Graham, 2010). It is meant as an interactive planned action model with phases that are not necessarily meant to be sequential, recognizing that implementation of evidence is iterative and often messy.

During three prescriptive phases of the model, facilitators assess barriers and support, then monitor the process and degree of use during implementation, and finally evaluate the impact of the project. The assessment phase includes understanding the **innovation**—the new evidence-informed practice, policy, or change in practice—its quality (appraising the evidence supporting the innovation), and other attributes. Innovations that are based on strong evidence, simple, easily tried, user friendly, compatible with current practice, and clear are more likely to be successful.

The assessment phase includes understanding the **potential adopters** of the innovation, such as practitioners, policy makers, patients, and other stakeholders. Adopters who are aware of the innovation have positive attitudes and intentions (perceiving fewer barriers and more facilitators), have the knowledge and skill necessary for the innovation, and are not concerned about the potential harm or work burden are more apt to adopt the innovation. Finally, the team or facilitator must assess the **practice environment,** the setting in which the change will occur. The practice environment includes parts of the implementation context such as the governing rules; cultural and social factors, such as local politics; power structures; resource availability; leadership approaches; peer groups; and other factors (Logan & Graham, 2010).

Based on a thorough assessment of the innovation, the adopters, and the environment, the facilitator and team can better target implementation interventions that maximize strengths and minimize barriers by using problem-solving and good management skills. However, Logan and Graham (2010) caution that the evidence about how to best target barriers and select effective implementation interventions continues to evolve. Facilitators and teams should be flexible and experimental when they try implementation strategies, such as using prompts and clinical cues as reminders, opinion leaders (e.g., well-respected, expert nurses on a unit) to influence peers, or audit and feedback of clinical behaviors. Throughout the implementation process, the facilitators must monitor both the initial and long-term use of the innovation. Sometimes adopters will adopt a new practice but return to old patterns.

During the final stage of the model, the facilitator and team evaluate outcomes related to the patient, practitioners, and system once the new evidence-informed practice has been sustained. The schema for the model indicates that the stages are connected and bidirectional, meaning that the stages are interactive and dynamic, and may not flow in a highly linear way (Logan & Graham, 2010). Multidisciplinary groups have used the OMRU model to guide a variety of practice innovations including speech pathology (Cunningham, Daub, & Cardy, 2019), pediatric health-care providers engaging in shared decision making (Boland, Lawson, Graham, et al, 2019), and critical care nursing (Tayyib & Coyer, 2017).

If the OMRU is used to implement the family presence in this chapter's clinical story, Mina, Jaspar, Alfredo, and Grace would all contribute to the implementation plan facilitated by their unit's clinical nurse specialist and a nurse researcher. The facilitators would appraise the evidence but invite the team to comment on what the evidence and innovation would mean to their work; how it relates to their values, worldviews, and prior experiences; what barriers they might anticipate; and what concerns they may have for the families and their work. Jaspar and other staff may express certain fears about having family present during such a trying event: this may pose a risk to the family's psychological well-being, or it may disrupt the efficient flow of a resuscitative effort. The team may even fear litigation if the outcome had not been good. These are all very important indicators of potential barriers.

Conversely, the facilitators would also recognize that some of the staff, such as Mina, Alfredo, and Grace, are important role models and champions for change if they believe families can safely be present and gain a sense of intimacy with their loved one during a resuscitative effort. Jaspar may voice that he was not convinced that it is a good idea for families to witness resuscitation, even if the evidence seems to point in that direction. The facilitators may probe his resistance and use this information to plan for others with similar feelings. The team also needs to identify what support (e.g., clergy, grief counselors) could be available to families and health-care providers involved in the resuscitation so that both have a sense of safety. Finally, they would assess the structure of the intensive care environment for feasibility barriers (e.g., to see whether there is enough room for the families near the bedside or chairs to sit in if someone became light-headed or could not stand).

During the preintervention phase, the team would likely engage many of the nurses and other professionals in education and discussion before starting a trial of the new policy; they may even use psychology professionals to role-play a simulated scenario to build the staff's confidence in supporting families. After trying to uncover all possible barriers and maximizing supports, they would decide on a clear start date for offering families the option of being present during resuscitation. The facilitators would be on hand to observe how the trial proceeded and to debrief the health-care team and family afterward to determine the intervention's degree of success or failure. Also, there may be additional changes, such as supplemental staff to support the family and those involved in resuscitation efforts. Facilitators would continue to monitor more episodes of family presence as they occur. To do this, they may conduct some guided telephone interviews with families of patients, survivors, and nonsurvivors, within a month or two of the event. These narrative stories could be analyzed to determine themes to help the team learn more about the experiences of families and health-care providers.

The nurses in this chapter's clinical story adopted the practice, and the outcomes for the family, nurses, physicians, respiratory therapy, and clergy were positive. They modified the published guideline somewhat when they realized that there was not enough space at the bedside in all patient rooms during resuscitation. But they resolved to make sure the family could touch, see, and talk to their loved one as soon as possible, and stay in the room if there was a safe nook for them to stand or sit in. The nurses also made sure they stayed near the family members to monitor and support their coping in the period following the resuscitation in case intervention was necessary.

Promoting Action on Research Implementation in Health Services (PARIHS/i-PARIHS)

In 1998, a group of nurse scientists from the United Kingdom involved in managing change and conducting research conceived the Promoting Action on Research Implementation in Health Services Framework, more commonly known as the **PARIHS framework,** to increase the uptake of evidence in various settings (Kitson, Harvey, & McCormack, 1998). Its purpose was to "serve as a practical and conceptual heuristic to guide and evaluate research implementation and practice improvement endeavors" (Rycroft-Malone, 2010, p. 110). **Heuristic** refers to a rule of thumb or structure for problem-solving. Unlike the Iowa model and OMRU, this framework does not describe the process, or how, of evidence implementation or practice improvement. Rather, the PARIHS framework originally focused on three key elements that the authors determined contribute to the success of evidence implementation: evidence, context, and facilitation (Fig. 5■4). Originally, the authors characterized each element on a continuum from low to high or weak to strong. You will read about the original framework and its revised version, as you will find that implementers will use both. They expressed the framework simply as an equation: $SI = f\ (E, C, F)$, where successful implementation (SI) is a function (f) of the level and type of evidence (E), the quality of the context (C), and the approach to facilitation (f) (Kitson et al, 2008). Successful implementation of evidence was more likely when the evidence and context are strong and expertly facilitated.

Each key element of the framework is further defined by subelements and descriptions of each on a low-to-high continuum. Evidence includes knowledge from research, clinical experience, patient preferences, and local data and information. An example of high clinical experience is expertise that others have critiqued, is

FIGURE 5■4 Promoting Action on Research Implementation in Health Services (PARIHS) framework. (Rycroft-Malone, J., & Bucknall, T. (Eds.). (2010). *Models and frameworks for implementing evidence-based practice: Linking evidence to action.* Oxford, United Kingdom: Wiley-Blackwell.)

consistent and accepted among groups, and is relevant and appropriately weighted in the decision-making process. At the other extreme, an example of weak clinical experience is a single anecdote that lacks any critical reflection and cannot be validated by others (Rycroft-Malone, 2010).

Context refers to the practice environment in which the change happens and includes the subelements of organizational culture, leadership, and evaluation practices. A culture on the high end of the continuum is characterized as a learning environment with decentralized decision making, mutually respectful relationships between the managers and staff, and facilitative leadership styles. Transformational (rather than autocratic) leaders who make roles clear and promote effective teamwork and structures are ranked on the high end of the leadership spectrum. The third subelement refers to mechanisms and structures for evaluation. Strong evaluation is characterized by many sources of information with straightforward feedback methods for individuals, teams, and the organization. The framework predicted "that a conducive context for evidence-based practice is where there is clarity of roles, decentralized decision making, staff are valued, transformational leadership, and a reliance on multiple sources of information on performance" (Rycroft-Malone, 2010, p. 119).

The third element of the PARIHS framework is **facilitation,** or "the process of enabling or making easier the implementation of evidence into practice" (Rycroft-Malone, 2010, p. 119). The method of facilitation depends on the characteristics of the evidence, the context, and the stakeholders. The mode of facilitation can vary from technical, "doing for," task-driven support to a more holistic, enabling, coaching approach. For example, "doing for" would be a facilitator who searches, appraises, and develops a list of strategies for evidence implementation and hands this over to a manager to enforce. An enabling facilitator would develop the skills in others, coaching and engaging the ideas of all stakeholders rather than making all of the decisions of implementation. Adept facilitators alter their approach based on their expert assessment of those involved, the qualities of the context, and the stage of the implementation process (see Box 5■2 for interdisciplinary tips).

In 2015, Harvey and Kitson revised the PARIHS framework and renamed it **i-PARIHS** (integrated PARIHS). I-PARIHS focuses more on evidence implementation as innovation and facilitation became the active ingredient that drives the process

---

BOX 5■2   **Interdisciplinary Rounds**

- Multiple disciplines such as psychology and sociology as well as other health-care fields have contributed to the development of frameworks, theories, and models.
- Most frameworks, theories, and models related to evidence implementation can be used by many disciplines and promote collaboration among disciplines.
- Seek out the perspectives of other disciplines to understand how worldviews may be influenced by discipline.

of engaging the recipients (or stakeholders) in the practice improvement, and they explicitly incorporated Roger's characteristics of innovation with the qualities of evidence to define *innovation*. They retained context as a key ingredient of implementation. They expressed the new framework as $SI = Fac^n(I + R + C)$ where Successful Implementation (SI) is a function of the Active Ingredient of Facilitation (Fac^n) and the nature of the Innovation (I), including the evidence, the Recipients' Engagement (R) and the quality of the Context (C) (Harvey & Kitson, 2015). Successful implementation is more likely to occur when (a) the scientific evidence is of high quality and strong. The new model incorporates Roger's characteristics of innovation and predicts that the change will be more likely if the recipients view it as compatible with professional and patient beliefs and as beneficial. The change can be trialed and observed, and it is designed to be less complex. As in the first version of PARIHS, a receptive health-care context for the innovation has supportive leadership, an organizational culture that welcomes change, and evaluation systems in place. Those who facilitate the innovation provide the "active ingredient" by selecting strategies that allow them to assess, align and integrate the other elements (Harvey & Kitson, 2015).

Jaspar, Alfredo, Grace, and Mina would work closely with a facilitator, such as a clinical nurse specialist (CNS), if they were to use the i-PARIHS framework to guide the implementation of the family presence initiative. The CNS would assess the qualities of the context, either through observations and insight or by using a formal context assessment tool to diagnose the strengths of the context as well as appraising the quality and strength of the evidence (Harvey & Kitson, 2015). Knowing that the evidence related to the effectiveness of family presence and its impact on families and health-care providers is positive yet still evolving, the CNS would need to gather local data from interviews of staff and families to assess their perspectives about the initiative.

In addition to the evidence, the facilitator would use any strengths he or she finds in the context, such as taking advantage of the decentralized decision making of the unit practice council and the staff's enthusiasm for learning from one another and the evidence. The CNS would enable the practice council by coaching them through the evidence selection and appraisal process if they need help. If the council is already skilled in appraisal and policy development, the CNS may focus more on supporting their teamwork rather than on technical tasks such as searching for evidence, organizing, and summarizing the evidence. The CNS would assess the recipients'/stakeholders' skills, knowledge, motivations, and perspectives as well as resources such as time, materials, funding, and availability of opinion leaders. Based on this assessment, the CNS might need to plan for greater staff support during resuscitation (e.g., determining how to delegate care during the resuscitation to ensure adequate staff and family support). During the outcome assessment process, the CNS would determine evaluations strategies available in a context. If they were strong, the CNS would focus more on helping staff reflect upon and refine their strategies. If these systems were lacking, the CNS would first develop the evaluation measurement. In fact, the CNS may enlist others and adapt and flex his/her approach based on the assessment and progress of the practice change.

The CNS may rely upon Harvey and Kitson's (2015) tools and checklist to design his/her approach to facilitation.

JBI

The last model examined in this chapter is the **JBI model** (Fig. 5■5). In the last chapter, you were introduced to the key elements of the JBI model. You learned JBI is an international organization that has comprehensively addressed evidence-based practice since its inception in 1996. The model describes how the institute and its global collaborating groups work together to get evidence into practice to improve global health. This goal sets the JBI model apart from the other models and framework presented in this chapter because the other models aim only at the local level. Despite its very broad purpose, the JBI model can be used to guide evidence implementation at a more local level, and provide the tools to allow you to think globally and act locally (Pearson, Wiechula, Lockwood, et al, 2005).

JBI revised the original model after more than 10 years in use, but it continues to focus on the same fundamental elements (Jordan, Lockwood, Munn, et al, 2018). To better understand the JBI model, picture it as a pie with five pieces, with evidence generation, synthesis, transfer, utilization, and enhanced global health in a circle clockwise (see Chapter 4 for definitions). At the center of the model is a "pebble of knowledge" that represents the breadth of legitimate knowledge types important to evidence-based health care that include evidence of feasibility, appropriateness, meaningfulness, and effectiveness of interventions. Each piece of the pie has subelements that further explain the model. JBI has developed methods and tools for each slice of the pie and its subelements to enhance the chance that evidence will make its way into routine practice.

The JBI model developers emphasize that different types of evidence are used to inform different types of questions, and the quality of the evidence varies in a way that is meaningful for the type of evidence (Jordon et al, 2018; Pearson et al, 2005). For example, questions of effectiveness of interventions are ideally answered by systematic reviews or meta-analyses of well-conducted, randomized controlled trials (you will learn more about these types of evidence in later chapters), whereas questions related to the meaning of interventions or phenomena to patients should not be answered with experimental evidence. Rather, these kinds of questions are best answered using narrative data from qualitative studies, ideally from systematic reviews or meta-syntheses of these types of studies. Similarly, questions of feasibility (i.e., physically, culturally, or financially possible within a certain context) and appropriateness (if an intervention fits or relates to the context) are also questions that are important to making clinical decisions.

At each stage of the JBI model, methods exist to make the concept operational. For example, at the synthesis stage, JBI has developed methods, software, and training to support the production of systematic reviews and an online library to distribute them. In addition, the library contains brief evidence summaries based on systematic reviews or other types of evidence. Guidelines are another type of synthesis. During the transfer stage, knowledge is actively transferred through

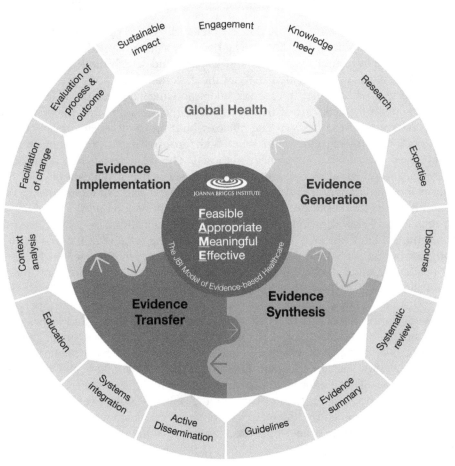

FIGURE 5■5 JBI Model of Evidence-based Healthcare. (From Jordan, Z., Lockwood, C., Munn, Z., Aromataris, E. (2019) The updated Joanna Briggs Institute Model of Evidence-Based Healthcare, *International Journal of Evidence-Based Healthcare, 17*(1), 58–71.)

dissemination, integration into knowledge systems, and education. The transferred knowledge must be implemented if evidence is to be of any value. Implementation processes include context analysis, facilitation, and evaluation of process and outcomes. Finally, the model schema shows that the movement from one element to the next is bidirectional and fluid. To support synthesis, transfer, and implementation, JBI has developed education, training, and tools, and more than 60 affiliated groups work together to make the model practical and useful to meet the goal of global health care through local efforts. The model acknowledges that culture, capacity, communication, and collaboration are overarching principles (Jordan et al, 2018; Pearson, 2010).

The group of staff nurses in this chapter's clinical story could use the JBI model tools to help them first know whether or not there is evidence to support family presence at resuscitation. Mina and Jaspar could search the JBI Database of Systematic Reviews to find evidence about the experience of family presence from the perspective of both health-care providers and the families. Because of JBI's unique attention to questions of meaningfulness, they could search for systematic reviews relevant to this question. The nurses would find a systematic review exists that would help them understand what both groups might experience if they implemented the program (evidence synthesis). The team could then summarize the systematic review into a shorter information sheet that includes a brief of the main methods and findings of the review so their fellow staff can more quickly and efficiently grasp the key aspects of the review and provide education and active dissemination of the knowledge (evidence transfer). Finally, they would need to embed the evidence through a process of assessing the context of the unit for the change, working with their leadership group to help identify potential barriers, and making baseline measurements of the way that families are cared for during resuscitation. They could use these baseline measurements and seek input from other staff and family members about what barriers exist to offer families the option to be present during resuscitation. In addition, Mina, Alfredo, Grace, and Jaspar each have a unique perspective about the initiative, which brings rich understanding to the potential ups and downs of the initiative. They would most likely develop multiple strategies such as speaking one to one with their fellow staff members, conducting role-playing educational sessions, and bringing an expert to the unit to discuss the best approaches to implementing the policy. Finally, after implementing the family presence initiative, the team would need to evaluate whether the barriers still exist, and then they should measure the impact of the project on families and staff (evidence implementation).

■ Summary

In this chapter, you were introduced to practical ways of using frameworks and models in everyday practice (Box 5■3). You learned about four quite different conceptual approaches to getting evidence into practice. The Iowa model focuses on step-by-step decision making when a problem, source of evidence, regulation, or other triggers prompt the beginning of a change process. Theories related to quality improvement could relate to this model. The OMRU is based on theories of planned action and diffusion of innovation. It directs facilitators to assess the qualities of the innovation, adopters, and practice environment before instituting the intervention; monitoring its use for adoption and sustainability; and finally evaluating

---

BOX 5 ■ 3 **Tools for Learning and Practice**

- Select two frameworks or models and apply them to an evidence implementation project; compare the way the conceptual approach steered the process.
- Work with a practice council or other clinical group to select a model to guide evidence implementation.
- Use online resources to help you understand frameworks and models for evidence implementation:
  - https://joannabriggs.org/jbi-approach-to-EBHC (description, links to articles, tools, and ongoing development of the model)
  - https://ktdrr.org/ktlibrary/ (a library of resources for knowledge translation and evidence-based practice in disability and rehabilitation care)
  - https://implementationscience.biomedcentral.com (a free, full-text online journal publishing ongoing development of frameworks, theories, and models)

the impact of the innovation on outcomes. The PARIHS/i-PARIHS framework diverges from these two models because it does not describe a process. Rather, it predicts successful implementation as a function of the evidence/innovation characteristics, the recipients and context with facilitation as the active ingredient. The JBI model describes the role of evidence generation, synthesis, transfer, and implementation in improving global health care. Finally, you learned that the nurses in the clinical story have unique worldviews based on their prior experiences, cultures, and family structures that shape their perspectives on nursing and patient care. These worldviews and the use of a particular model created distinct stories of implementing a family presence initiative at resuscitation.

CHAPTER QUESTIONS

1. Compare and contrast a theory, conceptual framework, and model. How might these three ways of thinking abstractly fit together?

2. How is a road map like a framework or model?

3. You are having coffee with a fellow student or colleague who thinks that theory, frameworks, and models are a waste of time and have nothing to do with practical nursing care. How might you argue that they can help you in daily nursing practice?

4. What are the essential pieces of each of the four models/frameworks discussed in this chapter?

(continues on page 70)

CHAPTER QUESTIONS (continued)

5. Which model or framework seems to fit your way of thinking best? Why?

6. What is the most important aspect of a framework or model?

7. Can you imagine different situations or contexts in which one model may fit better and another in which you might adapt another model? Explain.

8. Think about a recent practice change that occurred in your setting. Select one of the models or frameworks and apply it to what happened. Would the implementation process have gone differently if the model or framework had been used to guide implementation?

References

Aerts, D., Apostel, L., De Moor, B., et al. (2007). *World views: From fragmentation to integration.* Originally published in 1994 by VUB Press: Brussels. Internet edition by Clement Vidal and Alexander Riegler. Retrieved from http://www.vub.ac.be/CLEA/pub/books/worldviews.pdf

Boland, L., Lawson, M. L., Graham, I. D., et al. (2019). Post-training shared decision making barriers and facilitators for pediatric healthcare providers: A mixed-methods study. *Academic Pediatrics, 19,* 118–129. http://dx.doi.org.pnw.idm.oclc.org/10.1016/j.acap.2018.05.010

Cunningham, B. J., Daub, O. M., & Cardy, J. O. (2019). Barriers to implementing evidence-based assessment procedures: Perspectives from the front lines in pediatric speech-language pathology. *Journal of Communication Disorders, 80,* 66–80. https://doi.org/10.1016/j.jcomdis.2019.05.001

Harvey, G., & Kitson, A. (Eds.). (2015). *Implementing evidence-based practice in healthcare: A facilitation guide.* New York, NY: Routledge.

Iowa Model Collaborative. (2017). Iowa model of evidence-based practice: Revisions and validation. *Worldviews on Evidence-Based Nursing, 14*(3), 175–182. doi:10.1111/wvn.12223

Jordan, Z., Lockwood, C., Munn, Z., et al. (2018). Redeveloping the JBI model of evidence-based healthcare. *International Journal of Evidence-Based Healthcare, 16,* 227–241.

Kitson, A., Harvey, G., & McCormack, B. (1998). Enabling the implementation of evidence-based practice: A conceptual framework. *Quality and Safety in Health Care, 7,* 149–158.

Kitson, A., Rycroft-Malone, J., Harvey, G., et al. (2008). Evaluating the successful implementation of evidence into practice using the PARiHS framework: Theoretical and practical challenges. *Implementation Science, 3*(1). doi:10.1186/1748-5908-3-1

Logan, J., & Graham, I. D. (2010). The Ottawa model of research use. In J. Rycroft-Malone & T. Bucknall (Eds.), *Models and frameworks for implementing evidence-based practice: Linking evidence to action* (pp. 83–108). Oxford, United Kingdom: Wiley-Blackwell.

Mitchell, G. (2013). Implications of holding ideas of evidence-based practice in nursing. *Nursing Science Quarterly, 26,* 143–151. doi:10.1177/0894318413477139

Nilsen, P. (2015). Making sense of implementation theories, models, and frameworks. *Implementation Science, 10,* 53. doi:10.1186/s13012-015-0242-0

Pearson, A. (2010). The Joanna Briggs Institute model of evidence-based health care as a framework for implementing evidence. In J. Rycroft-Malone & T. Bucknall (Eds.), *Models and frameworks for implementing evidence-based practice: Linking evidence to action* (pp. 185–205). Oxford, United Kingdom: Wiley-Blackwell.

Pearson, A., Wiechula, R., Lockwood, C., et al. (2005). The JBI model of evidence-based health care. *International Journal of Evidence-Based Health Care, 3,* 207–215.

Rycroft-Malone, J. (2007). Theory and knowledge translation. *Nursing Research, 56*(4S), S78–S85.

Rycroft-Malone, J. (2010). Promoting action on research implementation in health services (PARIHS). In J. Rycroft-Malone & T. Bucknall (Eds.), *Models and frameworks for implementing evidence-based practice: Linking evidence to action* (pp. 109–135). Oxford, United Kingdom: Wiley-Blackwell.

Rycroft-Malone, J., & Bucknall, T. (2010a). Theory, frameworks, and models: Laying the groundwork. In J. Rycroft-Malone & T. Bucknall (Eds.), *Models and frameworks for implementing evidence-based practice: Linking evidence to action* (pp. 23–50). Oxford, United Kingdom: Wiley-Blackwell.

Rycroft-Malone, J., & Bucknall, T. (2010b). Using theory and frameworks to facilitate the implementation of evidence into practice. *Worldviews on Evidence-Based Nursing, 7.* doi:10.1111/j. 1741-6787.2010.00194.x

Tayyib, N., & Coyer, F. (2017). Translating pressure ulcer prevention into intensive care nursing practice. *Journal of Nursing Care Quality, 32*(1), 6–14. http://dx.doi.org.pnw.idm.oclc.org/10.1097/ NCQ.0000000000000199

Titler, M. (2010). Iowa model of evidence-based practice. In J. Rycroft-Malone & T. Bucknall (Eds.), *Models and frameworks for implementing evidence-based practice: Linking evidence to action* (pp. 137–146). Oxford, United Kingdom: Wiley-Blackwell.

Upton, D. J. (1999). How can we achieve evidence-based practice if we have a theory-practice gap in nursing today? *Journal of Advanced Nursing, 29,* 549–555.

Wilson, D., Heaslip, V., & Jackson, D. (2018). Improving equity and cultural responsiveness with marginalized communities: Understanding competing worldviews. *Journal of Clinical Nursing, 27,* 3810–3819. doi:10.1111/jocn.14546

Yancey, N. R. (2019). Evidence-based practice in nursing for teaching-learning: But is it really nursing? *Nursing Science Quarterly, 32,* 25–28. doi:10.1177/0894318418807929

CHAPTER **6**

Common Principles

Lisa Hopp

LEARNING OBJECTIVES

- Compare and contrast select models and frameworks for implementing evidence into practice.

- Using the principles common to select evidence implementation frameworks and models, construct a map to implement evidence in a particular context.

KEY TERMS

Complex problems
Complicated problems

*C*linical *Story*

It is a quiet night in the intermediate care unit. Libbie, Alin, Enrique, and Lindsay have just received the handoff report from the evening shift and are organizing how they will care for the 28 fairly stable, monitored patients for the night. In this unit, nurses exchange the shift report in the nurses' station and structure the oral report around patient problems. Two and a half or three hours may pass before a nurse enters some of the patients' rooms. Nurses may not see patients because of the time required for nurses who are due to end their shift to finish their chart reviews and documentation; for the handoff itself; and for the oncoming nurses to prepare medications, find supplies, and otherwise plan for their shift.

The four RNs are crowded around the medication area, waiting their turn to dispense the medications they need for midnight doses when suddenly they hear a crash at the far end of the hall. They rush toward the noise, and they find Mrs. W., a frail elderly woman, on the floor by the door to the bathroom. Lindsay quickly assesses Mrs. W.'s neurological status and finds that her pupils are equal, round, and reactive to light, but she is not responding to their verbal commands. In the fall, her IV line was been pulled out, and the puncture site is bleeding slightly. Libbie also notices that Mrs. W. has been incontinent of urine, and the floor is slick. Enrique checks her vital signs. Mrs. W.'s blood pressure is elevated, but her heart rate is regular and only slightly elevated, and she is breathing normally. The nurses stabilize her spine and roll her onto a lift board; Mrs. W does not show any response during the movement. While two nurses stay with the patient, Lindsay calls the physician and the night nursing supervisor. Enrique makes a quick check of the other patients.

Mrs. W. suffers a broken hip and concussion from the fall. Eventually she recovers but her hospital stay is over 3 weeks longer, and she is transferred to an acute rehabilitation center to recover more fully before returning home. She can no longer live independently because of a decrease in her functional ability, so she lives with her daughter.

The incident prompts a full study of what happened and must be reported as a sentinel event to The Joint Commission (the accrediting agency for the hospital). Lindsay, Enrique, Alin, and Libbie are distressed by the incident. The investigation of the incident reveals the nurse reporting off to Alin had not indicated that this patient was at high risk for a fall. The team wants to take a look at the procedures during shift changes and determine how they can better recognize risk to prevent patient falls and injury.

Think Before You Read

- What experience have you had using a conceptual model or framework to facilitate evidence-based practice change?
- What makes a model or framework useful to help shape practice change?
- What parameters will help you differentiate different models and frameworks?

Introduction

Conceptual models and frameworks are abstract representations of reality. They are useful because they can give us the big picture and guide our continued understanding of complex processes such as getting evidence into practice. In the previous two chapters, you learned about the debate between theorists and supporters of evidence-based practice, the value of theory, how to organize your thinking about models and frameworks, and some of the specifics of four models and frameworks of evidence implementation. These are the Iowa model, the Ottawa Model of Research Utilization (OMRU), the integrated Promoting Action on Research Implementation in Health Services (i-PARIHS) framework, and the JBI model (see Chapter 5 for descriptions and schema of each model). In this chapter, you will compare these four models/frameworks to better understand when to use a particular approach and examine their common principles to determine some universal features that are broadly applicable to your clinical practice (see Box 6■1).

In this chapter's clinical story, the four nurses face an all too common adverse event—a patient fall with injury. None of them was neglectful or uncaring, yet this patient fall may have been prevented. This is a real, concrete problem that can benefit from the application of a framework or model to uncover the best evidence and to put it into action.

On the surface, preventing falls in an acute care unit may not seem difficult. In fact, patients and their families fundamentally expect to be safe while in the

---

BOX 6■1   Analyzing Evidence-Based Practice Models and Frameworks

Before you buy a pair of shoes, you try them on for fit, style, comfort, and utility. Similarly, before you apply an evidence-based practice model or framework, you need to consider its fit and usefulness.

Consider the following factors:

- Who is intended to use it?
- What does the model or framework do?
- Where and at what level does the model or framework work best?
- What is its purpose?

When you have analyzed these factors, proceed to evaluate it based on the following criteria:

- Relevance
- Coherence
- Practicality
- Ability to structure messy or complex issues
- Fit with setting and user
- Effective visual representation
- Transferability to a variety of problems

hospital. But preventing falls is an example of a complex problem rather than a complicated problem, and there is a distinction. **Complicated problems** are usually made up of a series of simple problems. **Complex problems** tend to be unique, are associated with a great deal of uncertainty, and are less predictable. They cannot be solved with rigid rules; the essence of the problem lies within the patterns and relationships (Lindberg, Nash, & Lindberg, 2008). Theories, frameworks, and models can help capture complexity yet provide some structure to problem-solving.

In this chapter's clinical story, the four nurses are undoubtedly feeling responsible for the patient's fall. It is the unit's policy to "huddle" immediately after a fall to determine the details of what happened and to complete an incident report. Although these short debriefings help to capture the facts of the fall and may cause those involved to think about how to avoid the problem in the future, this method cannot address all of the multilevel issues related to preventing all falls. In fact, each fall presents unique issues and involves intersecting relationships, including the singular patient characteristics, the circumstances of the particular environment, the work load of the nurses, the processes of the unit (e.g., handoffs and placement of patients within the unit), the organizational supports and policy, and various other factors. Preventing all falls in all circumstances is a complex problem.

A Structure for Comparing Frameworks and Models

In the last chapter, you discovered you could compare models and frameworks using a simple journalist's approach. That is, you compare the who, what, where, when, why, and how of each. There are certainly more sophisticated methods to analyze theoretical ways of thinking, but this approach is practical and easy to apply. It will allow you to determine your preference for a particular model and its fit to a particular situation and to illustrate what is common and different among them. You may find one particular model or framework just makes sense to you so that you end up shaping your thinking to match that particular model. More likely, you will see that one framework or model will make more sense than another, depending on the nature of the problem, focus, setting, or other situational variable. Although each model is unique, there are some common principles that emerge with your analysis (see Table 6■1).

Who: Intended Users

Many frameworks and models are designed for multiple disciplines rather than for a single professional group. The four models discussed in Chapter 5 could be applied in any health profession. Despite this fact, some are more frequently used in nursing, whereas others are more commonly used in other disciplines. For example, the JBI model is appropriate for any group in health care and guides very diverse disciplines, including nursing, nurse midwifery, medicine, physiotherapy, radiological imaging, public health, and occupational therapy (Jordan, Lockwood,

TABLE 6■1 **Comparison of Four Evidence-Based Practice Models/Frameworks**

	Iowa	Ottawa	i-PARIHS	JBI
Who: Intended Users	Interdisciplinary or single discipline teams at unit or agency level; the Ottawa model can be extended to networks and the JBI model to an international collaborative network			
What: Function	A decision-support schema with three major decision points: determining the priority of the problem or knowledge-focused trigger, readiness of the evidence, and outcomes of a pilot implementation to change practice	Three iterative phases: (1) assessment of barriers and supports of the innovation, adopters, and practice environment; (2) monitor of the process and degree of use including barrier management; (3) evaluation of the impact on the patient, practitioner, and system	Successful implementation of evidence is a function of the active ingredient of facilitation on the combination of the characteristics of the innovation, recipients, and context. Skillful facilitators base their approach on their assessment of the innovation, the recipients and participants in the innovation, and the levels and characteristics of the context	Three phases beginning with synthesis of effect and meaning, moving to evidence transfer and utilization with tools for each phase; the goal is to improve global health through local implementation
Where: Settings	Units and systems	Individuals, units, systems, and networks	Units or groups of units, systems, networks, political/regulatory environments, etc.	Units, systems, centers, global collaboration
Where: Level of Intended Users	Meso	Micro Meso Macro	Micro to macro	Meso to macro
Why: Purpose	Descriptive and explanatory	Descriptive	Descriptive and explanatory	Descriptive

---

BOX 6■2 **Interdisciplinary Rounds**

- Negotiate using one of the models or frameworks to solve a complex clinical with a multidisciplinary team. Defend the team's choice to the chief operating officer of the institution (whose background is health-care administration).
- The quality assurance officer (who is not a nurse) does not believe that a model is necessary to address a clinical problem. Convince him.
- Ask someone from another discipline to tell you about a clinical problem and discuss how he or she would solve it. Explain how two of the models you studied would frame the problem. Negotiate a choice based on your shared evaluation of how well the model or framework would work to help you sort the problem, the evidence, and its implementation.

Munn, et al, 2018; Pearson, Wiechula, Lockwood, et al, 2005). The Iowa model has been very popular for nurse-sensitive evidence-based practice and quality improvement programs and in nursing curricula. The OMRU model has been used across nursing, medicine, and allied health. The PARIHS/i-PARIHS model has been most popular among nurse-driven evidence-based practice and research applications, but it is intended to be applicable within and across many disciplines (see Box 6■2).

What: Function of the Model or Framework

All four models under our consideration aim to enhance the implementation of evidence to improve patient outcomes. However, the functional aspects of each model are different. Each guides users to move evidence into practice in a different way. The Iowa model is a step-by-step decision aid with three key decision points: (1) whether the topic is a priority for the organization, (2) whether there is sufficient evidence to proceed, and (3) whether change is warranted based on a pilot implementation (see schema in Chapter 5). The model guides users through the common steps of the evidence-based practice process (identify the problem; form a team; systematically search, appraise, and summarize the body of evidence; design, pilot, evaluate the plan; and integrate and sustain practice changes). However, the model does not suggest specific evidence-based implementations strategies (the "how" of making practice change) to facilitate the change. Rather, steps of the pilot implementation are to "develop an implementation plan, prepare clinicians and materials, promote adoption and to collect and report post-pilot data" (Iowa Model Collaborative, 2017, p. 178). Some of these steps can align with implementation science interventions that you will learn about in later chapters. Examples of this alignment include stakeholder engagement (prepare clinicians), interactive education (prepare materials), and audit (collect post-pilot data) and feedback (report data). That being said, many clinicians find the format very friendly and useful in guiding their implementation ideas.

In contrast, the OMRU is an iterative model that directs users to first assess barriers to and supporters of the innovation as well as characteristics of adopters and the practice environment to target change processes. For example, if one barrier is a lack of equipment for the evidence-based innovation, the change process would include acquiring the appropriate equipment. The second phase of the model is to monitor the process and degree of use by managing barriers, facilitating transfer, and doing the follow-up that leads to initial and sustained adoption. The third phase is evaluation of the innovation's impact on patients, practitioners, and the health-care system.

The PARIHS/i-PARIHS framework explains how to assess the key elements (the innovation, participants, and context) and focuses on specific facilitation methods and strategies to promote the uptake of evidence into practice at multiple levels.

The JBI model functions through the array of tools for evidence synthesis (software, training, development, and dissemination of systematic reviews, evidence summaries, and guidelines) transfer (education, systems integration of evidence, and active dissemination) and implementation (context, facilitation, and evaluation).

Where: Levels and Settings

Generally, models are scoped for different levels of users such as the individual (micro), group or system (meso), or national/international level (macro). Some of the models and frameworks apply at all levels, whereas others are most suited for only one level. The Iowa model is best suited for teams working to influence clinical policy at the unit or within an agency (meso), rather than individuals using evidence to make nursing practice decisions (Titler, 2010). Individuals (micro), teams within a unit (meso), and even whole health systems or networks (macro) could use OMRU, because the potential adopters of the innovation include patients (if an individual practitioner uses the model), practitioners, and policy makers (if a team within a unit, system, or network of systems use the model) (Logan & Graham, 2010). It is best suited for teams who influence others to use evidence to impact patient, practitioner, and system outcomes.

With the revised i-PARIHS framework, Harvey and Kitson recognize the multiple contexts that exist that may require different approaches to facilitation and the assessment of different factors. They specifically identify micro to macro levels of context. They call these levels the "inner to outer contexts." You can think of these contexts as a concentric spiral from the inner (micro level, like a unit) to outer context (macro level, like the political context and regulatory environment) with levels in between. Each of these contexts has different characteristics that you need to assess and to evaluate their interactions with the implementation and facilitation strategies and iterations (Harvey & Kitson, 2015).

The JBI model is unique because its goal is to improve global health through international collaboration of all health-care disciplines. Even with the international focus, the intent is for implementation to occur at the local level and for it ultimately to impact global health (Jordan et al, 2018; Pearson et al, 2005). The JBI and its collaborating centers use the model to frame the work at the macro level (international) and to guide the activities of the center (meso). Because centers involve partner-clinical agencies, the model can apply at the unit level (micro) and at the health-care-system level (meso-macro). Nonetheless, it is perhaps best known for its unique approach at the macro level.

Why: Purpose

All four of models discussed in this book are descriptive, and all but the JBI model are also explanatory. That is, they explain the relationships among the concepts or stages in the process (Rycroft-Malone & Bucknall, 2010). The Iowa model and OMRU describe a process. OMRU describes three phases of moving evidence into practice: (1) assessment of barriers and supports, (2) monitoring of the process, and (3) use of evidence and evaluation of the impact (Logan & Graham, 2010). The Iowa model describes a series of decisions in the process of moving from problem trigger to evidence assessment (Iowa Model Collaborative, 2017; Titler, 2010). Both of these models can be used to guide quality improvement.

The JBI model is unique because of its scope and because of how the model uses available tools to make the key phases (evidence synthesis, transfer, and implementation) operational. It has been used to structure collaborative work including the formation of academic and clinical partnerships around the elements of the model. Individuals can also use it to structure their thinking about the flow of knowledge, from generation to utilization.

How Well: Evaluating the Usefulness

If you are just beginning to use theories, frameworks, and models to better understand nursing practice, you will want straightforward criteria for evaluating them. Even as you become more experienced, you will return to these criteria because they address how sensible and practicable the framework or model is for you. These criteria include the following:

- Relevance
- Coherence
- Practicality
- Ability to structure messy or complex issues
- Fit with setting and/or user
- Effective visual representation
- Transferable to a variety of problems

As when you read the first few pages of a new book, you will probably look at a model or framework to see if it attracts you in some way. This means it needs to be relevant to your practice and to how you use information to inform decisions. The model or framework needs to make sense—it must be coherent. Even though conceptual frameworks and models are a bit abstract by nature, they still need to be understandable and logical.

For a framework or model to be usable, it needs to be practical at some level. That does not mean that you will necessarily understand all of the concepts and their relationships at first glance, but you should be able to generate ideas about how to apply the model or framework without too much strain.

Frameworks and models should help you sort and understand complex problems. If a framework or model only makes your understanding muddier, it is not helpful. Conversely, a model can bring clarity and insight. For example, in this chapter's clinical story, if the nurses are to implement evidence-based changes, they will need to understand the context, those involved in the change, and the dimensions of the change itself. They could use the OMRU to help assess the barriers and promoters of the innovation, the adopters, and environment. Without this structure, they may not know how to begin the change process.

When you choose a model, it must fit the situation, the setting, the individual or team involved, and interpretation of both the problem and the model itself. This requires trying out a specific model or framework to determine whether it fits your needs, just as you might try out a lens prescription to be certain it improves your vision. The one that fits correctly will help you visualize and decipher an approach to the problem.

Most models are depicted in a visual schema or picture to help users see how the concepts relate to one another. This serves as a map, and you can use the diagram just as you might chart a trip. However, that picture needs to make sense.

Finally, to be useful a model or framework needs to work for a variety of problems. It may fit best in one context, but it should also be widely applicable to a variety of problems. For example, a question might arise from something that happens in the clinical arena (e.g., an increase in the incidence of falls) or from reading about a new approach in the literature (e.g., a systematic review about hourly rounding's effect on fall rates). Looking at your four options, you can see that the Iowa model is transferable to many situations that can arise from either of these triggers.

The nurses in this chapter's clinical story now begin to work with a team that includes a clinical nurse specialist, quality improvement nurse, physiotherapist, frontline nurses from several units, risk manager, and gerontologist. The team initially is overwhelmed at the prospect of sifting through the assessment, intervention, and evaluation aspects of this very important problem. Then Alin remembers studying the i-PARIHS framework in his senior capstone course; he and his team implemented a small-scale evidence-based practice innovation. He shares this experience with the team. In addition, the quality improvement nurse has used the Iowa model, and the gerontologist is familiar with OMRU. The physiotherapist is aware of the JBI model and has used some of the resources from the physiotherapy evidence summaries of JBI EBP Database. As they begin unraveling the solutions to the problem, they realize that different aspects of each model and framework influence their decisions.

After they formulate questions related to fall assessment and prevention, they consult with their hospital's library scientist (see Chapter 8 for question development and Chapter 9 for searching). A review of the JBI model reminds them that synthesis of evidence of effect and meaningfulness is necessary to understand the full scope of the problem and its solutions. When they transfer the knowledge from synthesized sources, they need concise summaries if they expect their colleagues to have time to attend to the key aspects of the evidence.

Using the i-PARIHS conceptual framework, they next assess the sources and strength of the evidence and the characteristics of the innovation as they plan. Then they use the Context Assessment Index (CAI) to evaluate the strengths and weaknesses of the inner context, including organizational culture, leadership characteristics, and evaluation practices (McCormack, McCarthy, Wright, et al, 2009). Based on these assessments, the team decides what type of facilitation (ranging from doing for to enabling others) is required for certain units. They select clinical nurse specialists from the pilot units to lead the facilitation efforts. Each unit has a unique subculture and leadership group, but they share the same evaluation processes.

Using the data from the CAI, the facilitators plan how to use facilitation tools and skills within and across the units to implement changes in risk assessment and fall prevention. One of the practice changes they plan to implement is bedside handoff. They realize this seemingly small shift in the location of the handoff report has reverberating consequences that will need skillful facilitation. They plan to use elements of the OMRU to further assess the barriers and supports for changing practice in the affected units. In addition, they will employ audit and feedback to use (JBI) and monitor (OMRU) the key best practices defined by the evidence. The solutions will undoubtedly reflect both the best available evidence as well as the multidisciplinary team's varied expertise.

The patients' preferences will also inform the project in at least two stages. As they are developing a plan to implement the results of the evidence, the team grapples with how they can ensure that nurses, physicians, and physiotherapists consider individual patient preferences. Throughout the project planning, Enrique voices his lingering guilt that the fall had a profound effect on the patient's subsequent functional ability, and he and Lindsay pursue more information on the patient experience of a fall with injury. They work with the librarian to find qualitative evidence of patients' experiences with a fall, and they advocate for including what they learn from this evidence in the implementation plan.

This commonplace clinical story illustrates how a critical incident can uncover a complex problem. The framework/model "mash-up" application should help you understand how elements of each model can bring light to the problem. You can see how the different models can influence how you see and approach the situation. However, it is best to use just one model to frame a complex problem and its solutions to bring coherence and structure to the process (see Box 6■3).

■ Summary

In this chapter, you learned about the common and distinguishing principles of the four sample models and frameworks. Each model or framework brings a unique

BOX 6■3 **Tools for Learning and Practice**

■ Explore the four models presented in Chapter 5 and this chapter using the Reference lists.
■ Search the bibliographic databases to find more models related to evidence and research utilization.
■ Conduct a Google search to find Web sites dedicated to the models and frameworks or search for illustrations of how they have been used:
  ■ https://jbi.global
  ■ i-PARIHS https://health-policy-systems.biomedcentral.com/ articles/10.1186/s12961-018-0392-z
  ■ https://ktdrr.org/ktlibrary/ktmodels.html
  ■ https://uihc.org/evidence-based-practice

perspective to implementing evidence into practice. It is your job to decide which model or framework best fits your particular problem, setting, and team. The evaluation framework can help you determine which one will work best. This chapter's clinical story shows that models and frameworks can bring clarity to complex problems.

CHAPTER QUESTIONS

1. Have you ever used a model or framework in how you think about a problem in your clinical work? If you have, how did it affect how you framed the problem? If you have not, why not?

2. Describe a complicated problem from your clinical experience. Describe a complex problem in your clinical experience. What characteristics differentiated the complicated from the complex? What impact did the complicated and complex problems each have on how you, a team, or the organization approached the problem? Was the solution successful? Why or why not?

3. Describe the key aspects of each of the four frameworks and models (Iowa, OMRU, i-PARIHS, and JBI). What do they share in common? What is particularly unique about each model?

4. Describe a recent complex problem or issue that you have experienced in your clinical setting. Which of the frameworks or models do you think would fit best? Why?

5. Think about a situation that would potentially benefit from using a model or framework to guide the implementation of evidence. What would you want that model or framework to do for you to be useful?

6. Can you imagine using one of the four models or frameworks in your clinical practice? Using the evaluation criteria, justify your answer.

References

Harvey, G., & Kitson, A. (Eds.). (2015). *Implementing evidence-based practice in healthcare: A facilitation guide.* New York, NY: Routledge.

Iowa Model Collaborative. (2017). Iowa model of evidence-based practice: Revisions and validation. *Worldviews on Evidence-Based Nursing, 14*(3), 175–182. doi:10.1111/wvn.12223

Jordan, Z., Lockwood, C., Munn, Z., et al. (2018). Redeveloping the JBI model of evidence-based healthcare. *International Journal of Evidence-Based Healthcare, 16,* 227–241.

Lindberg, C., Nash, S., & Lindberg, C. (2008). *On the edge: Nursing in an age of complexity.* Bordentown, NJ: PexusPress.

Logan, J., & Graham, I. D. (2010). The Ottawa model of research use. In J. Rycroft-Malone & T. Bucknall (Eds.), *Models and frameworks for implementing evidence-based practice: Linking evidence to action* (pp. 83–108). Oxford, United Kingdom: Wiley-Blackwell.

McCormack, B., McCarthy, G., Wright, J., et al. (2009). Developing and testing of the context of assessment index (CAI). *Worldviews on Evidence-Based Nursing, 6,* 27–35.

Pearson, A., Wiechula, R., Lockwood, C., et al. (2005). The JBI model of evidence-based health care. *International Journal of Evidence-Based Health Care, 3,* 207–215.

Rycroft-Malone, J., & Bucknall, T. (2010). Analysis and synthesis of models and frameworks. In J. Rycroft-Malone & T. Bucknall (Eds.), *Models and frameworks for implementing evidence-based practice: Linking evidence to action* (pp. 223–246). Oxford, United Kingdom: Wiley-Blackwell.

Titler, M. (2010). Iowa model of evidence-based practice. In J. Rycroft-Malone & T. Bucknall (Eds.), *Models and frameworks for implementing evidence-based practice: Linking evidence to action* (pp. 137–146). Oxford, United Kingdom: Wiley-Blackwell.

How to Do Evidence-Based Practice

In this unit, you will work through the evidence-based practice process step by step and relate it to the familiar nursing process. You begin with an overview of the process in Chapter 7 and then move to asking questions that lead to finding the best available evidence. You will be able to remember the process using a simple memory device of the 5 *A*s, meaning each step begins with an *A*: *A*sk, *A*cquire, *A*ppraise, *A*pply, and *A*ssess.

Just like assessing patients is an orderly process of probing, the evidence-based practice process begins with asking questions using a systematic approach. The second step is to acquire evidence by searching bibliographic databases or other sources of evidence where you will find the answers to your question if the evidence exists. This

(continues on page 86)

step relates to the diagnosis phase of the nursing process based on your assessment. After you establish a nursing diagnosis, you develop a plan by weighing your nursing care options and deciding what is important. This step in the nursing process relates to the important part of the process of appraising or weighing the quality of the evidence you find or using a system in which someone else has appraised the quality of the evidence. Next you apply the evidence just like you implement your nursing care plan. There are three chapters related to applying evidence because it happens at multiple levels—by individual nurses, health systems, and national groups. Finally, just as you evaluate the impact of your nursing interventions, you must assess the impact of evidence implementation.

CHAPTER 7

Overview of the Evidence-Based Practice Process

Lisa Hopp

LEARNING OBJECTIVES

■ Relate the definition of *nursing* with the characteristics of nursing and the nursing process.

■ Define *problem-solving* as fundamental to the nursing, research, and evidence-based practice processes.

■ List the steps of the research process.

■ Compare and contrast the research, nursing, and evidence-based practice processes.

■ Define each step of the evidence-based practice process.

■ Provide an example of how evidence might inform each phase of the nursing process.

KEY TERMS

Acquire	Expert consensus opinion
Apply	Magnitude
Appraise	Nursing
Ask	Nursing actions
Assess	Nursing process
Evidence-based practice	Nursing standards
process	PICO question

(continues on page 88)

KEY TERMS (continued)

PICo question   Research process
Preappraised evidence   Social contract
Problem-solving   Strength

Clinical Story

Ali is a student on a general surgical floor, and she has already received her assignment for the next day. She wants to be well prepared to provide care for a 70-year-old man who has had a bowel resection (removal and reconnection of part of the bowel). She will be caring for him on his first postoperative day. She anticipates he will experience postoperative pain. Although pain is just one issue that she will need to manage, she knows it will be one of her nursing care priorities. She thinks about how she will assess, diagnose, plan, implement, and evaluate her plan of care.

Because Ali wants to understand all aspects of caring for her patient's pain, she looks for a clinical practice guideline. She searches the Registered Nurses' Association of Ontario (RNAO) best practice guidelines first. She finds a comprehensive guideline on the assessment and management of pain that she can adapt for her patient's acute postoperative pain (RNAO, 2013). She plans to complete a comprehensive pain assessment when she first meets the patient and a standard quicker assessment to reassess his pain. Ali anticipates she will need to give the patient medication to relieve his pain, and she needs to be aware of possible adverse effects from the medication and how his other health problems may put him at higher risk for adverse reactions. Ali knows that she will need to make sure that the patient has adequate pain relief to be able to move and get out of bed to speed his recovery. She is aware that because her patient is older, he may react in a different manner than would a younger person to both the surgery and the analgesia. She reads the guideline to determine whether she might offer other interventions in addition to medications, such as music and relaxation, to help reduce the patient's pain. Also, she must carefully evaluate and document the patient's response to her interventions. Ali is confident her plan is well supported with the best available evidence and she is ready to adjust it as she cares for her patient the next day.

Think Before You Read

- What are some of the key clinical concerns that Ali must think about?
- What kind of knowledge might Ali rely upon to help her care for this patient?
- What general clinical questions could you formulate about postoperative pain management?

Introduction

Some might claim that evidence-based nursing practice is nothing more than providing good care. In part, they are right. Evidence-based practice is about doing the right thing, for the right patient, from the right person, at the right time, and in the right way to achieve the right outcome at the right cost (Royal Colleges of Nursing, as cited in Livesley & Howarth, 2007). But how do you know the right way to assess, diagnose, plan, implement, and evaluate your care? Evidence-based nursing practice is not something that happens *in addition* to the nursing process. Rather, evidence should inform all aspects of nursing care (Fawcett & Garrity, 2009).

In this chapter, you will review the definition of *nursing* and reflect on what nursing means to you. You will compare three processes, the nursing, research, and evidence-based practice processes, and relate them to basic problem-solving. Each step of the evidence-based practice process will be defined to prepare you to learn more about each phase in subsequent chapters.

Essence of Nursing Practice

Busy clinicians juggle many competing demands while caring for a caseload of patients in a complex environment. In this chapter's clinical story, Ali anticipates many potential problems that her postoperative patient may have in addition to recognizing the importance of pain relief. She realizes that although her patient's comfort is a priority in and of itself, pain relief is linked to other aspects of the patient's experience in the first postoperative day, such as being able to move to avoid complications of immobility.

The clinical story captures the essential features of nursing. The goal of Ali's care is to help the patient regain health through a caring relationship in which she attends to a range of responses including pain, limited mobility, challenges to nutritional and fluid intake, elimination, and the social and emotional impact of surgery. She plans to gather data, such as the patient's report of pain, to integrate into the decisions she makes to intervene and alleviate the patient's discomfort and to promote mobility. She has the obligation to find and use the best information to care for the patient correctly—to provide the highest quality and safest care by using evidence to inform her decisions (American Nurses Association [ANA], 2010) (Box 7■1).

Like Ali, you make many decisions, often simultaneously and perhaps without being fully aware of how you make these decisions. Think about what sets your care apart from what others do for and with patients. Then think about how you "know" and compare that with how others define the essence of nursing practice.

Definition of Nursing

The American Nurses Association (2010) defines **nursing** for nurses who practice in the United States. The current definition evolved from the first Social Policy

BOX 7■1   **Significance of Evidence-Based Practice**

- The American Nurses Association established the role of evidence-based practice in its 2010 Social Policy Statement; this policy statement ratifies using evidence to practice nursing as an expectation of every professional nurse in the United States.
- Registered nurses enter into a social contract with the public to use evidence to inform their nursing practice.
- Governing bodies in other countries such as the United Kingdom and Australia have explicitly committed nurses to using evidence in their practice.
- Evidence-based practice is integral to high-quality nursing practice; it is not an add-on or an academic exercise.
- Evidence informs each phase of the nursing process.

Statement written in 1980. The ANA states that "nursing is the protection, promotion, and optimization of health and abilities, prevention of illness and injury, alleviation of suffering through the diagnosis and treatment of human response, and advocacy in the care of individuals, families, communities and populations" (p. 3). When you become registered, you enter into a **social contract** with patients and families to uphold this definition of professional nursing. In the context of nursing, the code of ethics defines our social contract with the public, meaning the "profession's expression of the values, duties and commitments to the public" (p. 24). Through this social contract, society grants professional nurses the authority to practice.

Essential Features of Nursing

The ANA (2010) lists seven essential features of professional nursing. All of them relate to evidence-based nursing practice in some way if we heed the full definition of *evidence-based practice* (Table 7■1). For example, when nurses develop a caring relationship, they must embrace the patient's values and preferences and use effective interventions to facilitate health and healing. Similarly, when nurses influence public policy to promote social justice, they should advocate for decision makers to honor all patients' values and preferences and assure equal access to the treatments that work, regardless of the patients' ability to pay. If you think broadly and self-consciously, you will find a place for evidence in nearly every aspect of nursing.

Nursing Actions

When non-nurses discuss professional nursing, they generally talk about what nurses do. Nurses are known for **nursing actions.** Nursing actions are how nurses intervene to protect, promote, and optimize health and abilities. They act to prevent

TABLE 7■1 **Essential Features of Professional Nursing and Relationship to Evidence-Based Practice**

Essential Feature	Application to the Evidence-Based Practice Concept
Provision of a caring relationship that facilitates health and healing	Honoring patient preferences and values in shared decision making
Attention to the range of human experiences and responses to health and illness within the physical and social environments	Determining the applicability of evidence to an individual patient and his or her context
Integration of assessment data with knowledge gained from an appreciation of the patient or the group	Gathering individual or local data and situating them with evidence from the research of groups
Application of scientific knowledge to the processes of diagnosis and treatment through the use of judgment and critical thinking	Using clinical expertise and appraisal of the best available evidence of effectiveness to select the most appropriate nursing intervention
Advancement of professional nursing knowledge through scholarly inquiry	Using the evidence syntheses to identify gaps in knowledge and the need for further research
Influence on social and public policy to promote social justice	Advocating for policy that assures equal access to effective treatment and the incorporation of patient values and preferences in policy decisions
Assurance of safe, quality, and evidence-based practice	Questioning traditional practices and using the best available evidence to drive safe, high-quality care while discarding ineffective practices

From American Nurses Association. (2010). *Nursing's social policy statement: The essence of the profession.* Silver Spring, MD: Nursingbooks.org.

illness and injury; alleviate suffering; and advocate for individuals, families, communities, and populations to produce beneficial outcomes (ANA, 2010). These interventions are developed from knowledge gained from both theory and evidence (ANA, 2010).

The latest edition of the ANA's Social Policy Statement (2010) is the first time policy makers explicitly addressed the role of evidence-based practice in the definition of *nursing practice*. Previous editions in 1995 and 2003 did mention the role of research in informing nursing practice, but only the current edition features the role of evidence in all nursing actions (ANA, 2010). Now when nurses become registered, they enter into the social contract to use evidence to inform their actions.

Problem-Solving Processes

In daily practice, nurses are continually preventing and solving problems related to both the patient's experience and nursing actions. For example, Ali anticipated the patient would experience surgical pain. Her plan of care includes her plan for managing this potential problem. She uses the nursing process as a way to avert or modify the problem of acute pain related to the patient's abdominal surgery, and she uses evidence to inform each step of the process.

Problem-solving is a generic process that describes part of the thinking and doing of nursing practice. It is a step-by-step sequence of defining the problem, identifying the possible causes, generating possible solutions, selecting the best solution, implementing it, and evaluating the effect on the problem. Many disciplines use a problem-solving approach. In fact, people solve problems in their everyday life, but they do not pay close attention to how they approach problem-solving.

In contrast, evidence-based nursing does require close attention to the decision-making process by first considering the problem and its potential etiology, or cause; generating questions that focus on the effectiveness, feasibility, or appropriateness of interventions; and understanding the meaning of the patient's experience. As part of the process, you will ultimately choose an intervention or use what you learn from evidence of meaningfulness to guide how you address the problem. Finally, you will evaluate the effectiveness of your interventions and how your patient experienced your intervention. As you can see, problem-solving and evidence-based practice are closely connected (Fig. 7■1).

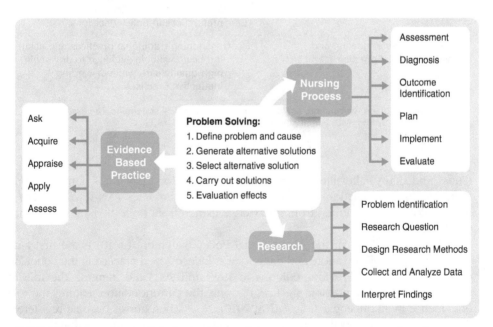

FIGURE 7■1 Concept map: Relating problem-solving, nursing process, research and evidence-based practice.

Nursing Process

Nursing's Social Policy Statement (ANA, 2010) defines the **nursing process** and links it with the definitions of *nursing* and *theoretical and evidence-based knowledge.* "Nurses use their theoretical and evidence-based knowledge of these human experiences and responses to collaborate with patients and others to assess, diagnose, plan, implement, evaluate care, and identify outcomes" (p. 14). This definition means that the nurse is obliged to use both theory and evidence to care for patients and to do the work of nursing. The nursing process employs critical thinking to assess, diagnose, identify outcomes, plan, implement, and evaluate. These actions may happen simultaneously or in a more sequential fashion (ANA, 2010).

The ANA has formed nursing standards for each phase of the nursing process. **Nursing standards** are an "authoritative statement by which the nursing profession describes the responsibilities for which its practitioners are accountable, the outcomes for which registered nurses are responsible, and by which the quality of practice, service, or education can be evaluated" (ANA, 2010, p. 42). In other words, a professional nurse has the responsibility to act competently in all six phases of the nursing process. In providing care, such as comfort measures to decrease pain, the nurse uses the best available evidence to inform how best to assess, intervene, and evaluate patient outcomes. You use evidence to understand how the patient experiences pain and discomfort.

Research Process

Ideally, research-based evidence will be available to answer the clinical question. Research-based evidence is stronger than other types of evidence because it is less susceptible to many types of bias if the research is conducted in a rigorous way. If research is not available, the nurse will need to seek out other sources, such as expert consensus opinion. **Expert consensus opinion** is formed when experts in an area of science discuss and come to an agreement about the best approach to a problem. The best expert consensus opinion would involve a systematic and rigorous method to determine a conclusion that is then exposed to public opinion or external critique.

The **research process** follows the basic problem-solving methodology. Investigators begin by posing a specific question related to a problem. For example, Good, Albert, Anderson, et al (2010) recognized that many people who have surgery have unresolved pain even though they receive IV medication through patient-controlled analgesia (patients trigger the IV dose on demand). They reviewed the literature to identify the unresolved issues related to successfully treating postoperative pain. They found questions remained about the effect on pain of combining relaxation and music during the immediate postoperative period. After narrowing their focus to this specific area, the authors designed a study to test hypotheses about the effect of patient teaching and relaxation plus music, both as single interventions and combined, on patients' pain ratings. They based these hypotheses on the

TABLE 7■2 **Comparison of Processes**

Problem-Solving	Nursing Process (ANA)	Research Process (Polit & Beck, 2008)	Evidence-Based Practice Process
Define problem and cause	Assessment	Problem identification and research question	Ask
Generate alternative solutions Select alternative	Diagnosis Outcome Identification Plan	Design research methods	Acquire Appraise
Carry out solution	Implement	Collect and analyze data	Apply
Evaluate effects	Evaluate	Interpret findings	Assess

From American Nurses Association. (2010). *Nursing's social policy statement: The essence of the profession.* Silver Spring, MD: Nursingbooks.org.

underlying mechanisms of how music and relaxation might work to decrease pain. They planned the methods of study so that they could detect differences among the treatments. Then they implemented the study with four groups of patients; an experimental condition was randomly assigned to each group to receive one of the experimental conditions or standard pharmacological care. Throughout the study, they carefully measured the same outcomes in all subjects, analyzed the results, and came to the conclusion that relaxation plus music therapy significantly decreased pain immediately after surgery, whereas patient teaching alone did not. Most single studies do not provide enough evidence to change practice, but you can see that the process of planning and conducting the research is systematic and logical.

The three processes—nursing process, problem-solving, and the research process—share parallel phases. For example, in all three, the first step is uncovering and naming the problem. In problem-solving, that is done by defining and stating the problem. In the nursing process, the problem is assessed and diagnosed. In the research process, the literature is reviewed, and the research question is stated (Table 7■2).

Evidence-Based Practice Process

The **evidence-based practice process** is problem-solving that begins by identifying the problem, asking specific questions, acquiring evidence based on the specific question, appraising the evidence for its quality, applying the evidence, and assessing the outcomes of the intervention. A memory device is the five 5 *As—Ask, Acquire, Appraise, Apply, Assess.* This sounds very neat and straightforward. However, putting evidence into action may not happen quite so tidily. Nursing practice and patients' responses to health and illness are complex. However, if you take time to understand each step, you will begin to master the process despite the complexity of your work.

Ask

It may seem obvious that to find an answer, you need to ask the right question. Therefore, the first step of the evidence-based practice process is to **ask,** or pose a clear question that will lead to the right evidence for the problem. As in the research process, the question drives the rest of the evidence-based practice process. It forms the blueprint for the search for evidence by pointing to keywords and maintaining the focus on the key decision that needs to be made to solve the problem. Similarly, in the nursing process you first assess the patient to determine the problem.

In the evidence-based practice process, the way you state the question depends on the purpose of your query. In future chapters, you will learn more about how to shape a general problem into either a **PICO question** (if you ask about the effectiveness of interventions) or a **PICo question** (if you want to understand the meaning of a patient's experience). This template approach ensures that you remember the important elements for specific, well-formed questions; each letter represents one part of the question. For questions of effectiveness (PICO), *P* represents *p*opulation; *I* equals *i*ntervention; *C* stands for *c*omparison intervention; and *O* is *o*utcome. For questions of meaning (PICo), *P* still represents *p*opulation; *I* refers to the phenomenon of *i*nterest; and *Co* means *co*ntext. When you use this simple memory device, you are more likely to develop solid, searchable questions.

The size of the problem will also influence how you ask the question. In the next chapter, you will learn more about scope and scale, two ways of thinking about the size of the question. For example, Ali may be interested in the best available evidence related to how patients experience acute, postoperative pain, and how to assess pain, intervene, and evaluate the effectiveness of her interventions. In this case, she would look for a very comprehensive source of evidence, such as a complete clinical practice guideline from the Registered Nurses' Association of Ontario or the American Pain Society. Alternatively, she may need information about only one very narrow part of her care, such as whether relaxation and music are likely to help limit the intensity and duration of pain during the immediate postoperative period. In this case, she may use evidence from a systematic review of all research trials that tested the effectiveness of these interventions. The size of these two problems is quite different. The way that Ali would seek evidence and use the evidence to inform her clinical decisions depends on how she asks the question.

Acquire

The next step of the evidence-based practice process is using the question to determine how to search for the evidence. That is, one **acquires** the best information that links the diagnosis of the patient problem with potential solutions. One needs to know where to look, how to access the source, and how to find the best available evidence. These are not trivial issues. Many nurses in the United States have limited access to the Internet at point of care, and a significant portion feel they do not have the right skills to search databases and time, among other barriers, remains a prevalent problem (Jun, Kovner, & Stimpfel, 2016; Melnyk, Fineout-Overholt, Gallagher-Ford, et al, 2012; Pravikoff, Tanner, & Pierce, 2005). Later in this book, you will find out more about the best way to approach the search process and when to seek the help of experts so you can avoid these barriers in your own practice.

The complexity or ease of the search process depends on the source you explore. As a novice, it may be helpful to know the best-bet resources: the places where it is easiest to find the best available evidence published in a thorough, yet efficient manner. In this chapter's clinical story, if Ali searches individual organizations for the practice guidelines, she can simply browse the sites for the pages that house the practice guidelines. She may only need to use a key phrase search such as "pain guideline" to find a short list of pages within the site. However, if she searched a larger database, such as the Guidelines International Network, a simple search using "pain" as the keyword would net more than 260 guidelines, far too many to sort them easily for relevance to her problem. She would need to use advance search tools or work with an expert, such as a librarian, to narrow the search. If she wanted to search for systematic reviews or individual research reports for information that was not adequately covered in the guideline, she would need to use bibliographic databases and a structured search employing the appropriate keywords and linkages.

Many students and bedside nurses find using bibliographic databases to be a significant barrier to using evidence in their practice. Practice leads to more confidence and expertise, and you should not be satisfied with a quick Internet search once you understand the importance of uncovering the best evidence. In some situations, you will need the help of a librarian or other expert to find the best information. In fact, librarians are integral members of strong evidence-based practice teams.

Appraise

The next step of the evidence-based practice process is to **appraise** the evidence; that is, critically evaluate the evidence for its quality. It is unlikely that you will find only a single source when you search for the best way to answer your question. In fact, if you settle for the first piece of information you find, you cannot be assured that it is the best available. Instead, you have to judge the quality of a variety of sources to determine what is truly the best available. In other words, nurses who use evidence to inform each aspect of the nursing process must be skeptical.

In cases of the effectiveness of interventions, one needs to evaluate both the **strength** and the **magnitude** of the evidence in the source. The strength of the evidence relates to the quality or believability of the evidence, whereas the magnitude of the evidence refers to the "so-what" factor, or how big an effect the intervention makes on the outcome. Similarly, when one appraises evidence of meaning, feasibility, or applicability, one evaluates the credibility of the source.

It may be easier to understand how important appraisal is if you examine a simple case of buying your next car. When considering your purchase, you will have criteria that are important to you. These might include cost, durability, appearance, fuel economy, comfort, and safety. Using these criteria, you can rate the quality of each car you are considering to help you make your decision. The difference among your choices may be large or small. When you judge the strength of quality of the cars, you rate each against your criteria, and the magnitude of the differences among the cars will help you finalize your decision, particularly if one costs a great deal more than another. You ultimately want to pick the one that is the highest quality for the best price. Selecting nursing interventions based on the evidence is quite similar. That is, you use a set of criteria to judge the quality and significance of the effectiveness of an intervention.

Some sources of evidence are **preappraised**. If this is the case, the guideline developers, reviewers, or publishers have already completed the hard work of evaluating the strength and magnitude of the evidence. However, you still need to understand what appraisal process the authors used to rate the evidence and if it was rigorous. In addition, you need to understand what the ranking system means. For example, you might choose to rely on the publication of a credible group, such as *Consumer Reports*, to conduct a thorough evaluation of the cars you are considering rather than completing the ranking yourself. *Consumer Reports* uses experts and a highly standardized approach to testing and rating the products it reviews ("How We Test," 2020). Not only do you save time by trusting the evaluation, you also benefit from the expert knowledge that backs the reports. Conversely, if you ask a salesperson in the showroom for an evaluation of a car that you are interested in, you may not receive a rigorous, unbiased rating of the cars—particularly if you ask about a car from another carmaker.

As the example shows, some preappraised evidence will save you time and produce a more expert ranking, whereas other sources might be biased. Later chapters discuss preappraised evidence, the systems used to rank strength and magnitude, and how to judge and use appraisal systems.

Apply

No matter how strong or large the effect, evidence is useless until put into action. To **apply** the evidence is to make it actionable. The way that evidence is applied can range in scope from influencing individual clinicians' decisions to national (and even global) health policy. Some of the largest challenges in the evidence-based practice movement relate to changing behaviors and application of the evidence. Systems are emerging that will ease and speed the integration of evidence into the everyday practice of health-care providers around the globe.

As an individual nurse, your goal is to use evidence to inform decisions throughout the nursing process. Once you have appraised and chosen the evidence based on its strength and magnitude, you need to decide how to use it.

In this chapter's clinical story, Ali wants to use the practice guideline to plan how best to assess the patient's pain and determine the appropriate intervention that will reduce the patient's pain while limiting side effects. She applies the evidence when she reviews the patient's record and sees that preoperatively, a nurse completed a comprehensive assessment of the patient's prior experiences, beliefs, and understanding of what to expect of his surgery. Ali knows the guideline made specific recommendations about tools to complete both comprehensive and ongoing assessments of pain intensity during the postoperative period. The guideline reinforced her understanding that the patient's self-report of pain is the ideal way to assess but that it requires the patient to be able to communicate (RNAO, 2013). She decides to use the numeric rating scale (rating pain intensity on a scale of 1 to 10) to assess the intensity of pain because it is valid, easy to use, appropriate to use with her patient who could communicate, and commonly used in the facility. Also, based on the guideline, Ali anticipates the pharmacological treatment and plans to offer music and/or relaxation as an adjunct to the medication. Ali feels confident about putting the evidence into action, especially when she realizes that the guideline developers preappraised the evidence and gave each of these recommendations their highest quality ranking. Although she has already planned to use the evidence to influence her own actions, she discovers the guideline also provides evidence and tools to help apply the evidence in nursing units, organizations, and even at the national level (RNAO, 2013).

Assess

As in the nursing, problem-solving, and research processes, the last stage of the evidence-based practice process is to **assess,** or evaluate, the outcomes. The method of assessment must be supported by evidence. That is, the measurement must be valid and reliable.

Some of the same tools are used to diagnose a problem and to evaluate the effect of interventions on outcomes. For example, Ali can use the same technique to assess her patient's level of pain before and after her interventions. However, additional tools can be used to assess whether the interventions worked or whether the interventions actually took place. In other words, one assesses and documents both the process and outcome of applying the evidence.

Process evaluation happens through an audit of whether the evidence-based interventions occurred. You may be part of an audit effort, or the quality team may conduct data collection. If quality officers or other facility staff audit and provide feedback about how frequently nurses use the evidence when providing care, then nurses have the opportunity to improve their care (Box 7■2). Although evidence is not always strong or well developed, audit and feedback remain common methods to enhance the uptake of evidence in practice (Cheater, Baker, Reddish, et al, 2006; Jamtvedt, Young, Kristofferson, et al, 2006; Landis-Lewis et al, 2020).

Ali uses the guideline to plan to reassess the patient's report of pain at the appropriate time after both the medication use (based on the predicted peak activity of the drug) and the introduction of music and relaxation, as well as when the patient changed his activity. She will document her assessments and evaluation in the record and advocate for other treatments if his pain is not adequately relieved (RNAO, 2013).

BOX 7■2   **Interdisciplinary Rounds**

- Librarians are part of the evidence-based practice team. Introduce yourself to the hospital or university library staff and discuss how you might work together to find evidence.
- Take a leadership role to work with librarians to identify best-bet resources and consult with an information technologist to make these online resources easily available on computers at the point of care.
- Evidence from many disciplines can inform nursing practice. Adopt an open, curious attitude when looking for evidence.
- Welcome and talk with members of other disciplines about how they use evidence to inform their practices.

Changing Practice Is Challenging

When you are new to nursing or to evidence-based practice, it is useful to deconstruct the process into its component parts. However, you will find that putting evidence into action is a messy process and often complex. Even when the issue and interventions seem quite straight forward, changing practice is challenging. You will find that although the steps of problem-solving, the nursing process, and the evidence-based practice process seem linear and can be neatly sorted on paper, in reality, they happen in cycles or in an iterative manner. Sometimes it will seem as though you take two steps forward and one step backward. However, that is often the nature of how people create change—in small steps, slowly nudging the process along. Despite the increased use of evidence in current nursing practice, more research is needed to better understand how to put evidence into action more reliably and more quickly (Box 7■3).

■ Summary

When you become a registered nurse, you enter into a social contract with the public to use evidence to inform your practice. The ANA and governing groups in other countries have developed standards of practice that explicitly state the role of evidence in nursing care. In this chapter, you were shown how the nursing, research, and evidence-based practice processes were all variations of problem-solving; they share parallel and common structures and functions. When deconstructed, the evidence-based practice process resembles the nursing process.

In future chapters you will read more about asking questions, acquiring and appraising the evidence that addresses the question, planning how to apply the evidence, and assessing the effect of putting the evidence into action.

BOX 7■3 **Tools for Learning and Practice**

■ Read the American Nurses Association's Social Policy Statement. Highlight statements relevant to evidence-based practice.
■ Ask your colleagues if they are aware of the explicit role for evidence in the statement.
■ Next time you care for a patient, ask yourself how you know what assessment techniques to use or what interventions you should use. Think about whether you know what evidence supports how you approached the patient.
■ Check your hospital's mission and goals to understand how the organization values evidence. Talk about the role of evidence-based practice with the formal and informal leaders in your unit and hospital.
■ Look around the clinical environment for "evidence of the evidence" in your organization. For example, look for how evidence is made explicit in policies, or if there are posters or other displays that transparently communicate the evidence and its quality.
■ Visit the library and explore what database, journal, and evidence resource subscriptions the organization maintains.
■ Think about a problem you recently had to deal with. Review the steps of the problem-solving and analyze how you defined the problem and its cause, generated alternative solutions, and selected from your alternatives and how you carried out and evaluated your solution.

CHAPTER QUESTIONS

1. What are the key words in the ANA's definition of *nursing?* How does this definition reflect what you do in your nursing practice?

2. What nursing standards require you to understand evidence-based practice?

3. Using the following hypothetical situation, think as an adult child. Generate a list of problems and their causes. Generate alternative solutions and discuss your thinking about selecting a solution and how you would evaluate the effectiveness of your solution:

   Your elderly parents have generally been healthy in the past and have lived independently in their own home. Your father has had a stroke and is unable to walk or complete the usual activities of daily living and has difficulty speaking. He needs ongoing intensive rehabilitation to recover more function. His insurance will not pay for inpatient rehabilitation. Your mother, though highly functional, cannot drive a car.

4. Using the same scenario, think as a nurse. Generate a list of nursing care problems and apply the nursing process to generate at least one diagnosis and a plan to intervene and evaluate the effect of your interventions.

CHAPTER QUESTIONS (continued)

5. Now think about what you know and don't know about intervening. How might the evidence-based practice process help you be more confident in your assessments or interventions? Make sure you can name each step of the evidence-based practice method.

6. Finally, how might you use the research process to fill in the gaps that you might not know how to handle?

7. How did your problem-solving, nursing process, evidence-based practice, and research steps relate to each other? How does thinking as an adult child versus thinking as a professional nurse compare?

8. What do you want to learn next about using evidence to inform your nursing actions?

References

American Nurses Association. (2010). *Nursing's social policy statement: The essence of the profession.* Silver Spring, MD: Nursingbooks.org.

Cheater, F. M, Baker, R., Reddish, S., et al. (2006). Cluster randomized controlled trial of the effectiveness of audit and feedback and educational outreach on improving nursing practice and patient outcomes. *Medical Care, 44,* 542–551.

Fawcett, J., & Garrity, J. (2009). *Evaluating research for evidence-based nursing practice.* Philadelphia, PA: F. A. Davis.

Good, M., Albert, J. M., Anderson, G. C., et al. (2010). Supplementing relaxation and music for pain after surgery. *Nursing Research, 59,* 259–269.

Jamtvedt, G., Young, J. M., Kristofferson, D. T., et al. (2006). Audit and feedback: Effects on professional practice and health care outcomes. *Cochrane Database of Systematic Reviews, 2006*(2). doi:10.1002/14651858.CD000259.pub2

Jun, J., Kovner, C. T., & Stimpfel, A. W. (2016). Barriers and facilitators of nurses' use of clinical practice guidelines: An integrative review. *International Journal of Nursing Studies, 60,* 54–68. https://doi.org/10.1016/j.ijnurstu.2016.03.006

Landis-Lewis, Z., Kononowech, J., Scott, W. J., et al. (2020). Designing clinical practice feedback reports: Three steps illustrated in Veterans Health Affairs long-term care facilities and programs. *Implementation Science, 15.* https://doi.org/10.1186/s13012-019-0950-y

Livesley, J., & Howarth, M. (2007). Integrating research evidence into clinical decisions. In J. V. Craig & R. L. Smyth (Eds.), *The evidence-based practice manual for nurses* (pp. 209–233). Edinburgh, Scotland: Churchill Livingston.

Melnyk, B. M., Fineout-Overholt, E., Gallagher-Ford, L., et al. (2012). The state of evidence-based practice in the US nurses: Implications for nurse leaders and educators. *Journal of Nursing Administration, 42*(9), 410–417.

Polit, D. F., & Beck, C. T. (2008). *Nursing research: Generating and assessing evidence for nursing practice* (8th ed.). Philadelphia, PA: Lippincott.

Pravikoff, D. S., Tanner, A. B., & Pierce, S. T. (2005). Readiness of U.S. nurses for evidence-based practice. *American Journal of Nursing, 105*(9), 40–51.

Registered Nurses' Association of Ontario. (2013). *Assessment and management of pain* (3rd ed.) (Nursing best practice guideline). Retrieved from https://rnao.ca/sites/rnao-ca/files/AssessAndManagementOfPain_15_WEB-_FINAL_DEC_2.pdf

Research and Testing. (2020). ConsumerReports.org. Retrieved from https://www.consumerreports.org/cro/about-us/what-we-do/research-and-testing/index.htm

Ask and Assess: Questioning

Lisa Hopp

■ List and define the elements of questions that address issues that are relevant to evidence-based nursing practice.

■ Using a clinical scenario, craft a PICO question about the effectiveness of a nursing intervention that includes all the elements of a properly framed question.

■ Using a clinical scenario, craft a PICo question about the meaningfulness of a patient-centered phenomenon that includes all the elements of a properly framed question.

■ Explain the usefulness of a PICO or PICo format to construct a question that leads to a successful search of the best available evidence.

■ Debate the role of questioning and curiosity in everyday nursing practice.

Attitude of inquiry	Iterative
Comparison	Meaningfulness
Context	Meta-paradigm
Environment	Narrative data
Health	Nursing
Intervention	Outcome

Person	Population
Phenomenon of interest	Qualitative research
PICo	Scale
PICO	Scope

Clinical Story

Amanda has had a busy day in a long-term acute care unit caring for five patients with a variety of medical problems, including heart failure, chronic obstructive pulmonary disease (COPD), and stroke. All of her patients are older than 70 years of age, have limited mobility, and have a decreased ability to care for themselves. Each patient had at least one IV infusion, and four required an IV medication. Despite the increased difficulty, Amanda administered 30 doses of medication safely and on time.

Completely exhausted at the end of her shift, Amanda still has many questions about her approach and the decisions she made during the day. She wonders if some of the IV drugs should have been pushed the way she did it. She thinks some of her patients could have been more mobile if she had the right equipment to help them. She wonders if the patient who was going to have heart surgery should have been bathed in a different way from what is normally done. These are just some of the questions that run through her mind as she drives home.

Think Before You Read

- Thinking about all of the types of patients and the systems of care that Amanda is managing, what is the array of questions she might ask to help her get through the day?
- How does the assessment stage of nursing process relate to the "ask" stage of the EBP process?
- What challenges face Amanda's ability to think about the evidence informing her practice in the midst of a very busy day?

Introduction

To find an answer, you must first ask a question. That seems self-evident. The evidence-based practice process welcomes and embraces a self-conscious curiosity about the daily decisions made by nurses. At its core, evidence-based practice requires an **attitude of inquiry.** As a practicing nurse, you should regard your practice with curiosity and a certain amount of skepticism. Conversely, you will become immobilized by indecision if you spend all day questioning every decision.

In evidence-based practice, the process is similar to following a treasure map; you must ask questions in a specific way to arrive at the necessary answers. In this chapter, you will learn how to develop different types of questions that point to evidence to inform your clinical practice.

What Is the Relationship Between Assessment and Questioning?

Before you can ask a question, you take stock of a situation. You may even do this instinctively. For example, by asking a teacher a question, you realized that there was a gap in your understanding. In nursing practice, this taking stock is known as "making an assessment." When nurses assess patients, they gather and organize information to identify a state of health or illness. In the evidence-based practice process, you will assess a situation to formulate a question.

Questions relevant to nursing practice arise from the concerns of the nursing **meta-paradigm:** person, health, environment, and nursing (Fawcett & Garrity, 2009, p. 5). The meta-paradigm is used to define nursing practice and provides a foundation on which to build a conceptual understanding of nursing concerns. Although the elements of the meta-paradigm and their use can be debated, think about them in broad terms to help organize the types of questions that are relevant to nursing practice.

Within the meta-paradigm, **person** refers broadly to the individual as well as families, groups, and communities. It also includes the integrated aspects of the biophysical, psychological, sociological, and spiritual person/family/community (Thorne, Canam, Dahinten, et al, 1998). **Health** can exist on a continuum as a person subjectively experiences and defines their own sense of wellness and illness along a spectrum (Thorne et al, 1998). **Environment** includes the immediate surroundings of the individual but can be expanded to incorporate sociopolitical and economical contexts of person (Thorne et al, 1998). **Nursing** is the "protection, promotion, and optimization of health and abilities, prevention of illness and injury, alleviation of suffering through the diagnosis and treatment of human response, and advocacy in the care of individuals, families, communities, and populations" (American Nurses Association, 2003, p. 6). To apply elements of the meta-paradigm to the clinical scenario, consider this: Amanda may have questioned how she could have helped (nursing) her elderly patients (person) become more mobile (health) in the busy long-term acute care facility (environment).

Elements of the meta-paradigm provide a structure to organize your thinking about clinical questions in broad terms. However, to develop more specific questions that align with appropriate types of evidence, you will use a particular format that incorporates elements of the meta-paradigm (Table 8■1).

Why Question?

When nurses reflect on their practice, they can discover better ways to care for patients. Reflection can lead nurses to consider alternative interventions, linking

TABLE 8■1 **Nursing Meta-Paradigm and PICO Questions**

Meta-Paradigm Element	Definition	Question Element	Example
Person	Individuals; families; communities; and the integrated aspects of the biophysical, psychological, sociological, and spiritual person/family/community	Population	Elderly people unable to move in bed
Environment	Immediate surroundings or sociopolitical or economical context of the person	Population (further specified) or context	Hospitalized in an acute care hospital
Nursing	Protection, promotion, and optimization of health and abilities; prevention of illness and injury; alleviation of suffering through the diagnosis and treatment of human response; and advocacy in the care of individuals, families, communities, and populations	Intervention Comparison	Repositioning with a slip sheet Repositioning using a "lift and push" technique
Health	How a person experiences wellness and illness along a continuum	Outcome	Incidence of pressure or shearing ulcers

care with outcomes and increased understanding of how the patients and families experience health and illness within a specific community or situation. By questioning practices in a self-conscious manner, nurses give themselves a chance to learn. Without this attitude of inquiry, their practice will more likely stagnate.

Questions need to progress from casual wondering to a specific search for particular information so that knowledge will transform into nursing action. In evidence-based practice, questions provide the basis for searching for the best available evidence, for understanding the patient or family experience, and driving the specific implementation and evaluation of nursing practice. The question is the point at which the evidence-based practice process begins, and the question drives the rest of the process—through finding the evidence, appraising the evidence, making decisions to implement, and finally evaluating the use of the evidence.

Scope and Scale of Questions for Evidence-Based Practice

In this chapter's clinical story, Amanda cared for patients with many different nursing care issues. Because of this variety, she might ask questions that vary in scope. **Scope** relates to the breadth of the question. It might also be defined in terms of setting, population, age-group, or other category. **Scale** relates to the how *much* of the scope one wishes to address. Amanda could think about the scope of questions related to the nursing care of adult patients who have limitations in mobility. Within this very broad scope, she might scale the question to include interventions that could help patients improve their mobility. Alternatively, she may scale the question to relate to how often patients with limited mobility may need to be turned to prevent pressure ulcers. The scale of these two issues is much different. The first is very large within the scope. To answer the question properly, Amanda needs to gather information about all interventions related to patient mobility and determine which interventions will improve the patients' condition. She also needs to investigate many kinds of mobility aids, such as gait belts, walkers, and canes, as well as methods of advancing mobility from bedrest to walking, and techniques for turning and moving patients in bed. The second question is much smaller in scale, and Amanda needs to focus only on turning frequency.

Finding the right scope and scale of the question will help you find the right information for the right patients. As you develop an effective question that leads you to a certain type of evidence, you may frequently change its scope and scale to reframe the question again and again in an **iterative** fashion. You will work and rework the question until you are satisfied that it asks what you want to know.

Elements of Questions of Effectiveness and Meaningfulness

Most leaders in the field of evidence-based practice agree that a structured approach will help you develop a well-built question. A proper question helps ensure a successful search of the literature. You begin by assessing the patient or situation. You deconstruct the problem into its smaller parts, and then you reconstruct the individual elements into a coherent question. Depending on the type of issue you are faced with, you will craft the question somewhat differently.

The kinds of questions that health-care providers ask depend on what is important to their practice. These differences in perspective have led to some debate related to what counts as legitimate evidence. Different disciplines and individuals have different ideas about the nature of evidence. Chapter 5 discussed the JBI model. The model's authors argued that health-care professionals engage in a variety of activities and decisions and interact with people in different ways. Therefore, their knowledge needs are diverse and the way they seek knowledge varies. When the authors described the model, they identified four categories of evidence—feasibility, appropriateness, meaningfulness, and effectiveness—and related questions that are particularly well suited for nursing practice (Jordan, Lockwood, Munn et al, 2018; Pearson, Wiechula, Court, et al, 2007). Feasibility questions are related to whether an intervention is "physically, culturally or financially possible within a given context" (Pearson et al, 2007, p. 86). Questions of appropriateness are similar but focus on how the intervention fits in the context. Finally, questions of meaningfulness and effectiveness are the types of questions that relate to how people experience an intervention or phenomenon and how well the intervention works to achieve an outcome (Pearson et al, 2007). Questions related to feasibility, appropriateness, and effectiveness can use a similar structure, but you will need to adapt the format somewhat to form meaningfulness questions.

Effectiveness Questions: PICO

When you want to find the best available evidence about the effectiveness of a nursing intervention, you will use the PICO format. **PICO** is an acronym and is an easy way to remember the important parts of the question.

- *P* stands for *p*opulation (person and perhaps environment in the meta-paradigm).
- *I* stands for *i*ntervention (nursing in the meta-paradigm).
- *C* stands for *c*omparison intervention (also nursing in the meta-paradigm).
- *O* stands for *o*utcome (health in the meta-paradigm).

Amanda can generate many PICO questions related to her patients' care. Questions come from surprising or unexplained events, unwanted outcomes, or even routine nursing care. Recall that Amanda wondered whether her elderly, chronically ill patients could have increased mobility. She begins by thinking, "I wonder what I could do to help my older patients get out of bed to walk in the hallway?" This is a worthy question, but it needs to be refined to help her create an efficient search for related evidence (Box 8■1).

Population

Amanda starts by focusing on the **population** ("person" and "environment" in the meta-paradigm). In PICO, *population* is defined as the group of people that is of concern in the question. This group may be related by a disease, a health condition, risk profile, the environment in which they exist, age-group, or any combination of these factors. As you define the population by introducing more factors, you limit the scope and scale of the question. To define the population for Amanda's question, she begins very broadly with "elderly people." But this definition would not specifically target elderly patients in the hospital with limited mobility who also have special needs. Amanda begins to narrow the population of the question to "elderly patients with limited mobility." However, although she is specifically interested in the environment of a long-term acute care setting, this may narrow the question too much and may eliminate helpful evidence. She may need to revisit the issue of environment after she begins to explore the literature. Once she finds some

BOX 8■1   **Significance of Questioning**

- Being curious about your practice leads to questioning and having an attitude of inquiry.
- Wondering about the "rightness" of your practice provides an opportunity to learn and to advance the practice of others.
- Questions should come from everyday nursing practice issues and therefore are real and meaningful to clinical work.
- Questions are of large and small scope and scale and therefore their answers can affect groups of people (patients, nurses, systems) or individuals.
- A pluralistic acceptance of different types of evidence requires adaption of the PICO (population, intervention, comparison, outcome) to the PICo (population, phenomenon of interest, context) format for asking questions.
- A guide to asking PICO and PICo questions helps to focus the question.
- The PICO or PICo question drives the entire evidence-based practice process and keeps you focused on the problem.
- The elements of the question lead to generating keywords and synonyms to form a search strategy and/or to use to consult with a librarian.

evidence, she can make a judgment about how well the evidence relates to the specific setting. You will find that as you develop your questions, you may need to revise and refine as you test the breadth of the evidence.

Intervention

After population, address the **intervention** ("nursing" in the meta-paradigm). An intervention is the nursing treatment or action that is the focus of the question. Amanda considers a variety of interventions such as gait belts to assist walking, walkers, lift devices, physiotherapy consultation, or even prompts that remind nurses to help patients increase movement. She settles with a fairly general intervention, such as a transfer aid, or a very specific intervention, such as a transfer sling that will help her assist patients' transfer out of bed.

Comparison

If you are interested in comparing one intervention against another, you will include a **comparison** intervention in your question. The comparison may be to any other nursing intervention or it may be to taking no action at all. In her question, Amanda can compare using a transfer belt against a transfer sling, or she may be interested in comparing a slip-sheet to a lift device. However, comparisons are not essential to the evidence-based practice process. A comparison may not be necessary if you are interested in effectiveness regardless of the testing of any other intervention.

Outcome

Finally, you specify the **outcome**(s) ("health" in the meta-paradigm) that you want to know about. The outcome is the specific effect(s) of the intervention or what matters to the nurse and patient. It is what the nurse would use to evaluate whether the intervention had a beneficial or harmful effect on the patient, nurse, or organization. When developing her question about increased patient mobility, Amanda needs to address issues related to her patients' safety; how quickly patients mobilize; or complications of immobility, such as venous thromboembolism, pressure ulcers, fatigue, or discomfort. Like the other elements of the question, the degree of specificity or generality of the outcome will influence the scope and scale of the question and the breadth of your search.

Creating a PICO Question

After you determine the four important items, you glue the pieces together to form a complete PI(C)O question. Most questions of effectiveness can take the following form: What is the effectiveness of [insert intervention] versus [insert comparison, if there is one] in patients with [insert population/environment] on [health outcome]? When thinking about patient mobility, Amanda can ask, "What is the effectiveness of a transfer sling (I) versus a transfer belt (C) in elderly patients in long-term acute care (LTAC) with impaired mobility (P) on patient comfort and incidence of nurse back injury (O)?" Another question Amanda might develop is "What is the effectiveness of using a turn schedule (I) versus an audible public address reminder (C) on the incidence of pressure ulcers (O) in elderly patients in LTAC who require turning (P)?" She could also generate many questions related to the effectiveness of various interventions for her elderly hospitalized patients with impaired mobility. Following the PICO model, Amanda starts with broad questions and develops more specific questions to focus her search. You can use these sample questions to help you formulate your own questions related to the effectiveness of interventions (Table 8■2).

Meaningfulness Questions: PICo

Nurses have broader concerns than merely the effectiveness of interventions. Leaders in evidence-based nursing practice have advocated for a pluralistic view of what counts as evidence (Jordan et al, 2018; Pearson et al, 2007; Rycroft-Malone, Seers, Titchen, et al, 2004). Legitimate evidence arises from many sources including both quantitative and qualitative research. If we claim that as nurses, we are person centered, then we must care about how people experience their health. As a result, we are interested in the **meaningfulness** of health-related phenomena. Pearson et al (2007) define *meaningfulness* as "the extent to which an intervention or activity is positively [or negatively] experienced by the patient. Meaningfulness relates to the personal experience, opinions, values, thoughts, beliefs and interpretations of patients or clients" (pp. 86–87).

Evidence-based health care recognizes that patient preferences and values are important to decision making. Nurses and other health-care providers can use evidence of meaningfulness from **qualitative research** to help understand patient preferences and values. Qualitative research is a "systematic, subjective methodological approach used to describe life experience and situations and to give them meaning" (Burns, Gray, & Grove, 2016, p. 20). Certainly it is inappropriate to seek meaningfulness

TABLE 8∎2 **PICO Questions of Effectiveness**

General question: What is the best way to care for urinary catheters in patients with a stroke?

Narrower question: What is the best way to remove catheters in patients who have had a stroke and who have a urinary catheter?

	Element	Definition	Example
P	Population	Who in what circumstance is at the center of the issue?	Adult patients after stroke with an indwelling catheter
I	Intervention	What is the intervention of interest?	Clamping the catheter before removal
C	Comparison	What is the alternative intervention (if there is one)?	Gravity drain before removal
O	Outcome	What are the benefit(s) or harm(s)?	Time to first void Incidence of urinary tract infection

Final PICO: What is the effectiveness of clamping versus gravity drain prior to removal of an indwelling urinary catheter in patients after a stroke?

knowledge from quantitative or experimental studies because meaning comes from the story, the **narrative data** gathered through qualitative research or discourse. According to Sandelowski (1994), a leading American qualitative research expert, "narratives are generally understood to be stories with a certain dynamic structure and shape directed toward achieving wholeness, or health" (p. 23).

To accommodate meaningfulness in the development of your question, you will adapt the PICO format to the **PICo** approach for questions related to meaning. That is, *P* still reflects the *p*opulation of interest but *I* refers to the phenomenon of *i*nterest and *Co* refers to the *co*ntext (Lockwood, Porrit, Munn, et al, 2017).

Phenomenon of Interest

Phenomenon of interest is the part of the patient's experience that you want to understand. Although they can vary in scope, the phenomena of interest tend to be broad. Like her curiosity about the effectiveness of the nursing interventions, Amanda has questions about many phenomena related to the meaning of the patients' experiences. She wonders about the meaning of impaired immobility, the experience of being dependent on someone else for mobility, or losing independence in general. If one of her patients has acquired a pressure ulcer, she will want to understand the meaning of having a pressure ulcer or being in pain.

When you consider the phenomenon of a patient's experience, the words associated with that experience must have meaning to the patient and be part of the patient's vocabulary. You would not ask the question about the patient's experience using a term that has meaning only to nursing or another health-care professional. For example, you would not ask the question, "What is the meaning of the experience of continuous lateral rotation?" The term "continuous lateral rotation" has meaning for professionals. Instead of using unfamiliar terms, you need to find what the patient calls that experience. The patient may experience the treatment as helplessness (a more negative response) or comfort (a more positive response), but the experience is wholly of the patient, not the nurse. You may think that the treatment is effective and helpful, but it may mean something entirely different to the patient.

Context

Context is important in how a phenomenon is experienced; it is the surroundings of the phenomenon or person. A patient experiences comfort while hospitalized in an intensive care unit differently from how he or she experiences comfort at home under usual circumstances. The context may be the environment, particular cultural factors, the community, the setting, or a health problem. In this chapter's clinical story, if Amanda wants to know about an elderly patient's experience of helplessness, she could use the general context of an acute care hospital unit. Alternatively, she can specify the context as the patient's experience within a particular health problem, such as the recovery phase from a stroke that leaves residual paralysis. Finally, she may combine both contexts to determine the patient's experience during acute care hospitalization and the recovery phase from a stroke that leaves residual paralysis.

Creating a PICo Question

As with effectiveness questions, you may find it helpful to use a template approach for your meaningfulness questions. For example: How do patients [insert population] experience [insert phenomenon] in the context of [insert context]? You can imagine a variety of questions for Amanda's practice (Table 8■3).

Much like the research process, the question posed to the evidence-based practice process drives the rest of the course of action. The next section shows how Amanda prepares to take her questions to the next phase—searching.

Taking Questioning to Searching

The next step in the evidence-based practice process is to search for and find the best available evidence. This is the first job for your newly formed question. Regardless of whether you will consult a librarian or if you will construct your own evidence search, you need to deconstruct the question to identify keywords related to each element. Even if you are consulting with a librarian, you will need to know what synonyms are most likely associated with each element of your question. You will want to approach the librarian with a clear idea of what you want to know; it is best to go well prepared (Box 8■2).

Consider Amanda's next question: "What is the effectiveness of using a turn schedule versus an audible public address reminder on the incidence of pressure ulcers in elderly hospitalized patients who require turning?" To begin her search for appropriate evidence, Amanda should begin by unpacking her PICO question

TABLE 8■3 **PICo Questions of Meaningfulness**

General question: What is it like to experience a stroke?

Narrower question: What does it mean to lose motor function after a stroke?

	Element	Definition	Example
P	Population	Who in what circumstance is at the center of the issue?	Patients with a stroke
I	Phenomenon of Interest	What is the patient-centered experience you want to understand?	Loss of control over movement
Co	Context	What is the environment, particular cultural factors, timing, community, setting, or health problem influencing the situation?	Early phase of hospital-based rehabilitation

Final PICo: How do people experience losing control of movement in the early phase of a stroke while they remain hospitalized for rehabilitation?

BOX 8■2 **Interdisciplinary Rounds**

- Questions provide a common ground for collaboration among disciplines.
- Multiple disciplines may have an interest in the same interventions and phenomena.
- Librarians are key to successful searches for the best available evidence.
- Take your PICO or PICo question to consult with your librarian and generate keywords and their synonyms.

Example
A nurse on a long-term acute care unit takes the following PICO question to the library scientist: What is the effectiveness of a bladder-training program on incontinence in female patients recovering from a stroke?

The keywords and phrases include "bladder training," "urinary incontinence—control and prevention," "bladder retraining," "bladder program," "bladder management," "prompted voiding," "continence care," "incontinence," "continence," "urinary continence," "stroke," "cerebral vascular accident."

again. Then she should determine synonyms for each of the *P, I, C, O* elements. For the population, Amanda would use the keywords "aged," "elderly," "older adult," or other related term. For the intervention of "turn schedule," she would need to think about all words that could be used to describe a reminder system representing a schedule. These might be short phrases such as "turn clock" or "reminder clock." For her comparison, she could use terms such as "audible signal," "public address," or "audible reminder." Finally, for the outcome, she would use "pressure ulcer,"

BOX 8■3 **Tools for Learning and Practice**

- Ask yourself what you need to know to provide the best possible nursing care to your patients. Think through a typical day and ask yourself, "Do I know what the best evidence is to . . . ?" "How do I know if this is the right thing to do?"
- Move from big questions to smaller questions (think of pouring all your questions through a funnel), particularly when you are a novice.
- Think about each element of a good question and identify what you want to know.
- Use a PICO approach for effectiveness questions or PICo for questions of meaning to help you build each part of the question.
- Glue the elements together to create a full question.
- Use this format to formulate effectiveness questions: What is the effectiveness of [insert intervention] versus [insert comparison, if there is one] in patients with [insert population/environment] on [health outcome]?
- Use this format to formulate meaningfulness questions: How do patients [insert population] experience [insert phenomenon] in the context of [insert context]?
- Tear the question apart again to identify keywords and their synonyms.
- Practice writing questions and ask someone else to make sure the questions contain all of the correct elements.
- Find out the names of your librarians, their contact information, and the process for working with them.
- Take your question, keywords, and synonyms with you when you meet with the librarian.

"decubitus ulcer," "pressure sore," and other terms. Although developing a list of synonyms is time consuming, the next step in the process is easier if you have synonyms for each element of the question. If you carefully use the most meaningful terms to represent what you want to know, your selection of key terms for the search will be easier and more effective (Box 8■3).

■ Summary

Finding the right answers requires the right questions. Questions relevant to nursing practice emerge from reflection on your daily work and relate to the meta-paradigm. The PICO and PICo formats will help you construct questions that will likely lead to effective searches and to the best available evidence of effectiveness of interventions and meaningfulness of patient experiences, respectively. If you adopt an attitude of curiosity and inquiry, you will find an abundance of questions as you think more self-consciously about your practice. With a little practice, you will be able to form questions that lead to effective searches and interpretation of the evidence.

CHAPTER QUESTIONS

1. What is meant by an "attitude of inquiry"?

2. Where do questions about nursing practice come from?

3. What is the purpose of asking questions in a particular format before proceeding with the evidence-based practice process?

4. Examine a typical day in your nursing practice. What types of questions can you ask about your day?

5. What do PICO and PICo represent?

6. Identify the *P, I, C* (if identified), and *O* in the following questions:
   a. What is the effectiveness of 2% chlorhexidine-impregnated wipes versus a traditional soap-and-water basin bath on the incidence of surgical site infections in adult patients who receive cardiothoracic surgery?
   b. What is the effect of using bar coding on medication errors in patients receiving oral medications in an acute care medical-surgical hospital?
   c. What is the effectiveness of using moisture-barrier products versus not using a moisture barrier on the rate of skin breakdown in incontinent, bed-ridden patients?

7. Develop a PICO or PICo question to fit the following issues:
   a. How well a smoking-cessation program works in adults with at least a 20-year pack-a-day history of smoking
   b. The impact of various dressings for IV catheters on phlebitis
   c. How a patient with end-stage heart failure experiences hopefulness

8. Identify what element is missing in the following questions and then improve them:
   a. What is the experience of family presence?
   b. What is the effect of open visiting hours?
   c. What is the optimal frequency of assessing risk for pressure ulcers?
   d. Do pressure-reducing mattresses work?

9. What are key terms that you would ask your librarian to use to search for evidence related to this question: What is the effect of suctioning a tracheostomy every 2 hours versus on an as-needed basis on secretion clearance in patients with a new tracheostomy?

References

American Nurses Association. (2003). *Nursing's social policy statement* (2nd ed.). Silver Spring, MD: Author.

Burns, N., Gray, J. R., & Grove, S. K. (2012). *Understanding nursing research: Building an evidence-based practice* (6th ed.). St. Louis, MO: Saunders-Elsevier.

Fawcett, J., & Garity, J. (2009). *Evaluating research for evidence-based nursing practice*. Philadelphia, PA: F. A. Davis.

Jordan, Z., Lockwood, C., Munn, Z., et al. (2018). Redeveloping the model of evidence-based healthcare. *International Journal of Evidence-Based Healthcare, 16*, 227–241. doi:10.1097/XEB000000000000139

Lockwood C., Porrit K., Munn Z., et al. (2017). Systematic reviews of qualitative evidence. In E. Aromataris & Z. Munn (Eds.), *Joanna Briggs Institute reviewer's manual.* Retrieved from https://reviewersmanual.joannabriggs.org/

Pearson, A., Wiechula, R., Court, A., et al. (2007). A re-consideration of what constitutes "evidence" in the healthcare professions. *Nursing Science Quarterly, 20*, 85–88. doi:10.1177/0894318406296306

Rycroft-Malone, J., Seers, K., Titchen, A., et al. (2004). What counts as evidence in evidence-based practice? *Journal of Advanced Nursing, 47*(1), 81–90.

Sandelowski, M. (1994). We are the stories we tell: Narrative knowing in nursing. *Journal of Holistic Nursing, 12*, 22–33. doi:10.1177/089801019401200105

Thorne, S., Canam, C., Dahinten, S., et al. (1998). Nursing's metaparadigm concepts: Disimpacting the debates. *Journal of Advanced Nursing, 27*, 1257–1268.

CHAPTER 9

Acquire and Diagnose: Linking the Problem With Finding Best Sources of Evidence

Kim Whalen

LEARNING OBJECTIVES

- Distinguish among types of summarized sources of evidence.
- Generate keywords for searching.
- Conduct a bibliographic database search using Boolean operators.
- Identify the best available resources for locating evidence.
- Describe how to communicate and partner with a librarian or information scientist.

KEY TERMS

Bibliographic databases
Boolean operators
Centre for Reviews and
  Dissemination (CRD)
Citation chasing
Clinical practice guidelines
Cochrane Library

Critical appraisal
Cumulative Index to Nursing
  and Allied Health Literature
  (CINAHL)
Embase
Google Scholar
Hand searching

Interlibrary loan
JBI Evidence-based Practice
  (EBP) Database
Keywords
Literature review
MEDLINE
MeSH subject headings
Peer-reviewed journals
Primary source
PubMed

PubMed Central
PubMed Central's Clinical
  Queries
Secondary sources
Standardized subject
  headings
Systematic review
Truncation
Wildcards

Clinical Story

Mark is in his final semester of his BSN program, and he is excited to participate in the capstone project that focuses on improving hand hygiene among nurses at the local community hospital. The team plans to conduct a literature review to locate the best available evidence, summarize their findings, and propose an educational intervention to the nursing leadership team at the hospital. To begin, Mark and his teammates read their project outline and start to divide up their tasks. One teammate suggests using Google, Bing, or another Internet search engine to gather all the information they need for their literature review. Because of the extensive research that he completed for his nursing theories course, Mark knows not to rely only on Internet sources, and he suggests they meet with their nursing librarian, Mrs. Daniels. She can provide advice on using journals and bibliographic databases available through their university library and help them identify the search strategies that can improve their search results from the databases and from the Internet. Mark quickly e-mails Mrs. Daniels to set up a time for them all to meet.

Think Before You Read

- Before you learned about evidence-based practice, how would you seek information to help you with a problem that you are not sure how to solve?
- If you think about how you ask a question to find the best available evidence, how might you break up the question to search for evidence?
- How might you communicate with a librarian in order to be the most efficient you can be in the search process?
- What type of evidence sources would best help Mark and his team with the problem they want to solve?

Introduction

Seeking the best available evidence for clinical decisions is like a treasure hunt: you need a map to help you hunt for the most valuable prize. You use your question and the structured search strategy as your map to search for the best available evidence. Remember, the ideal evidence is the highest quality information that answers your question.

Whether you are preparing an academic paper or simply trying to find the answer to a clinical question in the middle of your clinical day, you need to develop some basic search skills and know when to seek help from a professional knowledge seeker: your librarian. Before beginning your search, you must be clear about what type of information you need. For example, if you have a very narrow question, you should start your search with clinical practice guidelines or a high-quality systematic review. If you are unable to find your answer in either option, you will need to search for individual articles and primary source documents. In this chapter, you will learn the differences between types of information; the basics of conducting a search of bibliographic databases; where to search for clinical practice guidelines, systematic reviews, and primary sources; and the importance of forming a partnership with professional librarians.

Sources of Evidence

With health-care information being published in books, journals, magazines, news-papers, bibliographic databases, and the Internet at such a rapid pace, staying on top of the latest findings can be difficult. When you are a busy clinician, making many decisions every day, the ideal source of evidence is one in which someone else has completed the difficult work of searching, appraising, and synthesizing the evidence. To be efficient in your search, you need to be able to distinguish among many types of evidence, know where to find the "best-bet" sources of evidence, and know how to get to those sources.

You may be familiar with the term **literature review.** It is often the first step in writing a paper or developing a research proposal. Its purpose is to summarize information from various authors and sources. Literature reviews help you to understand background issues and determine the scope of literature available. They also help to uncover gaps in the literature or areas in which further research should be conducted. However, because they lack the rigor of other types of reviews, you should not directly inform your clinical decisions with casual literature reviews. Authors of literature reviews usually do not explicitly communicate the methods they used to find their information, nor do they use a highly structured approach to the search strategy or explain how they selected the information included in the literature review.

Another type of review is a **systematic review.** This is a very different source of evidence from a casual literature review. Systematic reviews may include meta-synthesis or meta-analysis of evidence on a topic. They involve "the application of scientific strategies, in ways that limit bias, to the assembly, critical appraisal, and synthesis of all relevant studies that address a specific clinical question" (Cook, Mulrow, & Haynes, 1997, p. 376). Qualitative systematic reviews summarize study findings without using statistics; therefore, they are known as meta-syntheses. Meta-syntheses combine summary statements, or themes, from multiple studies. A meta-analysis, or quantitative systematic review, uses statistical methods to summarize study findings, and, according to Pearson, Wiechula, Court, et al (2005, p. 212), "key outcomes of the meta-analysis are the measure of effect, the confidence interval and the degree of heterogeneity of the studies synthesized." Although systematic reviews are a better place to start looking for answers to clinical questions than original studies written about within individual journal articles, systematic reviews have not been developed for every clinical question.

Clinical practice guidelines are another form of synthesized evidence designed to provide comprehensive recommendations about the diagnosis, management, or treatment of a particular condition or clinical question. Based on systematic reviews and adapted to local circumstances and values, guidelines assist practitioners and patients with making decisions about care. High-quality clinical practice guidelines represent the synthesis of the best available evidence, clinical expertise, and consumer and stakeholder input. In addition, they contain practical tools to help you use the evidence. Many organizations, governments, and health-care specialty societies produce and publish clinical practice guidelines.

During your time in school, or during your nursing practice, there will be occasions when you will conduct your own primary research. Literature reviews, systematic reviews, and clinical practice guidelines are different from articles describing primary research because they all offer analysis of already completed work by others, they are not describing new research. Despite that, all reviews should be conducted with the same rigor that is applied to a primary research project. In this chapter, you will learn how to develop an effective search strategy to identify relevant evidence for a literature review. You will also learn about the resources to use for efficiently locating evidence including clinical practice guidelines, systematic reviews, and primary research articles (Box 9■1).

Begin With a Good Question

With all the health-care information available, where do you begin? The previous chapter stressed that the first step in locating the best available evidence is the development of a focused PICO or PICo question (Table 9■1). In this chapter's clinical story, Mark and his capstone project team begin by brainstorming their assignment and identifying their *p*opulation, *i*ntervention, *c*omparison, and *o*utcome. The team was charged with improving hand hygiene among nurses at the local community hospital. They were also charged with developing an educational program that would increase adherence to the hospital's hand hygiene protocol among nurses. As a result of the assignment, the team initially asks, "What impact does an

BOX 9■1 **Significance of Acquiring the Best Sources of Evidence**

- Use of incomplete or out-of-date information could affect patient safety.
- Gaining experience in identifying the best available information resources will make you a more effective and efficient researcher as well as nurse.
- A thorough search will provide the best available evidence for an informed clinical decision.
- Clinical practice guidelines, systematic reviews, and other types of synthesized evidence are important information tools.
- Individual articles describing primary research studies are also important, but used independently do not always provide the best available evidence.
- Hospital and university librarians, also known as library scientists, are available to help you access the information you need—take advantage of their expertise and assistance.

TABLE 9■1 **Development of PICO Question**

General question: What is the best way to get nurses at the community hospital to properly wash their hands?

Narrower question: What is the best way to increase nurses' adherence to the community hospital's hand hygiene protocol?

	Element	Definition	Example
P	Population	Who is at the center of the issue?	Nurses in a community hospital
I	Intervention	What is the intervention of interest?	An educational program
C	Comparison	What is the alternative intervention (if there is one)?	A marketing campaign
O	Outcome	What is the benefit(s) or harm(s)?	Increase adherence to the current hand hygiene protocol

Initial PICO: What impact does an educational program (I) or marketing campaign (C) have on community hospital nurses' (P) adherence to the hospital's hand hygiene protocol (O)?

Final PICO: What is the effectiveness of offering a mandatory training session or posting written marketing materials throughout the hospital on improving adherence to the hospital's hand hygiene protocol among nurses on the ICU floor?

educational program (I) or marketing campaign (C) have on community hospital nurses' (P) adherence to the hospital's hand hygiene protocol (O)?" After a bit of discussion, the team decides to further focus their question to ask, "What is the effectiveness of offering a mandatory training session (I) or posting written marketing materials throughout the hospital (C) on improving adherence to the hospital's hand hygiene protocol (O) among nurses on the ICU floor (P)?"

While developing the PICO question, the team may find that they are interested in comparing a very specific type of educational program, a mandatory in-person session, or an online seminar to a very specific type of marketing campaign, an email reminder system, or print posters displayed throughout the hospital. Rephrasing and refining the research question will result in a more effective search.

Generating Keywords

While rephrasing their question, the team develops a list of **keywords** and phrases to use to search the library's bibliographic databases and the Internet. Although it seems simple, selecting useful keywords is often the most time consuming and difficult part of an effective search (Hartzell, Fineout-Overholt, Hofstetter, et al, 2015; Timmins & McCabe, 2005). Mark's team begins by generating synonyms and related terms for each PICO element. For example, for the outcome of "adherence to the hand hygiene protocol," they think about all the other words and phrases used to describe a hand hygiene protocol. These include words such as "handwashing" or "policy," or phrases such as "hand washing," "hand sanitation," "hand cleaning," and "hand hygiene." For the intervention of educational program, they list words and phrases such as "seminar," "workshop," "inservice," "orientation session," "in-person workshop," and "online workshop." Armed with their PICO question and a set of synonyms, keywords, and phrases for each element of the question, the team is ready to move on.

Setting Limits

Before implementing their search, Mark and his team agree on the types of information resources they will search during their research. One of Mark's teammates thinks information found on the Internet would be sufficient. However, other teammates are concerned about finding quality health-care information within books, journals, magazines, trade publications, newspaper articles, dissertations, and library bibliographic databases. It is important for the team to agree on the types of information resources appropriate for their assignment. At the same time, the team must focus on accessing the best available evidence to answer their question.

Popular magazine articles, newspaper articles, and trade publications are valuable information resources but more practical in nature. They are typically not written by researchers or experts, nor do all of the articles go through a rigorous review process before publication. Useful for current awareness of health-care issues, procedures, equipment, and professional events, these types of publications are not sufficient resources for Mark's capstone assignment. Although books and textbooks are also valuable sources of information, it is more appropriate for Mark and his team to search scholarly journals and other sources of peer-reviewed evidence for their assignment. Scholarly **peer-reviewed journals** publish results more quickly than books and textbooks. They report original research findings as well as synthesized analysis like systematic reviews and clinical practice guidelines to professionals within the field. Before being published, most scholarly articles are approved through a peer-review process. This process involves multiple reviewers who hold advanced degrees within the discipline, teach within the field, are experts in the profession, and are very knowledgeable about the topic. Each reviewer evaluates the article, the research conducted, and the findings represented to determine whether the article warrants publication within that specific scholarly journal. Scholarly journals are often referred to as peer-reviewed, juried, refereed, or academic journals.

Scholarly peer-reviewed journals publish primary sources of information as well as secondary sources of information. A **primary source** is one created by the witness of the event. Taylor (2007) defines primary sources as those that have not been edited, interpreted, condensed, or evaluated by someone else. She states, "Primary sources also present original thinking and observations, such as the original research used to write journal articles reporting on original scientific studies, experiments, or observations" (p. 38). An article written by a nursing student in a doctor of nursing practice (DNP) program summarizing the results of her online survey of nurses about their preferred method of hand sanitation in their academic health center would be a useful primary source for Mark's assignment.

Secondary sources report on the work of others, not on the author's own original research findings. Although often easier to find, secondary sources need to be critically appraised to ensure that the information presented maintains the integrity of the original research findings and it has not been misinterpreted or altered (Hartzell et al, 2015; Taylor, 2007). Literature reviews, systematic reviews, and clinical practice guidelines are considered secondary sources of information because they synthesize previously reported findings of others. A quantitative systematic review, also described as a meta-analysis, analyzing the research conducted on educational interventions found most influential in improving the rate of hand washing among hospital staff is an excellent secondary source for Mark's assignment (Box 9■2).

It is important that Mark and his teammates know the parameters of their assignment to discern if they can use both primary and secondary sources of information. If they are unable to use secondary sources, they can use the references cited or bibliography published within a literature review or systematic review to locate primary sources identified by the review's authors. **Citation chasing,** the term used to describe the process of using references or a bibliography to identify other relevant evidence, is an efficient and important step in the information gathering process. Mark and his team must also know if there is a time limit on the information they can use for their assignment. Some assignments require sources used to be published within the last 5 or 10 years; some assignments have no publication time limits. Keep in mind that limiting a search by time frame can help control the amount of information retrieved but it can also eliminate seminal, groundbreaking pieces of information that were published outside of the time frame. Other limitations include limiting information published by language or by publication type. Limiting the search to only the information published in English or to only those studies conducted in the United States can help control the amount of information identified

---

BOX 9■2 **Interdisciplinary Rounds**

Reading multiple articles on a specific topic can seem overwhelming. Imagine being handed a stack of articles on a specific topic and having to take the time to appraise the studies conducted, analyze the reported findings, and compare the results. A goal of evidence-based practice is to synthesize the best available evidence so that students, clinicians, and patients can effectively access the information available and efficiently put the information to use.

Example

A patient asks two different orthopedic nurses for information on the treatment of rotator cuff tears. Both nurses enjoy regularly reading nursing journals and both had read recent articles on the topic. One journal contained an article reporting that rotator cuff tears are best repaired through all-arthroscopic surgery. Another journal published an article reporting that cuff tears are best repaired with mini-open surgery. Yet another journal, not read by either of the two nurses, contained an article on the success of nonoperative treatments for rotator cuff tear repair. Which article or articles would be the best evidence to share with the patient?

Reading individual articles and independent primary sources of information can yield different reported results. Synthesized evidence, including systematic reviews, provides a summary of individual articles and primary sources of information related to a specific topic. Some systematic reviews use statistics to summarize findings and limit bias, whereas others create summary statements describing study findings. Systematic reviews appraise the studies conducted and the findings reported, and compare the results. Searching for a systematic review of the best treatments for rotator cuff tears would provide both the patient and the nurses with the best available evidence on the subject.

---

but can also eliminate key findings from the global health-care community (Adorno, Garbee, & Marix, 2016). Limiting a search by publication type can focus findings only on scholarly peer-reviewed journal articles and eliminate information published within magazines, trade publications, and other sources. After confirming the assignment, Mark and his team use their knowledge of the project and the required quality of information to determine which, if any, publication type limits what they want to apply to their search.

Get Ready, Get Set

Scholarly peer-reviewed primary and secondary sources of information are most readily located within the **bibliographic databases** made available by academic and public libraries as well as from government and professional organizations on the Internet. Bibliographic databases contain abstracts (a synopsis of the article), and some contain the full text of articles including graphics, images, tables, and charts. Many databases are subscription based, so a fee must be paid to access them. Bibliographic databases commonly used by nursing students include Cumulative Index to Nursing and Allied Health Literature (CINAHL), MEDLINE, PubMed, PubMed Central, the Cochrane Library, Embase, and the JBI EBP Database.

Although bibliographic databases are offered by various vendors, the user-friendly interfaces are designed in a similar way. Searches can be focused on a specific subject term or expanded through the use of keywords and phrases. Specific subject terms, otherwise known as **standardized subject headings,** were developed by the Library of Congress to organize large subjects logically into categories. Medical subject headings, known as **MeSH subject headings,** were designed as a controlled vocabulary for medicine by the United States National Library of Medicine. Arranged in an alphabetical and hierarchical structure, MeSH subject headings allow for more organized and accurate searching. According to the United States National Library of Medicine's National Center for Biotechnology Information, the MeSH heading of "hand disinfection" is defined as "the act of cleansing the hands with water or other liquid, with or without the inclusion of soap or other detergent, for the purpose of destroying infectious microorganisms" (National Center for Biotechnology Information [NCBI], 2020). Based on the definition, Mark and his team could choose to start their search using the MeSH subject heading for "hand disinfection" instead of the other keywords and phrases including handwashing and hand sanitation they had been considering (see Box 9■3 for links to find subject headings).

In addition to a search using subject headings, the team should also search bibliographic databases using multiple keywords and phrases. Keywords and phrases can be combined using the **Boolean operators** AND, OR, and NOT to broaden or narrow a search. These operators can be used within most bibliographic databases as well as with most Internet search engines. Mark and his team could choose to search using the search string handwashing OR "hand washing" OR "hand disinfection" OR "hand sanitation" OR "hand cleaning" OR "hand hygiene." This string will locate all the articles that contain at least one of these words or phrases (Fig. 9■1). Adding the Boolean operator AND will narrow the search. The team could then search using the string (handwashing OR "hand washing" OR "hand disinfection" OR "hand sanitation" OR "hand cleaning" OR "hand hygiene") AND nurse. Placing

---

BOX 9■3　**Subject Heading Sources**

■ Library of Congress Subject Headings (http://id.loc.gov/authorities/subjects.html)
■ MeSH Subject Headings (https://meshb.nlm.nih.gov/search)

FIGURE 9■1 (A) Using the OR Boolean operator (results will include articles with both keywords or phrases). (B) Using the AND Boolean operator (results will include articles with both keywords and phrases).

quotation marks around a phrase ensures the results will include the entire phrase together and not each word separately. Like a mathematical equation, the parentheses enclosing a set of words and phrases allow the results within the parentheses to be combined with additional words and phrases outside the parentheses. The result of the search string with the AND nurse would locate all the articles that contain at least one of the listed handwashing words or phrases as well as the word *nurse.* Adding the NOT operator eliminates specific keywords or phrases from the search and should only be used by experienced searchers. When used incorrectly, the NOT operator can eliminate key pieces of information that contain the unwanted words (Adorno et al, 2016). Incorporating Boolean operators with subject headings, keywords, and phrases will shape the search strategy and result in the identification of more relevant information results.

Additional tools that can assist in shaping a search include **truncation** and **wildcards.** A truncation symbol, typically an asterisk (*) in bibliographic databases, can be applied to the end of the root of a keyword to retrieve all the words beginning with that root. Nurs* would identify articles that include the word "nurse," "nurses," "nursing," and so on. Wildcards, typically a question mark (?) in bibliographic databases, can be inserted within a word to retrieve all the words with alternate spellings. Randomi?ed would identify articles that include the word spelled "randomized" or "randomised."

As previously discussed in this chapter, bibliographic databases are designed to enable a search to be limited by many elements including scholarly (peer-reviewed) journals, publication type, publication date, and published language. Limits also can include age-groups, gender, inpatients, or outpatients. Though the same database might be accessed from a different publisher or vendor (EBSCO, ProQuest, and Ovid are common bibliographic database vendors), databases are structured so similarly that once Mark and his team identify their best search strategy within one database, they should apply a similar strategy to the other bibliographic databases and Internet sources. Multiple search attempts should be tried before the best search strategy is identified and multiple information resources should be searched before the evidence gathering is complete. In the meantime, do not give up—developing an accurate and appropriate search strategy can take some work.

Now Search

Clinical Practice Guidelines

Mark and his team start their search for information with a search of the synthesized evidence. If you are interested in knowing all aspects of care, often your first search should be for a comprehensive clinical practice guideline. Quality clinical practice guidelines are often built on systematic review findings. As with all sources of evidence, however, you need to be a good, critical consumer, as clinical practice guidelines vary a great deal in their rigor.

It is difficult to know whether a clinical practice guideline might have useful information embedded in it; therefore, always consider searching practice guideline sources first (Box 9■4). Mark's project covers a question in which evidence will not likely be available within a guideline. The team should then focus their search on systematic reviews and peer-reviewed journal articles.

Databases of Systematic Reviews

Systematic reviews, another form of synthesized evidence, might provide the ideal evidence needed for this assignment (Box 9■5).

BOX 9■4   Clinical Practice Guideline Database and Internet Sources

- Canadian Medical Association's (CMA) subsidiary Joule (https://joulecma. ca/cpg/homepage)
- National Guideline Centre (NGC) commissioned by National Institute for Health and Clinical Excellence (NICE) (https://www.rcplondon.ac.uk/projects/ nice-guidelines-developed-ngc)
- Registered Nurses' Association of Ontario (RNAO) (https://rnao.ca/bpg/ guidelines)
- TRIP Database (https://www.tripdatabase.com/)
- U.S. Preventive Services Task Force (USPSTF) (https://www. uspreventiveservicestaskforce.org/Page/Name/recommendations)
- Many professional organizations including the American Academy of Pediatrics and American Diabetes Association develop and publish evidence-based clinical practice guidelines. Search the Web site of relevant associations for guidelines or links to journal articles which might include the guideline text.
- Guidelines are often published as articles within journals, so bibliographic databases should be searched. CINAHL has a limiter titled "Publication Type" that enables you to limit results to "Practice Guidelines" and MEDLINE also has a "Publication Type" for "Practice Guideline."

BOX 9 ▪ 5 **Systematic Review Subscription Databases and Internet Resources**

- Centre for Reviews and Dissemination (CRD) (https://www.york.ac.uk/crd/)
- DynaMed (https://www.dynamed.com/home)
- Essential Evidence PLUS—Daily POEMS (Patient-Oriented Evidence That Matters) (https://www.essentialevidenceplus.com/content/poems)
- Cochrane Library (https://www.cochranelibrary.com/)
- JBI (https://joannabriggs.org/)
- PubMed Central's Clinical Queries (https://www.ncbi.nlm.nih.gov/pubmed/clinical)
- UpToDate (https://www.uptodate.com/home)

The Cochrane Library

The **Cochrane Library** is a collection of the following databases:

- The Cochrane Database of Systematic Reviews (CDSR)
- Cochrane Central Register of Controlled Trials (CENTRAL)
- Cochrane Clinical Answers (CCAs)

The Cochrane Library is viewed as one of the most comprehensive collections of systematic reviews, controlled trials, and evidence-based health-care sources (Box 9▪6). There is a cost to subscribe to the Cochrane Library, so Mark's team will need to check for availability at their library.

JBI EBP Database

The **JBI Evidence-based Practice (EBP) Database** contains peer-reviewed systematic reviews, evidence summaries, best practice information sheets, and evidence-based recommended practices. There is a cost to subscribe to the JBI EBP Database.

Additional Subscription Resources

Busy clinicians sometimes have access to additional synthesized resources not available within university libraries. Essential Evidence PLUS with its Daily POEMS (Patient-Oriented Evidence That Matters) database makes brief summaries of research available to clinicians at the bedside via mobile devices. UpToDate and DynaMed are other resources available to clinicians that synthesize evidence and provide answers to clinical questions and treatment recommendations at the bedside. Check with your university or hospital librarian to find out what synthesized resources are available to you.

Additional Resources Containing Systematic Reviews, Literature Reviews, and Primary Source Articles

Systematic reviews might also have been published within journals accessible through bibliographic databases, so the search for synthesized information is not over. Mark and his team move on to search other bibliographic databases for systematic reviews,

BOX 9■6 **Search Tips for the Cochrane Library**

Tip 1—As Mark and his team have already identified the appropriate MeSH subject heading of "hand disinfection," they can use this to target their search. Selecting Cochrane's Advanced Search will enable the team to search using the Medical Terms (MeSH) option. Limiting the search to only those pieces of information with the predetermined MeSH "hand disinfection" subject heading will lead to very targeted results.

   Tip 2—To make sure you've located the best available evidence, try another search with keywords and phrases. The Cochrane Library's Advanced Search option incorporates a useful Boolean operator structure, multiple search boxes with an AND operator in between, within the interface. Limiting results to those with the keywords and phrases only in the abstract or only in the title, abstract, or keywords can also be useful. A targeted search, as in the example below, incorporates a combination of keywords, phrases, and limiters. It is not necessary to use truncation symbols, the placement of * after the root of the word, in this database.

handwashing OR "hand washing" OR "hand disinfection" OR "hand sanitation" OR "hand cleaning" OR "hand hygiene"		in	Title, Abstract, or Keywords
AND	Intervent OR educat OR workshop OR seminar OR train	in	Title, Abstract, or Keywords
AND	nurse	in	Title, Abstract, or Keywords

   Tip 3—Search for evidence in a few different ways, with different keywords, phrases, and limiters before moving on to another resource.

BOX 9■7 **Additional Sources Containing Systematic Reviews, Literature Reviews, and Primary Source Articles**

■ CINAHL (https://www.ebscohost.com/nursing/products/cinahl-databases)
■ Embase (https://www.elsevier.com/solutions/embase-biomedical-research)
■ Google Scholar (https://scholar.google.com/)
■ MEDLINE (https://www.nlm.nih.gov/bsd/medline.html)
■ PubMed (https://www.ncbi.nlm.nih.gov/pubmed/)
■ PubMed Central (https://www.ncbi.nlm.nih.gov/pmc/)

literature reviews, and primary source articles (Box 9■7). Remember, many of the most commonly used bibliographic databases for evidence-based nursing practice require a subscription for access.

- **CINAHL,** the **Cumulative Index to Nursing and Allied Health Literature,** is available by subscription through most nursing school libraries. Subscriptions to CINAHL vary in coverage and cost. The most basic CINAHL subscription through EBSCO indexes over 5,300 English-language journals published since 1976 and provides the full-text of 70 journals. The most comprehensive CINAHL subscription through EBSCO, CINAHL Complete, indexes over 5,400 English-language journals published since 1937 and provides the full-text of over 1,300 journals (see Box 9■8 for search tips).
- **MEDLINE,** created by the United States National Library of Medicine, is also available by subscription through most nursing school libraries. MEDLINE subscriptions vary in coverage and cost. The most basic MEDLINE subscription through EBSCO contains over 25 million abstracts from 5,200 worldwide journals. The most comprehensive subscription, MEDLINE Complete, contains the full text of over 2,200 journals published since 1916.
- **Embase** contains over 32 million records from over 8,200 journals from over 95 countries published since 1947. Viewed as one of the most global sources of abstracts and full-text articles, Embase has limited availability in U.S. nursing school and hospital libraries.

Free Resources

In addition to subscription-based resources, there are some free Internet resources that contain peer-reviewed scholarly journal citations, abstracts, full-text articles, systematic reviews, and other quality health-care information. However, keep in mind that many free Internet resources do not provide access to the full text of articles. Rather, you will only be able to view or download abstracts or article citations. **PubMed** is a free Internet resource made available since 1996 by the U.S. National Institutes of Health (NIH) and managed by the National Center for Biotechnology Information (NCBI) at the National Library of Medicine. PubMed provides access to over 30 million citations and abstracts for biomedical literature and links to the full text of articles available on a publisher Web site or with PubMed Central. **PubMed Central**, a companion database to PubMed, is a free, full-text archive of over 5 million full-text records from participating journals, publisher Web sites, scholarly societies, and other Internet sites. PubMed Central has been available since 2000. You can also supplement your search of subscription-based bibliographic databases by using the Internet search engine **Google Scholar.** Google Scholar search results include information freely available from the Internet, so the results only include abstracts of articles found within subscription-based bibliographic databases. You must use caution and understand that results will not be comprehensive and often do not freely link to the full text of journal articles. Again, check with your university or hospital librarian to find out what Internet resources he or she recommends for your research.

BOX 9■8 **Search Tips for CINAHL**

Tip 1—As do the Cochrane Library, JBI EBP Database, and other database interfaces, CINAHL's interface offers Basic Search and Advanced Search options. CINAHL's Advanced Search option incorporates a useful Boolean operator structure, multiple search boxes with an AND operator in between, within the interface. Using the Advanced Search interface, searches can be limited to scholarly (peer-reviewed) journals, the journal subset of nursing journals, or the publication type of practice guidelines or systematic reviews. Searches can also be limited by publication date, language, and many other useful elements.

Tip 2—CINAHL offers the ability to search using CINAHL subject headings, a subject heading system very similar to MeSH subject headings. When using the EBSCO host interface, place a checkmark in the "Suggest Search Terms" box and place the phrase "hand hygiene" in the search box. CINAHL will direct you to use the CINAHL subject heading of "handwashing" instead of the MeSH heading of "hand disinfection." The CINAHL search can be expanded to include results for the "handwashing" subject heading as well as its first layer of narrower terms. Narrowing to "Major Concept" will return only those results in which the "handwashing" subject heading is the major topic. No matter which vendor provides your access to CINAHL, practice using CINAHL subject headings to target your search.

Tip 3—Try using the Advanced Search option to combine CINAHL subject headings with keywords and phrases. Also try limiting results to those with the keywords and phrases only in the abstract instead of throughout all text. A targeted search, such as the example below, incorporates a combination of subject headings, keywords, phrases, truncation symbols, and limiters.

Handwashing (make sure to have selected handwashing as the Major Concept)		in	No need to add a limiter
AND	Intervent* or educ* or workshop* or seminar* or train*	in	Abstract
AND	nurs*	in	TX All Text

Tip 4—Do you notice how similar the search example above looks to the search example for the Cochrane Library? Once you figure out a search string that returns relevant results, use a similar structure to search other resources.

Tip 5—Search for the information needed in a few different ways, with different keywords, phrases, and limiters before moving on to another resource.

Mark's team can also search for free full-text systematic reviews via **PubMed Central's Clinical Queries** interface. In addition, internationally developed systematic reviews can be found at the highly respected **Centre for Reviews and Dissemination (CRD),** made available from the National Institute for Health Research (NIHR) and the University of York. Keep in mind that not every review is available in full text on the Internet, so work with your librarian to access the full text from another source.

Tracking Search Results

While Mark and his team search bibliographic databases and the Internet, they should also keep track of the search terms they used and the corresponding results. Keeping track of the most useful search string developed and the limits applied within each database will ensure that the same effective search can be reproduced in another database. Tracking the number of relevant articles located from a specific database, an Internet source, or a specific journal will make it easier to revisit the most useful resources again, if needed.

If you find many relevant articles have been published within a specific journal, it is a good idea to **hand search** that journal. Since not all search strategies or bibliographic databases are perfect, hand searching is the process of looking through the table of contents of multiple issues, and at times multiple years of issues, of a specific journal to make sure that your database search has not missed other relevant articles. Hand searching can be done by physically flipping through the print copies of a journal and reading the table of contents or by accessing the Web site of the journal publisher and skimming the table of contents of the issues listed. Journals often publish special issues in which multiple articles related to a topic are included. Hand searching lowers the chance of overlooking relevant articles in that key issue or key journal.

Library Services

As Bird (2003) states, "Unfortunately, there is no single super discovery tool that will, by itself, search all the relevant literature for health care" (p. 58). A comprehensive search requires searching multiple sources of information to locate the best available evidence. If you find an abstract or citation mentioned on the Internet or within the references list or bibliography of a journal article, check to see if your library subscribes to the full text of the journal within a bibliographic database or in print. Believe it or not, there are still some peer-reviewed nursing and health-care journals available only in print. If your library does not have the journal in electronic or print form, ask if a copy of the article is available through **interlibrary loan.** Interlibrary loan is a system where university libraries, public libraries, and hospital libraries share the full text of articles, books, and other sources of information with one another. Most university libraries will acquire the full text of articles for students for free or a nominal fee. Hospital libraries vary in their ability to provide interlibrary loan services to their clinicians, staff, and patients, so check with your hospital librarian to see what is available to you.

Diagnosing the Quality

Developing a successful search strategy and retrieving the full-text information is just part of the evidence-based practice process. The next step is the **critical appraisal** of the evidence once it's found. That means you need to judge if the information is relevant, and valid, and if the findings will help you answer your question. McKibbon and Marks (1998) point out, "Despite the peer review process, not all research studies published in journals are methodologically sound, and some may be more sound than others" (p. 69). As you get more comfortable with creating a search and more knowledgeable about the best resources for locating evidence related to nursing practice, you will become more efficient in your knowledge-gathering skills. Nonetheless, as you will find in Chapter 11, it is your job to always be a critical consumer of the information gathered.

Student–Librarian Partnerships

Many researchers would agree that after you have identified your research topic or developed your PICO question, your next step should be to contact your librarian (Boss & Williams 2014; Gerberi & Marienau 2017; Timmins & McCabe 2005). In this chapter's clinical story, Mark is wise to suggest a meeting with the school's nursing librarian. Librarians and information scientists are trained to assist with identifying relevant keywords, phrases, and subject headings. They are educated in the organizational structure of bibliographic databases and the Internet and are knowledgeable in using Boolean operators, truncation, and wildcards to locate relevant electronic information. They are also trained to identify relevant electronic and print resources and have the ability to acquire needed resources from others. Partnering with a librarian will result in a more effective search and more efficient information retrieval.

Visit your university or hospital library's Web site to find out the best way to contact your librarian. Many librarians prefer that students, especially a team of students like Mark's, make an appointment to meet. This ensures that the librarian and the group are available and prepared for the meeting. At the initial meeting with your librarian, be prepared to discuss your project and the types of evidence resources that you need to ideally address the problem. Bring your PICO or PICo question and an initial list of synonyms and keywords that you know might relate to the question's key components. In most cases, do not expect your librarian to do the searching for you; he or she will help fine-tune your search strategy and introduce you to the resources that will enable you to locate the best available evidence (Box 9■9).

■ Summary

The best available evidence can be found in many forms. There will be times when a synthesized form of information, including a systematic review, a clinical practice

BOX 9■9 **Tools for Learning and Practice**

■ Locate your hospital or university library's list of available information resources. Look for sources of synthesized information as well as primary sources of information. Spend about 10 minutes in each resource, becoming familiar with the interface and doing a quick search to see what kinds of information can be retrieved.

■ Use Google to search the Internet for "clinical practice guidelines" and "systematic reviews." Explore the sites. Pay particular attention to the original author and the professional organization, publisher, or overall source of the information. Take note of the domain from which the information is available, for example, .edu, .gov, .com, .org.

■ Search the Internet for PubMed Central Clinical Queries and bookmark the site for later use.

■ Search the Internet for the U.S. National Library of Medicine for Medical Subject Headings (MeSH). Use the MeSH Browser to search the controlled vocabulary for a term used to describe a research interest of yours. Bookmark the page for later use.

■ Find out the name of the hospital or university librarian who can work with you to locate information. Contact him or her to set up a time to talk or meet face-to-face.

guideline, a Best Practice Information Sheet, or a summary of the evidence, will be the best evidence. Other times, a handful of individual journal articles, or just one journal article, will be the best available evidence. Evidence can be found within bibliographic databases, Internet resources, journals, magazines, and books. Evidence can also be found by having conversations with experts within the field. Through practice you will learn how to wade through the wealth of information that exists, and ultimately identify and access the best available evidence for your question. In the meantime, contact your hospital or university librarian for help along the way.

CHAPTER QUESTIONS

1. Why is it important to be able to identify the best available evidence? Describe how you use evidence to make clinical decisions.

2. Name at least two types of synthesized evidence.

3. Define what a systematic review is. Explain the difference between a meta-synthesis and a meta-analysis.

4. Explain how a systematic review is different from a literature review.

(continues on page 134)

CHAPTER QUESTIONS (continued)

5. What is a primary source of evidence?

6. Generate keywords, phrases, and MeSH subject headings to use for researching evidence for the following:

   a. The effect complementary medicines have on the treatment of chronic pain

   b. What diet and exercise interventions work best for adults with type 2 diabetes

   c. Effective treatments for pressure ulcer prevention in hospitalized older adults

7. What is the definition, also known as scope note, for the MeSH subject heading of "Health Literacy"?

8. What are the three common Boolean operators used to structure a search?

9. How would you use a truncation symbol, the asterisk, with the keyword "nurse" to ensure that the information in your search results would contain the keywords "nurse," "nurses," and "nursing"?

10. How would you use the question mark (?) wildcard to find information containing the phrases "complimentary medicine" and "complementary medicine"?

11. List the bibliographic databases, Internet resources, and print resources available through your hospital or university library that contain the best available evidence for the questions listed in question 6.

12. Identify the names of the librarians and information scientists within your university or hospital library who can work with you to find the information you need. How can they help you find the evidence needed to answer your question?

References

Adorno, M., Garbee, D., & Marix, M. L. (2016). Improving literature searches. *Clinical Nurse Specialist, 30*(2), 74–80.

Bird, D. (2003). Discovering the literature of nursing: A guide for beginners. *Nurse Researcher, 11*(1), 56–70.

Boss, C. M., & Williams, B. (2014). Conducting a literature review. In C. Hedges & B. Williams (Eds.), *Anatomy of research for nurses* (pp. 97–109). Indianapolis, IN: Sigma Theta Tau International.

Cook, D. J., Mulrow, C. D., & Haynes, R. B. (1997). Systematic reviews: Synthesis of best evidence for clinical decisions. *Annals of Internal Medicine, 126*, 376–380.

Gerberi, D., & Marienau, M. S. (2017). Literature searching for practice research. *AANA Journal, 85*(3), 195.

Hartzell, T. A., Fineout-Overholt, E., Hofstetter, S., et al. (2015). Finding relevant evidence to answer clinical questions. In B. M. Melnyk & E. Fineout-Overholt (Eds.). *Evidence-based practice in nursing & healthcare: A guide to best practice* (pp. 40–70). Philadelphia, PA: Wolters Kluwer Health.

McKibbon, K. A., & Marks, S. (1998). Searching for the best evidence. Part 1: Where to look. *Evidence-Based Nursing, 1,* 68–70.

National Center for Biotechnology Information (2020). MeSH: Hand disinfection. Retrieved from https://www.ncbi.nlm.nih.gov/mesh/?term=hand+disinfection

Pearson, A., Wiechula, R., Court, A., et al. (2005). The JBI model of evidence-based healthcare. *International Journal of Evidence-Based Healthcare, 3,* 207–215.

Taylor, T. (2007). *100% information literacy success.* Clifton Park, NY: Thomson Delmar Learning.

Timmins, F., & McCabe, C. (2005). How to conduct an effective literature search. *Nursing Standard, 20*(11), 41–47.

CHAPTER 10

Appraise and Plan I

All Evidence Is Not Created Equal

Leslie Rittenmeyer

- Explain the purpose of critical appraisal of evidence.
- Explain the skill sets needed to carry out critical appraisal activities.
- Discuss the critical appraisal of qualitative evidence.
- Discuss the critical appraisal of quantitative evidence.

Animal-assisted therapy (AAT)
Bias
Credibility
Critical appraisal
Critical Appraisal Skills Program (CASP)

Dependability
Rapid critical appraisal
Skill set
Transferability

C *linical Story*

Kristin is in her last semester of a baccalaureate nursing program. She is planning a required clinical preceptorship. Nicole, a team leader on the inpatient psychiatric unit of the local community hospital, has agreed to be her preceptor. Nicole and Kristin have discussed their observation that many patients on the psychiatric unit seem to experience high levels of anxiety, regardless of their diagnosis. Kristin remembers reading about the use of animal-assisted therapy (AAT) to reduce anxiety in patients with Alzheimer's disease, and wonders whether this treatment might be as effective in other contexts. She shares her thoughts with Nicole, and, after discussing it with their evidence-based practice faculty mentor, they begin to search for the evidence. Taking a pluralistic approach, they focus their search on two PICO questions: "How effective is AAT as compared to other group therapies in reducing anxiety in persons with a mental health diagnosis?" and "How is animal-assisted therapy experienced by patients and practitioners in the area of mental health"?

After completion of their search, they found two systematic reviews, an array of effectiveness studies, and one qualitative study. They know the next step in the process, after question development and searching for evidence, is the critical appraisal process.

Think Before You Read

- What is the difference between being critical and using critical appraisal skills?
- What do you need to think about in order to determine whether you can trust a source of evidence?
- Can you ask the same questions to determine the trustworthiness of a source of evidence, no matter the type of evidence? Why or why not?
- What happens to the evidence-based practice process if you skip the appraisal step? Does it make a difference?
- What challenges do you anticipate in using critical appraisal in your everyday nursing practice?

Introduction

In the evidence-based practice environment, it is expected that clinicians possess basic knowledge of research methods and the skills to critically appraise sources of evidence to determine their usefulness for practice. Knowledge of evidence-based practice is now considered a baccalaureate degree competency by the American Association of Colleges of Nursing (AACN), and most schools integrate these concepts and skills into their curricula. This speaks well for the future generation of nurses who will be well versed in the processes of evidence-based practice.

When you want to access information about a particular clinical problem, you would most likely start with a literature search, just as Kristin and Nicole did in this chapter's clinical story. Following that, you would probably identify reports that you believe would be helpful in answering your questions. However, once you have them, what do you do with them? Do you read them and just assume that the conclusions are accurate, or do you introduce some healthy skepticism into the process? A healthy skeptic would ask the following questions:

- How do I judge the quality of the research?
- How much confidence can I have that the evidence is of high enough quality to merit suggesting practice change?
- When should I be seeking further evidence?
- What criteria should I use to make these judgments?

These are all appropriate questions, and each can be answered by applying the step of **critical appraisal** to the evidence-based practice process. Critical appraisal is a process in which evidence is systematically evaluated to judge its quality and trustworthiness in informing practice change.

Whether you are a student or a practicing clinician, you need to develop critical appraisal skills. Studies are often subject to **bias.** For example, bias can come from distortions in the research process, the ways in which data are collected, number of participants, or how data are analyzed. This is true in both quantitative work and qualitative work, and there is a danger of bias when the study is conducted in a way that might lead to a particular conclusion. Good researchers attempt to minimize bias by applying certain research methods. Unfortunately, some research work is conducted with more rigor than are others, and you will have to decide whether the studies you are appraising are trustworthy and reliable enough to inform your practice.

The focus of this chapter is to help you become a skeptic by providing you the skills to make a competent critical appraisal. Be aware that there are many tools to guide critical appraisal. Katrak, Bralocerkowski, Jassy-Westropp et al (2004) conducted a systematic review of critical appraisal tools, and found at that time that there were 121 published instruments to conduct reviews. For the purpose of illustration, the focus of this chapter is on two groups of tools: (1) the JBI critical appraisal checklists (the tools designed to align with specific study types that users can use to perform appraisals); and (2) the Critical Appraisal Skills Program (CASP). Both groups of tools are explained in more depth later in the chapter. These two appraisal systems have been selected because of their reliability and validity, and they are user friendly and readily available for students and clinicians alike.

How to Begin

There are some **skill sets** that you must develop to implement a systematic critical appraisal. A skill set comprises techniques you need to carry out a task. In the case of critical appraisal, a basic understanding of research language, methodologies, and methods is needed. In addition, an understanding of basic statistics is helpful in the evaluation process. Different research paradigms call for different skill sets. For example, criteria for appraising research carried out in qualitative methodologies are different from the criteria for appraising research conducted in quantitative methodologies. This is further complicated by the fact that there are differences in criteria for appraising research from different types of quantitative studies, for example, randomized controlled trials (RCTs), case control studies, cohort studies, diagnostic test studies, prognostic studies, and economic studies. There are also tools to appraise the quality of systematic reviews and clinical guidelines. It is most important that the appraisal criteria in the tool match the research design.

For you to assess your own skill set for doing critical appraisal, Tables 10■1 and 10■2 provide a short description of the most common quantitative and qualitative study designs, and Box 10■1 provides a list of common statistical concepts that you should know. The content from your baccalaureate research course should be adequate to allow you to do a basic critical appraisal. It is very important that you maintain your basic research skills so that you can gather and appraise information that informs your clinical decisions. To inform your clinical decisions with the best available evidence, you need to be able to judge the quality of that evidence for application to your practice.

Critical Appraisal Tools

Feeling confident in their basic research and statistical knowledge base, Kristen and Nicole are ready to explore the tools they will use to conduct their critical appraisal. With the help of their evidence-based practice mentor, the students are able to identify the skill set they need. As was stated earlier, it is important that you use an appraisal tool that asks the right questions for the particular research methodology. It is also important to keep in mind that no matter which tool is used, the purpose of critical appraisal is threefold:

1. To assess whether the study is valid or of high enough quality to consider using to inform practice change
2. To determine whether the results fit into a local context (your own)
3. To judge whether the results will help your patients

JBI Appraisal Checklists and CASP Critical Appraisal Tools

Melnyk and Fineout-Overholt (2005) discuss a method they refer to as **rapid critical appraisal.** They contend that clinicians should be able to quickly appraise evidence to determine its validity and applicability to practice, and critical appraisal approaches should be user friendly so that busy clinicians can swiftly appraise a piece of research. The JBI supports this stance and developed critical appraisal checklists with about 10 questions to assess a particular type of evidence. These checklists can help students and clinicians develop skills in critical appraisal, allowing them

TABLE 10■1 **Selective Quantitative Study Designs**

Quantitative Study Designs	Description
Systematic review	The application of strategies that limit bias in the assembly, critical appraisal, and synthesis of all relevant studies on a particular topic
Meta-analysis (quantitative)	Use of statistical methods to pool the results of independent studies
Meta-aggregation	Qualitative analysis of a group of individual studies in which the findings of the studies are pooled
Randomized controlled trial	A true experimental design in which there is randomization, control, and manipulation
Cohort study	A form of longitudinal study that is used to examine associations of exposure to disease; can be retrospective or prospective (observational study design)
Case control study	A study design that uses patients who already have the disease and looks back and analyzes if there are characteristics of these patients that differ from those who do not have the disease (observational studies)
Case series / case report	A case series or report (also known as a clinical series) is a research design that tracks patients with a known exposure, given similar treatment, or examines their medical records for exposure and outcome; can be retrospective or prospective (observational studies)
Cross-sectional study	A cross-sectional study involves data collected at a defined time, providing a snapshot of a disease in the population (observational studies)
Diagnostic study	A study design that evaluates the accuracy of a diagnostic test
Prognostic study	A study that measures the possible outcomes of a disease and the frequency in which they occur

to quickly exclude papers that are of inadequate quality to inform practice so they can focus on the salient factors of high-quality research. The JBI checklists provide appraisal criteria for a variety of study designs. These are easily accessible for free on the JBI Web site (search for the JBI and look for EBP resources). Although providing an example of the complete array of appraisal tools for all research designs is beyond the scope of the chapter, Box 10■2 lists JBI's available tools. Later in the chapter, Kristin and Nicole will use the appropriate appraisal tool for their study on the Effects of Animal-Assisted Therapy on Anxiety Ratings of Hospitalized Psychiatric Patients (Barker & Dawson, 1998).

TABLE 10■2 **Selected Qualitative Study Designs**

Selected Qualitative Study Designs	Description
Phenomenology/ hermeneutics	A study design that aims to describe the meaning of a phenomena for persons (either through participant voice or text)
Grounded theory	An inductive study design that uses systematic procedures to arrive at a theory (either through participant voice or text)
Participatory action research	A study design in which researchers and the study participants enter into an equal partnership to study a problem and then plan action based on the research findings, resulting in a difference in the lives of the participants
Ethnography	A research method whose major aim is to study persons in their cultural context
Focus group	A research method that asks groups of persons about their opinions, attitudes, and beliefs about a particular topic

BOX 10■1 **Statistics to Review**

- Mean (X)
- Standard deviation (SD)
- Odds ratio (OR)
- Risk
- Relative risk (RR)
- Confidence interval (CI)
- Numbers needed to treat (NNT)
- Mean difference (MD)
- Weighted mean difference (WMD)
- Standardized mean difference (SMD)

The **Critical Appraisal Skills Program (CASP)** from the United Kingdom provides a set of tools appropriate for critical appraisal of both quantitative and qualitative methodologies. These tools are part of the Oxford Centre for Triple Value Healthcare LTD portfolio. The aim of CASP is to enable both students and clinicians to develop the skills to find and make sense of research evidence, helping them to put knowledge into practice. The CASP tools can be easily downloaded from the CASP Web site (https://casp-uk.net/casp-tools-checklists/), and Box 10■3 lists the available CASP tools. A little later, Kristin and Nicole will use the CASP Tool to appraise their qualitative study.

BOX 10■2 **JBI Critical Appraisal Tools**

Analytical Cross-Sectional Studies
Case Control Studies
Case Reports
Case Series
Cohort Studies
Diagnostic Test Accuracy Studies
Economic Evaluations
Prevalence Studies
Qualitative Research
Quasi Experimental Studies
Randomized Controlled Trials
Systematic Reviews
Text and Opinion

Retrieved from https://joannabriggs.org/critical-appraisal-tools

BOX 10■3 **Public Health Resource Center CASP Critical Appraisal Tools**

■ Systematic Reviews
■ Randomized Controlled Trials
■ Qualitative
■ Cohort Study
■ Case Control
■ Diagnostic
■ Economic Evaluation
■ Clinical Prediction Rule

Retrieved from https://casp-uk.net/casp-tools-checklists/

Appraisal of Quantitative Research

When designing a study, researchers make well-thought-out decisions about what methods they will employ to decrease the possibility of bias. Box 10■4 reviews the key items a researcher may consider when designing a study. When the design of the study is well thought out, there is less chance that the study will be flawed in some way, therefore making the results suspect.

The first step in the critical appraisal of quantitative studies is to identify what research design was used so you can choose the correct appraisal tool. (See Table 10■1 for a description of various research designs.) Once you have chosen the appropriate tool, you can then proceed to evaluate the study or systematic review. If you are working with another person, both of you should appraise the study

> BOX 10■4 **Planning a Good Research Study**
>
> ■ Possible threats to external and internal validity
> ■ The sources of possible bias
> ■ The best design to measure the research question
> ■ The sampling strategy to be employed
> ■ Possible legal/ethical concerns
> ■ Appropriate data collection methods
> ■ Methods needed to test reliability and validity of instruments
> ■ Correct statistical methods for data analysis

independently. This creates a system of checks and balances, making the process transparent and open. Kristin and Nicole are ready to appraise their study on the effects of **animal-assisted therapy (AAT)** on anxiety ratings of hospitalized psychiatric patients. Remember that no matter what appraisal tool you use, it must match the research design of the study. Table 10■3 demonstrates the appraisal criteria and how Kristen and Nicole apply the appraisal process to a systematic review and Table 10■4 illustrates critical appraisal of an observational study.

Appraisal of Qualitative Research

Qualitative evidence plays an important role in informing clinical decision making. It is also valuable in informing health services policy and planning. The data from qualitative work show how individuals and groups perceive health and health-related phenomena. Qualitative methodologies provide insights into topics that are difficult to measure quantitatively. Whereas quantitative paradigms attempt to control and predict, qualitative paradigms attempt to illuminate meaning and promote understanding.

Just as appraising quantitative evidence for quality, it is equally important to be able to judge the quality of qualitative evidence. Traditionally, the concepts of reliability, internal validity, and external validity are used to judge the quality of quantitative evidence. Lincoln and Gruba (1985) suggest that the words *dependability, credibility,* and *transferability* are more suited to qualitative paradigms. Whereas the quantitative word *reliability* speaks to achieving the same results time and time again, in the qualitative world, **dependability** speaks to whether the results are logical, transparent, clearly documented, and of consistent similarity in the quality of results achieved. **Credibility** refers to proof that the researcher made every effort to report an honest representation of the true voices of the participants. Finally, **transferability** refers to the degree to which the results of the study can be applied to other contexts or situations.

After updating their skill set to appraise qualitative research, Kristin and Nicole are ready to appraise their qualitative research article. They use the CASP criteria for qualitative research (Critical Appraisal Skills Programme, 2018). Table 10■5 illustrates how Kristin and Nicole apply the CASP criteria to their qualitative study.

TABLE 10■3 **Example of JBI Critical Appraisal of a Systematic Review**

Is the review question clearly and explicitly stated?	The review question is an essential step in the systematic review process. A well-articulated question defines the scope of the review and aids in the development of the search strategy to locate the relevant evidence.	**The review question was clearly articulated in the review. The objective of the review was to summarize the evidence from randomized clinical trials (RCTs) on ATT.**
Were the inclusion criteria appropriate for the review question?	The inclusion criteria should be identifiable from objectives, and match the review question(s).The necessary elements of the PICO should be explicit and clearly defined.	**Studies were included if they were RCTs on the effects of AAT and the study included at least one treatment group in which AAT was applied.**
Was the search strategy appropriate?	A systematic review should provide evidence of the search strategy that was used to locate the evidence.	**Evidence of a comprehensive search strategy was articulated in the report and was comprehensive, including all international databases. Hand searching and reference checking were also done.**
Were the sources and resources used to search for studies adequate?	A systematic review should attempt to identify "all" the available evidence and, as such, there should be evidence of a comprehensive search strategy.	**There was a clear attempt to identify all of the available evidence. The search strategy was well documented in the report.**
Were the criteria for appraising studies appropriate?	The systematic review should present a clear statement that critical appraisal was conducted and provide the details of the items that were used to assess the included studies.	**Three review authors independently assessed the quality of the articles using Cochrane's criteria list for methodological quality.**

TABLE 10■3 **Example of JBI Critical Appraisal of a Systematic Review** (continued)

Was critical appraisal conducted by two or more reviewers independently?	A key characteristic to minimize bias or systematic error in the conduct of a systematic review is to have the critical appraisal of the included studies completed independently and in duplicate by members of the review team.	**Yes; three independent reviewers from the research team.**
Were there methods to minimize errors in data extraction?	Strategies to minimize bias may include conducting all data extraction in duplicate and independently, using specific tools or instruments to guide data extraction and some evidence of piloting or training around their use.	**Ten review authors described the summary from each article based on the recommended structured abstracts.**
Were the methods to combine studies appropriate?	A synthesis of the evidence is a key feature of a systematic review. The synthesis that is presented should be appropriate for the review question and the stated type of systematic review and evidence it refers to.	**Although the goal was to perform meta-analysis when possible, a meta-analysis could not be performed because of heterogeneity by difference of outcome measurement. The evidence was summarized.**
Was the likelihood of publication bias assessed?	A comprehensive search strategy is the best means by which a review author may alleviate the impact of publication bias on the results of the review.	**Publication bias was a factor. Although there was no linguistic restriction in the eligibility criteria, the authors searched studies with only English and Japanese key words. The review reported on a relatively small and heterogeneous sample of studies.**

(continues on page 146)

TABLE 10■3   Example of JBI Critical Appraisal of a Systematic Review (continued)

Were recommendations for policy and/or practice supported by the reported data?	Ideally, a review should present recommendations for policy and practice. Where these recommendations are made, there should be a clear link to the results of the review.	The researchers state that although further accumulation of RCT data is necessary, AAT may be effective treatment for the following diseases and symptoms: cancer and/or advanced life-limiting illnesses that affect mental status, impaired circulatory function with mechanical assistance, autistic spectrum disorders involving communication skills.
Were the specific directives for new research appropriate?	The systematic review process is recognized for its ability to identify where gaps in the research, or knowledge base, around a particular topic exist.	The researchers set a future research agenda for studies of cure effects by ATT. They felt that the quality of the studies was poor in many cases.

From Critical Appraisal Tools I Joanna Briggs Institute https://joannabriggs.org/critical-appraisal-tools

Kamioka, H., Okada, S., Tsutani, K., et al. (2014). Effectiveness of animal-assisted therapy: A systematic review of randomized controlled trials. *Complementary Therapies in Medicine, 22*(2), 371–390. https://doi.org/10.1016/j.ctim.2013.12.0

TABLE 10■4   Example of a JBI Appraisal Checklist of an Analytical Cross-Sectional Study/Observational Study

Were the criteria for inclusion in the sample clearly defined?	Clear inclusion and exclusion criteria that were developed prior to recruitment. The inclusion criteria and exclusion criteria should be specified.	The inclusion criteria were stated. There were 230 patients referred to recreational therapy and able to complete the State-Trait Anxiety Inventory.
Were the study subjects and the setting described in detail?	The study sample should be described in sufficient detail so other researchers can determine whether it is comparable to the population of interest to them.	The study included patients hospitalized with a psychiatric diagnosis. The diagnosis was specified. There were few data other than that.

TABLE 10■4 **Example of a JBI Appraisal Checklist of an Analytical Cross-Sectional Study/Observational Study** (continued)

Was the exposure measured in a valid and reliable way?	The study should clearly describe the method of measurement of exposure. The validity of exposure measurement relates to whether a current measure is appropriate.	Instruments were scored twice for accuracy by one of the authors using the scoring keys for the State-Trait Anxiety Inventory. A mixed-models, repeated measure analysis was used to compare pre- and posttreatment differences in anxiety scores between and within the AAT condition and the therapeutic recreation therapy condition by diagnostic category.
Were objective, standard criteria used for measurement of the condition?	It is useful to determine whether patients were included in the study based on either a specific diagnosis or definition. This is more likely to decrease the risk of bias. The group may also be matched by key characteristics	All participants were hospitalized with a psychiatric diagnosis.
Were confounding factors identified?	A high-quality study will identify the potential confounding factors and measure them when possible. This can be difficult where behavioral, attitudinal, or lifestyle factors may impact the result.	The authors did not speak specifically to confounding factors. They did speak to allergy to dogs, fear of dogs, and dislike of dogs as a factor.
Were strategies to deal with confounding factors stated?	Strategies to deal with effects of confounding factors may be dealt with in the study design or in data analysis.	Participants were excluded from the study if they had any of the above.
Were the outcomes measured in a valid and reliable way?	A recognized, validated tool was used for measuring the outcomes. For example, when measuring a patient's level of consciousness, the Glasgow Coma Scale is a widely recognized tool.	The study utilized the state scale of the State-Trait Anxiety Inventory to measure patients' level of anxiety before and after AAT and recreational therapy. The internal consistency for the state scale of the State-Trait Anxiety Inventory is high: median alpha coefficient is 0.93. Construct validity is supported by studies showing that the state scale scores are higher under stressful conditions.

(continues on page 148)

TABLE 10■4 **Example of a JBI Appraisal Checklist of an Analytical Cross-Sectional Study/Observational Study** (continued)

Was appropriate statistical analysis used?	There are several statistical analyses available; the one(s) chosen were appropriate to the data being presented.	F test and P values were used to show significance of change over time.
Was the dropout rate significant?	Generally, a dropout rate of 15% or less is considered insignificant. A rate of 20% or greater is considered to significantly impact the validity of the study.	Although the N for this study was 230, only 50 participants completed a pre- and posttreatment measure for both types of sessions. Failure to complete all four measures was primarily due to time conflicts with medical treatments and patient discharges. A power analysis of the magnitude of differences between the change scores for AAT and therapeutic recreational therapy indicated that larger samples would be needed to achieve an 80% power level at an alpha of 0.05: of 300 patients with psychotic disorder, 125 patients with substance disorders, and 61 patients with other disorders. The fact that only 50 participants completed all four tools out of 230 is a major limitation of the study. Their findings are in line with this limitation, suggesting only promise for the intervention and the need for more research.
Was the rate of patient follow-up adequate?	At least 80% of patients were followed up.	There was no statement that patients were followed up after completion of the study.

From Critical Appraisal Tools I Joanna Briggs Institute https://joannabriggs.org/critical-appraisal-tools

Barker, S., & Dawson, K. (1998). The effects of animal-assisted therapy on anxiety rating of hospitalized psychiatric patients. *Psychiatric Services, 49*(6), 797–801.

TABLE 10■5 **Example of a Qualitative Study Utilizing CASP Criteria**

Was there a clear statement of the aims of the research?	Consider: ■ The goal of the research ■ Why it is important ■ Its relevance	The aim of the study was articulated: to explore how animal-assisted therapies and interventions create a positive effect on a person's mental health and well-being during psychotherapy.
Is the qualitative methodology appropriate?	Consider: ■ If the research seeks to interpret or illuminate the actions and/or subjective experience of research participants	This study used an existential conceptual framework in conjunction with the biophilia hypothesis. Thematic analysis was employed. The methodology was appropriate to the research question.
Is it worth continuing?	Two over-reaching questions to decide whether the research is worthy of appraisal	YES
Was the research design appropriate to address the aims of the research?	Consider: ■ If the researcher has justified the research design (e.g., have they discussed how they decided what methods to use?)	The research design was appropriate to address the aim of the study. The researcher justified the research design and explained why the design was chosen.
Was the recruitment strategy appropriate to the aims of the research?	Consider: ■ If the researcher has explained how the participants were selected ■ If they explained why the participants whom they selected were the most appropriate to provide access to the type of knowledge sought in the study ■ If there was discussion around recruitment (e.g., why some people chose not to take part)	The researcher used a purposive sample that is appropriate for this type of research. Participants were chosen because they had knowledge of the phenomena and had provided a therapeutic service using animals.

(continues on page 150)

TABLE 10■5   **Example of a Qualitative Study Utilizing CASP Criteria** (continued)

Were the data collected in a way that addressed the research issues?		In-depth, one-to-one interviews were used in order to produce detailed qualitative data. The interviews were semi-structured. Interviews were reported with participant consent.
Has the relationship between researcher and participants been adequately considered?	Consider whether clear: ■ If researchers critically examined their own role, potential bias, and influence during: 　■ formulation of research questions 　■ data collection, including sample, recruitment, choice of location 　■ How the researchers responded to events during the study and whether they considered the implications of any changes in the research design	The researcher admits to having a particular personal interest and outlook on working with animals. The author described this as possible research bias.
Have ethical issues been taken into consideration?	Consider: ■ If there are sufficient details of how the research was explained to participants for the reader to access whether ethical standards were maintained ■ If the researcher has discussed issues raised by the study (e.g., issues around informed consent or confidentiality or how they have handled the effects of the study on the participants during and after the study) ■ If approval has been sought from the ethics committee	Ethical standards were discussed. There was a clear explanation of informed consent and how confidentiality would be maintained. Ethical approval was obtained through the British Psychological Society.

TABLE 10■5 **Example of a Qualitative Study Utilizing CASP Criteria** (continued)

Was the data analysis sufficiently rigorous?	Consider: ■ If there is an in-depth description of the analysis process ■ If thematic analysis is used. If so, is it clear how the categories/themes were derived from the data? ■ Whether the researcher explains how the data presented were selected from the original sample to demonstrate the analysis process ■ If sufficient data are presented to support findings ■ To what extent contradictory data are taken into account ■ Whether the researchers critically examined their own role, potential bias, and influence during analysis and selection of data presentation	There was an in-depth discussion of the data analysis procedure. The data analysis method was appropriate for the research design. Data analysis was done using thematic analysis. It was clear how the themes were derived.
Is there a clear statement of findings?	Consider: ■ If the findings are explicit ■ If there is adequate discussion of the evidence both for and against the researchers' arguments ■ If the researchers have discussed the credibility of their findings (e.g., triangulation, respondent validation, more than one analyst) ■ If the findings are discussed in relation to the original research question	The findings were explicit and flowed from the themes and were supported by participant narrative. The findings were discussed in relation to the original research question.

(continues on page 152)

TABLE 10■5   **Example of a Qualitative Study Utilizing CASP Criteria** (continued)

How valuable is the research?	Consider:	
	■ If the researcher discusses the contribution the study makes to existing knowledge or understanding (e.g., do they consider the findings in relation to current practice or policy or relevant research-based literature?) ■ If they identify new areas in which research is necessary ■ If the researchers have discussed whether or how the findings can be transferred to other populations ■ If the researchers considered other ways the research may be used	Although this study had a limitation of a small sample size, it provided a roadmap for further research on a more global scale, where the results would produce more consensus on the effectiveness of animal-assisted therapy. The author suggests that animal-assisted therapies ought to be utilized more often and can be embedded into other therapeutic techniques such as cognitive behavioral therapy.

From CASP (2018). ©CASP, Creative Commons. *CASP checklists.* https://casp-uk.net/casp-tools-checklists/

Wood, S. (2016). Anyone's best friend: A qualitative exploration of the positive influences of animal assisted therapy on mental health and well-being (Unpublished undergraduate project). Manchester Metropolitan University. Manchester, United Kingdom. Retrieved https://e-space.mmu.ac.uk/id/eprint/617866

Making a Decision

Once you have appraised your evidence, how do you decide whether the study is of high enough quality to trust? Research is conducted in the real world and is therefore not always perfect. For a variety of reasons, research designs must adapt to certain problems in the process, and small compromises in quality are sometimes made. The question that drives the decision to use a study is whether the study is good enough or trustworthy enough to use in clinical decision making. This returns to the notion of best available evidence. A study that does not meet any or meets only a few of the critical appraisal criteria would obviously be rejected, but if there are weaknesses found in some of the criteria and the researchers acknowledge the limitations, then the study might still be useful. An example is the study on AAT in the psychiatric setting that Kristen and Nicole appraised. During the appraisal process, they identified limitations in the study. The fact that only 50 participants out of 230 completed the tools on both interventions surely reduces the validity and reliability of this study. However, the fact that the researchers acknowledged the limitations and their recommendations were appropriate for the study's limitations

---

BOX 10■5 Interdisciplinary Rounds

You would like to be able to receive some support when doing a critical appraisal. You have read about journal clubs and think this is a good way for clinicians to improve their critical appraisal skills. How would you go about organizing such a group?

- Who could be involved?
- How often would you meet?
- What is involved in a journal club?
- How would you decide where and when to meet?
- What goals would you have for this journal club?
- How would the research be chosen?
- How would you choose your tools for appraisal?
- How would you know the journal club is meeting its goals?

BOX 10■6 Tools for Learning and Practice

- Locate the JBI Web site and find the critical appraisal tools.
- Locate the CASP Web site and download the appraisal tools.
- Locate the CINAHL and search the database. Find one quantitative research report and one qualitative research report and find the correct JBI or CASP tools. Try appraising each report. You might want to work with a partner or group at first.
- Write down the things that caused you the most difficulty when doing an appraisal. Discuss these with your instructor.

---

still allowed for this study to provide some useful information. An additional consideration is whether the findings of a particular research project will work in a particular context or setting. Are the recommendations feasible to carry out in your context? Are there resource limitations in your context? Finally, and most important, will it help your particular patient? To address these issues, clinical expertise comes into play. These can be difficult decisions for novice clinicians, but asking for advice and help is useful in gaining experience (Boxes 10■5 and 10■6).

■ Summary

Critical appraisal is an important step in the evidence-based practice process. Clinicians need to maintain a skill set that allows them to critically appraise evidence to judge its ability to inform clinical decisions. A basic understanding of research language, methodologies, and methods is adequate to carry out a good critical appraisal. A good critical appraisal is also possible to do rapidly. Students and clinicians such as Kristin and Nicole can raise good clinical questions, search for the evidence, and appraise its quality. This leads to a clinician who is informed by the best available evidence and therefore making decisions that achieve better patient outcomes.

CHAPTER QUESTIONS

1. What started Kristin and Nicole on the search for more information?

2. How did they focus their search for evidence?

3. What skill sets do you need to carry out a good quantitative or qualitative critical appraisal?

4. What are the three main purposes of the critical appraisal process?

5. How would you explain appraisal to a fellow student?

6. What does it mean when someone says that the critical appraisal tool must match the study design?

7. Compare reliability, external validity, and internal validity in quantitative paradigms to dependability, credibility, and transferability in qualitative paradigms?

References

Barker, S., & Dawson, K. (1998). The effects of animal-assisted therapy on anxiety rating of hospitalized psychiatric patients. *Psychiatric Services, 49*(6), 797–801.

Critical Appraisal Skills Programme (CASP) (2018). CASP qualitative checklist. Retrieved from https://casp-uk.net/casp-tools-checklists/

Kamioka, H., Okada, S., Tsutani, K., et al. (2014). Effectiveness of animal-assisted therapy: A systematic review of randomized controlled trials. *Complementary Therapies in Medicine, 22*(2), 371–390. https://doi.org/10.1016/j.ctim.2013.12.016

Katrak, P., Bralocerkowski, A., Jassy-Westropp, N., et al. (2004). A systematic review of the content of critical appraisal tools. *BMC Med Research Methodology, 4*(22). doi:10.1186/1471-2288-4-22

Lincoln, Y. S., & Gruba, E. G. (1985). *Naturalistic inquiry.* Beverly Hills, CA: Sage.

Melnyk, B., & Fineout-Overholt, E. (2005). Rapid critical appraisal of randomized controlled trials (RCTs): An essential skill for evidence-based practice (EBP). *Pediatric Nursing, 31*(1), 50–53E.

Wood, S. (2016). Anyone's best friend: A qualitative exploration of the positive influences of animal assisted therapy on mental health and well-being (Unpublished undergraduate project). Manchester Metropolitan University. Manchester, United Kingdom. Retrieved from https://e-space.mmu.ac.uk/id/eprint/617866

CHAPTER 11

Appraise and Plan II

Pre-Appraised and Synthetic Sources of Evidence

Lisa Hopp

- Explain what an evidence hierarchy is and discuss different approaches to rating the quality and substance of an evidence source.

- Discuss the rigor of various evidence sources.

- Differentiate various types of pre-appraised sources of evidence according to their purpose, scope, and usefulness to busy clinicians.

- Discuss the advantages and disadvantages of using pre-appraised, digested sources of evidence.

- Assess a source of evidence for its transparency and rigor.

- Select and defend a pre-appraised source of evidence as best available evidence.

Case-controlled study
Cohort study
Digested evidence
Evidence hierarchies
Expert opinion
Grading of Recommendations
  Assessment, Development,
  and Evaluation (GRADE)
  Working Group

Homogeneity
Levels of evidence
Levels (or grades) of
  recommendations
Meta-analysis
Narrow confidence
  intervals
Observational study
Pre-appraised evidence

(continues on page 156)

**Randomized controlled trial
(RCT) with concealed
randomization
Rigor**

**Synopses
Syntheses
Transparent**

Clinical Story

When Jacob arrives at his medical-surgical unit one evening, his patient is a
frail, elderly woman who has been on his unit for a week with dehydration
caused by a urinary tract infection and subsequent septicemia. She needs
frequent blood draws and IV medications. It has become increasingly difficult to
obtain and maintain venous access. The resident physician decides to insert a
multilumen central line to ensure access. Jacob is quite new to the unit and
has not yet assisted with a central line insertion. However, he knows the unit
has had a recent increase in bloodstream infections related to these catheters
and that a multidisciplinary team revised the unit's policy relating to catheter
insertion. He needs quick information that he can trust to make sure he knows
key aspects of nursing care during the procedure. He wants a concise
reference of the evidence to feel confident about his role and, in particular, the
main interventions related to keeping the patient safe.

Jacob logs on to a computer in the central nurse's station and accesses the
"evidence and policy resources" icon on the desktop; it takes him to a search
page. He completes a basic search using the phrase "central venous line
insertion" to find what he needs to know to assist with the procedure. He
notes that the policy reflects the approval of a multidisciplinary panel (medical
director, infectious disease team, quality improvement group, and nursing). He
finds the policy has an embedded link to a brief evidence summary. The policy
lists his responsibilities, and the linked evidence provides the information he
needs—a description of the type of evidence supporting the summary and key
points to guide him just before he gathers the equipment he needs for the
procedure. He also notices that a grade level (A, B, C, D or 1, 2, 3, 4) follows
each recommendation. One of the recommendations that stands out is
"maximum sterile barrier conditions and aseptic techniques are recommended
in the procedure (grade A)." In addition, he reads that 2% chlorhexidine is
superior to other skin-cleansing solutions (level 2) and that ultrasound-guided
catheterization is recommended (grade A). The policy emphasizes that the
assisting nurse can stop the procedure if these criteria cannot be met. Just
minutes later, he heads to the room armed with the insertion kit and
confidence in the knowledge he needs to keep the patient safe during the
procedure.

·

Think Before You Read

- What are some barriers to using evidence in everyday nursing practice?
- What factors shape your decision about whether or not you will use a piece of evidence?
- How do you determine whether a piece of evidence lives up to the definition of being "evidence-based"?
- Reflect on how you have used information in the past. Did you sometimes default to what was easy to find and read?

Introduction

Critical appraisal is at the heart of evidence-based practice. That is, to properly employ the evidence-based practice process, you must be able to judge the strength and quality of the information you use to make decisions. In the previous chapter, you learned how to use specific tools to guide you in judging different types of research. You discovered that you need to use the right tool for the job. Although some appraisal questions are generic, others must match the design of the research to sensibly and fairly judge a particular study. These tools are very useful when you need to evaluate the quality of individual research reports. However, it may not be possible to appraise individual studies when you are making rapid decisions on the job. Even if you are an experienced expert, time constraints can affect your ability to be thorough in the middle of providing nursing care. A good solution for this dilemma is to use evidence sources in which someone else has already done the hard work of searching, appraising, and summarizing the evidence. Pre-appraised, digested sources of evidence are ideal for use at the point of care.

In this chapter, you will learn where to locate pre-appraised sources, how to judge their quality, and how evidence hierarchies can speed the process of appraising the strength of evidence that you can use during your busy clinical practice.

Pre-Appraised and Digested Sources of Evidence

Reader's Digest specializes in condensed material, giving you the most important points of an article concisely. In fact, maybe you have heard someone say, "Just give me the *Reader's Digest* version!" That means you want to get right to the heart of the issue and focus on the key points. When making simultaneous decisions in the midst of care, clinicians often need to use the *Reader's Digest* approach to find answers quickly and efficiently. However, they also need to be confident that the evidence that supports those answers is the best available evidence. **Pre-appraised evidence** is literature that an author or a group of experts has already reviewed and evaluated the evidence against quality indicators. **Digested evidence** is a source that an author or group of authors has carefully read, selected, and summarized; the most essential parts have been condensed into a shorter version, so it is easier to read and understand quickly. **Synopses,** short abridged summaries of the evidence, can be very useful digests for busy clinicians who may only have a few moments to get to the heart of the matter. **Syntheses** refer to systematic reviews of quantitative or qualitative evidence that follow explicit methods of search, appraisal, and analysis of the evidence. Synopses of syntheses are particularly strong sources of evidence when they are brief, pre-appraised, and guided by rigorous methods.

You can recognize pre-appraised evidence by looking for a rating system and an explanation of the meaning of the rating. Many systems exist, so you need to look for a key to the ranking. Usually a rating of I, 1, or A is better than II, 2, or B; however, some systems are the opposite, meaning a IV may be better than a I. You can see how these different rating systems can be confusing, especially if you do not look at the key accompanying the evidence.

When evidence is packaged so that clinicians can more easily search and obtain a bottom-line recommendation, both physicians and nurses with advanced preparation are more likely to find the right answer to questions in the first 2 minutes of searching (Coiera, Westbrook, & Rogers, 2008). In some cases, 2 minutes may be the maximum amount of time you have. One observational study of resident physicians showed that many skipped searching for evidence for most questions they had, but if they did search, they spent only 2 minutes looking for answers. Most commonly, they asked another colleague for answers (Ramos, Linscheid, & Schafer, 2003). Other studies have shown that advanced practice nurses in primary care and nurses in hospitals are no different from their physician colleagues; they favor asking a colleague over searching an electronic database (Codgill, 2003; McCaughan, Thompson, Cullum, et al, 2005; Pravikoff, Tanner, & Pierce, 2005). Melnyk, Fineout-Overholt, Gallagher-Ford, et al (2012) confirmed that nurses value evidence-based practice but they need online resources, mentors, and better tools to help them implement best practices.

Clinicians consult other trusted colleagues because they believe one another, and it is a handy way to find an answer. But the quick consultation of a nearby coworker cannot be relied on for the validity of information in the same way that a published source of evidence can be. The ideal source is one that is as easy to access as a colleague but has already been judged for its quality (Box 11■1).

In this chapter's clinical story, Jacob consults a source of evidence on the desktop computer in his unit (i.e., the point of care) instead of asking a nearby colleague. He uses a simple search and quickly finds a brief summary of the evidence. In addition, he can quickly judge the quality of the best practice recommendations based on a simple A, B, C, or D rating or 1 to 4 level of evidence, although he needs to understand these rankings to determine how confident he can be in the evidence. Jacob soon discovers he needs to know just how good the evidence is when he must defend the approach he thinks is right to protect the patient from possible adverse consequences of the central line insertion.

> BOX 11■1 **Significance of Pre-Appraised and Digested Evidence**
>
> ■ Most frequently, clinicians consult one another when they have a question about clinical practice; although convenient, it is difficult to know how trustworthy any one clinician's opinion or recommendation may be.
> ■ Busy clinicians need access to brief summaries and synopses of evidence they can trust as high quality.
> ■ When clinicians use a system that allows easy searching, they are more likely to find the best answer in the first 2 minutes of searching.
> ■ Many evidence hierarchies exist; you need to understand the meaning of the hierarchy to know what an evidence rank means.
> ■ Pre-appraised, digested evidence should be both transparent and rigorous to allow the clinician to trust the source.

Evidence Hierarchies

In the previous chapter, you learned that all evidence is not equally robust, credible, or trustworthy. Whether the best available evidence originates from quantitative or qualitative research, from local data, or from text and opinion, you need some method to rank your confidence and trust in the information you use to guide decisions. **Evidence hierarchies** are systems used to rank evidence statements according to certain criteria. They help you determine the amount of confidence you can have in a particular recommendation or source of evidence. However, many different hierarchies exist, and it is easy to become confused. Some hierarchies rank the **level of the evidence** based on the design of individual studies or systematic reviews of several studies. In quantitative research, the level of evidence increases when the research design controls more extraneous variables. In qualitative research, the level of evidence increases when the credibility and dependability of the methods and the researcher's interpretations increase. Others combine the type of study with the magnitude of the effect or the degree of variability of results to determine rank. Still others are based on the quality of the information as well as the ease and feasibility of using the evidence.

Some hierarchies are based on the assumption that all evidence relates to the effectiveness of interventions, ignoring the idea that clinicians have a range of questions whose answers require different study designs. For example, if a hierarchy ranks a meta-analysis (a systematic review with a statistical summary of many individual studies) as the highest level of evidence, this system is not relevant for questions about the meaning of a symptom or experience in individuals with a certain condition. Questions of meaning need to be answered with study designs that produce narrative data, the words that people use to describe an experience.

Because there are many hierarchies, you need to locate the explanation of the hierarchy when you see a rating associated with a source of evidence or a particular recommendation. The following are three systems that you may encounter when you evaluate evidence-based guidelines or individual sources of evidence. Each system has a unique approach.

Grading of Recommendations Assessment, Development, and Evaluation Approach

The soundness of the research methods used to answer any question is key to any rating system. However, an evidence rating system for effectiveness questions can include other factors as well. These factors include the relative importance of individual outcomes, the magnitude of effect, and the balance of harm and benefit (Guyatt, Oxman, Vist, et al, 2008). The **Grading of Recommendations Assessment, Development, and Evaluation (GRADE) Working Group** is an international group of evidence-based medicine experts who have spent many years creating a rating system that takes all of these factors into consideration. They aim to provide a standard system that guideline developers can use to grade the certainty of the evidence and the strength of recommendations that clinicians without strong backgrounds in critical appraisal can understand. Although this system stems from medicine, many disciplines have contributed to the debate and the system is used for multidisciplinary guidelines. The rankings for the certainty or quality of evidence in the GRADE approach may simply be high, moderate, low, and very low (Table 11■1) and the strength of the recommendations as just two categories (for or against) with clear definitions. However, a rigorous, transparent approach to appraisal of study designs and methods, consistency of results, directness of the measurement of results, potential for bias, precision and importance of outcomes, and size of the effect all influence the ultimate grade of evidence (GRADE Working Group, 2019; Guyatt et al., 2008). You should have the greatest confidence in evidence with a "high" ranking because the source has the least possibility for bias,

TABLE 11■1 GRADE Working Group Classification of the Quality of Effectiveness Evidence

Quality Rating	Definition
High	Further research is very unlikely to change confidence in the estimate of effect
Moderate	Further research is likely to have an important impact on the confidence in the estimate of effect and may change the estimate
Low	Further research is very likely to have an important impact on the confidence in the estimate of effect and is likely to change the estimate
Very low	Any estimate of effect is very uncertain

Adapted from Guyatt et al (2008).

addresses the most important outcomes (e.g., mortality and highly morbid conditions), and has a large impact. Lower rankings can indicate a problem with some type of bias, inclusion of less important outcomes, or a smaller impact. Many international guideline groups have already adopted this approach, including the World Health Organization, Agency for Healthcare Research and Quality, the Scottish Intercollegiate Guidelines Network, and the European Respiratory Society, among many others (GRADE Working Group, 2019).

JBI Levels of Evidence and Grades of Recommendations

JBI has developed a unique method to rank levels of evidence and recommendations. JBI embraces many types of evidence as both legitimate and important when answering questions relevant to enhancing global health. Therefore, it has created four parallel hierarchies for four different types of questions. The rating systems relate to questions of feasibility, appropriateness, meaningfulness, and effectiveness (Joanna Briggs Institute, 2013b; Jordon, Lockwood, Munn, et al, 2018).

In Table 11■2, you see the top level of evidence for each category refers to a meta-synthesis or meta-analysis of the most trustworthy primary research. As in many other evidence hierarchies, JBI ranks a systematic review that nets a meta-synthesis or meta-analysis of the ideal findings or evidence as the most reliable and believable source of evidence. Recall that *systematic review* is a general term, meta-syntheses are systematic reviews of qualitative evidence, and meta-analyses are systematic reviews that include statistical analyses of quantitative data. Systematic reviews rank highest because of their exhaustive, systematic search and rigorous appraisal and the judicious selection of the evidence included in the systematic review (Joanna Briggs Institute, 2013b). Meta-syntheses and meta-analyses rely on methods that ensure rigor at multiple stages of the conduct of systematic reviews. Although a discussion of these techniques is beyond the scope of this book, there is good consensus among the many evidence hierarchies that this type of evidence ranks highest.

When you examine the JBI system of ranking levels of evidence, you will find that level 1 is the highest level and rankings decline to 4, the lowest level. For questions that are best answered with qualitative evidence (i.e., feasibility, appropriateness, and meaningfulness), meta-syntheses are still listed as level 2 and level 3a. However, for level 2, the trustworthiness of evidence contained in the meta-synthesis is not as high as level 1. Instead of being unequivocal, the evidence in a level 2 meta-synthesis is credible, meaning the findings are plausible but could be challenged. For level 3a, the meta-synthesis uses text and opinion rather than qualitative studies; this text and opinion may come from papers produced by scientific organizations or other non–research-based sources. Level 3b is a single qualitative research study of high quality (Joanna Briggs Institute, 2008). Finally, level 4 is evidence from expert opinion.

The evidence leveling for questions of effectiveness is similar to many other hierarchies. At level 1, two types of evidence rank highest: (1) a meta-analysis of

TABLE 11■2   **JBI Levels of Evidence**

Level of Evidence	Feasibility	Appropriateness	Meaningfulness	Effectiveness
1	Meta-synthesis of research with unequivocal synthesized findings	Meta-synthesis of research with unequivocal synthesized findings	Meta-synthesis of research with unequivocal synthesized findings	Meta-analysis (with homogeneity) of experimental studies (e.g., RCT with concealed random assignment) OR one or more large experimental studies with narrow confidence intervals
2	Meta-synthesis of research with credible synthesized findings	Meta-synthesis of research with credible synthesized findings	Meta-synthesis of research with credible synthesized findings	One or more smaller RCTs with wider confidence intervals OR quasi-experimental studies (without random assignment)
3	a. Meta-synthesis of text/opinion with credible synthesized findings b. One or more single research studies of high quality	a. Meta-synthesis of text/opinion with credible synthesized findings b. One or more single research studies of high quality	a. Meta-synthesis of text/opinion with credible synthesized findings b. One or more single research studies of high quality c. Observational studies (without control group)	a. Cohort studies (with control group) b. Case-controlled studies
4	Expert opinion	Expert opinion	Expert opinion	Expert opinion, or physiology bench research or consensus opinion

RCT = randomized controlled trial
Adapted from Joanna Briggs Institute (2013b). Levels of evidence. Retrieved from https://joannabriggs.org/jbi-approach.html

randomized controlled trials (RCTs) with homogeneity of experimental studies, or (2) one or more large experimental studies with narrow confidence intervals. To understand why these types of evidence rank highest for questions of effectiveness, you need to understand more about these study designs.

A **meta-analysis** is a secondary research method that statistically pools data from multiple studies to produce a single statistic of effectiveness. Meta-analyses are highly regarded because they carry safeguards against bias, they should only combine data from well-designed and well-conducted studies, and they follow a research protocol. In addition, they are more generalizable, and you can have greater confidence in the answers because the researcher combines data from more than one study. **Homogeneity** means that the results of each of the individual studies combined in the meta-analysis do not vary widely. Statistical methods can judge whether the results are homogeneous, and the author should address this in the publication.

In an **RCT with concealed randomization,** participants are blindly assigned to a group (treatment or control). The RCT is stronger when those blinded include the person who allocates participants to the groups, the participants themselves, those who administer the treatment and collect data, and those who analyze the data. An example of a very rigorous approach to blinding is a study comparing two types of insulin administered by a subcutaneous injection. The control and experimental participants receive prefilled syringes that look identical, a computer program assigned the groups, the nurses providing the instructions do not know the group assignment, blood glucose data are gathered via computer associated only with a number, and the statistician who analyzes the data knows only which data belong to group A and B but is unaware of what each group means. Depending on the type of treatment, not all of those involved in the study can be blinded to group allocation.

Narrow confidence intervals is a statistical term that means how precisely the statistic estimates the true population value and to what degree of probability you can be sure of the estimate. In other words, it represents the "noise" around the estimate (Fig. 11■1). If the confidence interval is wide, the results are less precise and more noise exists in the study, meaning other known and unknown factors are making it difficult to determine the true result. Many factors can contribute to the size of the confidence interval, but the smaller the confidence interval, the more confident you can be in the result. Traditionally, most meta-analyses use a 95% confidence interval, meaning that you can be 95% confident that a true value is between the two ends of the interval. For example, in the RCT using two types of insulin, if the mean difference between glucose levels is 50 mg/dL with a 95% confidence interval of 45 to 55, then the average true difference in the effect of the two insulin treatments is 50 mg/dL. In addition, if you were to repeat the experiment again and again, 95% of the time the difference will fall between 45 and 55 mg/dL and 5% of the time the difference will be greater. If, instead, the 95% confidence interval was 49 to 51 mg/dL, the estimate was more precise and less noisy.

If you put all these factors together—a meta-analysis, homogeneity, concealed randomization, and a narrow confidence interval—you have the most powerful

FIGURE 11■1 Confidence intervals and precision. (A) The wider confidence interval around the mean difference in glucose level means the estimate is less precise and more noisy (represented by the wider width of the interval around the mean). (B) The narrower confidence interval around the mean difference in glucose level means the estimate is more precise and less noisy (represented by a narrower interval around the mean).

evidence of the effectiveness of an intervention. If you have only one study instead of a meta-analysis, you still have strong evidence, but your ability to generalize is lessened. Level 2 in the JBI hierarchy refers to one or more smaller RCTs with wider confidence intervals, meaning less precision and generalizability.

Three subcategories of single studies make up level 3. Each subcategory has the potential for more bias and less confidence in the results. However, many times these study types are the only feasible way to pursue an answer. **Cohort studies** with a control group are studies in which researchers follow an experimental cohort, or group of people, with something in common. They compare the cohort to another group whose members are otherwise similar, except for the factor that is being investigated. Researchers often use this design when they cannot feasibly or ethically manipulate the experimental conditions. For example, a cohort-controlled study might be a study of the effect of secondhand smoking on the incidence of asthma. The experimental cohort is a group of children who live in middle- to upper-class households with smokers who smoke one to two packs of cigarettes per day and expose the children to smoke at least 10 hours per day. The control group is children of the same age and similar socioeconomic status, but they live with nonsmokers. The researchers follow both groups from birth to 18 years of age and compare the number of children in each group who develop asthma. Obviously, it would not be ethical to randomly assign children to a smoking and nonsmoking family, but the question is important to the public health, and a cohort with control study allows researchers to obtain data and draw relevant conclusions in an ethical manner. However, there is greater risk of bias because the researchers have less control over other factors that may coincide with the children's smoking exposure status. Perhaps the families who do not smoke also have other healthy habits that could explain a difference in asthma rates. If the researchers could randomly assign children to smoking and nonsmoking families, they could assume other factors, like healthy eating or exercise habits, would occur at the same random rates in both the experimental and control groups. Without random assignment, researchers cannot assume similar rates in both the cohort and control groups. Despite this, they could strengthen the study design by measuring these healthy habits in both groups to see if there is a difference that contributes to the asthma outcome. Still, cohort-controlled designs rank lower because of the greater chance of bias.

In a **case-controlled study,** researchers select cases (those with a particular outcome) and the control group (those without a particular outcome) and compare the participants' history of exposure. In the asthma study example, the researchers are comparing 18-year-olds with asthma to those without asthma to see whether there is a difference in family smoking habits since birth (DiCenso, Guyatt, & Ciliska, 2005).

Level 3c evidence concerns **observational studies** without a control group. These studies include different types of studies in which researchers simply observe what happens and take measurements. These studies can be fraught with bias because of lack of control over other variables that can influence outcomes. Conversely, sometimes an observational study may be the only feasible design, or it is a way to explore a relationship before using a more rigorous but expensive study design. For example, before doing a cohort-controlled study, researchers may have investigated the relationship between the incidence of asthma and secondhand smoke exposure by surveying households and counting how many children had asthma in smoking and nonsmoking households.

For all questions, **expert opinion** is ranked the lowest (level 4), but it does count as a legitimate source of evidence. In fact, not all hierarchies will include expert opinion in their rankings. When you are faced with no research evidence that ranks above expert opinion, you still need to make a decision. If expert opinion is the best available evidence, you need to use this type of evidence with caution. However, many nursing interventions have no stronger evidence than level 4 (expert opinion), yet we have incorporated these interventions into common practice. For example, there is no evidence beyond expert opinion that tells us how frequently we should turn patients who are unable to move themselves to prevent a pressure ulcer from forming. However, expert opinion supports turning these patients at least every 2 hours and more frequently if signs of skin breakdown such as redness occur or they are high risk (Registered Nurses' Association of Ontario, 2005, 2011). Of course, there are interventions that nurses can employ to prevent pressure ulcers in addition to turning patients. There are many studies and systematic reviews that examine the effectiveness of different types of bed surfaces but none that have examined turning frequency alone. But if a highly controlled study is never conducted to compare turning frequencies, expert opinion may remain the best evidence that we will ever have to support the turning frequency of patients who are confined to their beds and unable to move themselves.

As do other organizations, JBI also has a system to rank recommendations. These **levels (or grades) of recommendations** incorporate the evidence that underpins the recommendations, as well as the appropriateness and relevance of the evidence to practice. The approach to grades of recommendations adapts the GRADE approach discussed above. A "strong" recommendation incorporates the following: there is clear, desirable effects that outweigh undesirable effects, the evidence is of adequate quality, there is a benefit or no impact on resources, and the values, preferences, and patient experience are taken into account. A weak recommendation means the following: the desirable effects appear to outweigh the undesirable, although this may not be clear, there is evidence supporting its use but the evidence may not be high quality, and patient values, preferences, and experience may not have been taken into account (Joanna Briggs Institute, 2013a).

In this chapter's clinical story, Jacob uses a policy with embedded evidence summaries much like the pre-appraised evidence summaries from the JBI collection called JBI EBP Database. The summary includes a list of recommendations and associated grades. In addition, the evidence that supports the recommendations is ranked according to levels of evidence. Jacob's evidence summary is based on a strong level of recommendation (strong support and based on the highest level of evidence) and level II evidence (an evidence-based practice guideline) (Sivapuram, 2019).

Keeping this information in mind, when Jacob opens the insertion kit, he is pleased to find chlorhexidine cleansing swabs. However, he finds a small sterile barrier that will only partially cover the patient during insertion. In addition, there is no portable ultrasound machine in the room to help guide the insertion process. Jacob expresses his concerns to the physician about the lack of a full barrier and an ultrasound machine. The resident physician insists that they continue the procedure, as she is certain she can maintain a sterile field with the smaller barrier, and, considering her other responsibilities, she is unwilling to wait for a new, full-sized barrier and an ultrasound machine to be delivered to the unit. Jacob, knowing he has the support of medical and nursing leadership in his unit, informs the resident physician they must stop the procedure until these standards can be met. He further supports his decision by telling the physician that high-level evidence supports his stance. The resident physician interrupts the procedure, but Jacob can tell she is a bit impatient and not pleased about this turn of events.

The 6S Pyramid: Syntheses and Synopses

In addition to determining the quality and significance of evidence and recommendations, ease of use is an important, practical determinant of whether clinicians will use an evidence source. DiCenso, Bayley, and Haynes (2009) proposed a hierarchy of pre-appraised evidence that ranks sources based on the degree of synthesis and summary. At the peak of the 6S pyramid is the ideal—a clinical decision support system in which evidence is filtered for quality, concisely summarized, and continually updated with emergent research and is linked to the electronic medical record (Figure 11■2). One example is a system that takes in all of the patient assessment data, uses algorithms to determine the patient's condition (e.g., risk for bloodstream infection related to a central line), and creates recommendations for interventions (e.g., full barrier precautions, aseptic technique, ultrasound guidance). This would happen at the point of care, seamlessly and automatically. Unfortunately, few systems such as this exist (DiCenso et al, 2009).

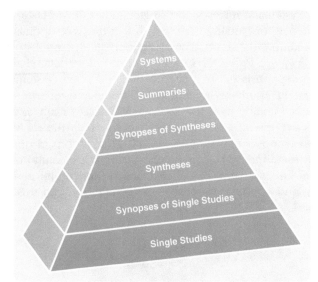

FIGURE 11■2 6S pyramid. DiCenso et al (2009) adapted the 4S pyramid by adding two additional levels to the hierarchy. Systems = clinical decision support system, where evidence is filtered for quality, concisely summarized, and continually updated as new research emerges and is linked to the electronic medical record or clinical practice guidelines. Summaries = pre-appraised, filtered for excellence, and based on the systematically developed and transparent. Synopses of syntheses = brief summary of key elements of a synthesis such as a systematic review; synopses of single studies = brief summary of key elements of single study; single studies = original studies without filtering or pre-appraisal. (With permission from BMJ Publishing Group Ltd.)

The next level in the 6S pyramid is summaries. These are summaries of evidence that are pre-appraised, filtered for excellence, and systematically developed and transparent; the authors explicitly detail the methods they used to ask, acquire, appraise, and synthesize the evidence. DiCenso et al (2009) include clinical practice guidelines (CPGs) in this level of the pyramid. However, they emphasize the following: "A CPG should be based on comprehensive searches and appraisal of the literature (ideally current systematic reviews, if they exist), and each recommendation should be accompanied by levels of evidence" (p. 100). If the methods of the summaries are not clear, it is difficult to know whether the source is truly based on the best available evidence. In this chapter's clinical story, Jacob uses an evidence summary from the JBI Database system (Sivapuram, 2019). This system falls in the category of summaries in the 6S pyramid because the methods of finding the summaries and the evidence that supports the recommendations are clear, and the summaries are regularly updated.

The next level in the 6S pyramid is synopses of syntheses. These are brief summaries of systematic reviews. You can find synopses of syntheses in the Cochrane Nursing Care Field systematic review summaries published in journals such as the *International Journal of Nursing Practice, AORN Journal, Clinical Nurse Specialist, Neonatal, Paediatric & Child Health Nursing,* and many others. You will also find summaries of both systematic reviews and single studies at McMaster University's Nursing+, Best Evidence for Nursing Care, which is a free, pre-appraised synopsis online service. In addition, there are abstracting journals that publish synopses of syntheses, such as *Evidence-Based Nursing*. If you need more detail than a synopsis of a synthesis or no synopsis exists, you can find the actual systematic reviews published in general literature or in libraries of systematic reviews such as the Cochrane and Campbell libraries and JBI Evidence Synthesis. Finally, if no syntheses exist, you can seek synopses of individual studies found in the same abstracting journals that publish synopses of syntheses, or individual reports of original studies that have not been pre-appraised. Remember, you must use caution when using this pyramid; make sure you find evidence that has undergone a rigorous and transparent filtering and appraisal process to be certain you can trust the source (DiCenso et al, 2009).

Judging the Quality of Pre-Appraised Sources

The advantage of using pre-appraised sources is that you can more quickly determine a source's quality and strength, which helps you decide whether you should use the evidence and the appropriate level of confidence you can have in the source (Box 11■2). However, you must still evaluate whether the pre-appraised source can be trusted. Once you have established that the methods of the pre-appraised sources are solid, you can quickly screen content for its quality (see Box 11■3 for tips and best bet sources).

BOX 11■2 Interdisciplinary Rounds

- All health-care disciplines need evidence in a form that is easy to use and trustworthy.
- Search for high-quality synopses and summaries of syntheses in any discipline that relates to your clinical problem or question.
- Regardless of the disciplinary source, make sure you understand the ranking system or hierarchy for the evidence you consider using.
- Some systems of evidence are created for many disciplines and others are aimed at more singular audiences.
- Ask colleagues from other disciplines what pre-appraised and digested evidence sources they use.
- Be ready to support your decisions when other professionals challenge your position; understanding the level of evidence and degree of confidence in the evidence may affect how vigorously you argue the point.
- Having ready access to evidence at the point of care that is pre-appraised and summarized may foster a culture of evidence-based decision making among all disciplines.

BOX 11■3 **Tools for Learning and Practice**

Free Pre-Appraised, Digested Evidence Sources

- https://www.tripdatabase.com—The Turning Research Into Practice (TRIP) is an easy-to-use, free tool to search across several databases. It uses a color-coded method of identifying the quality of evidence and you can filter evidence to find summaries of systematic reviews or clinical practice guidelines. The search process is not exhaustive, but it is somewhat transparent. The focus is on both medical and nursing decisions.
- https://rnao.ca—Registered Nurses' Association of Ontario Nursing Best Practice Guidelines are based on transparent methods and a rigorous approach, using tools to help with implementation. Each guideline has a short summary with grades of evidence for each recommendation.
- https://jbi.global—JBI provides brief synopses of systematic reviews called "Best Practice Information Sheets" that are freely available at 6 months after publication date.

Subscription-Based Pre-Appraised, Digested Evidence Sources

- https://jbi.global/ebp#database—JBI EBP Database is a subscription-based service of nursing and health-care disciplines. Evidence sources include summaries as well as systematic reviews of evidence of effectiveness as well as feasibility, appropriateness, and meaningfulness. Systematic reviews are highly transparent.
- https://bestpractice.bmj.com/info/us/—BMJ Best Practice is a product of the *British Medical Journal* publication that uses an explicit approach to searching and the GRADE evidence rating system. The majority of evidence relates to medical rather than nursing decisions.
- http://www.ebscohost.com/dynamed—Dynamed uses an explicit and comprehensive approach to the search and appraisal of evidence with regular, ongoing updates. It is more heavily oriented toward medical practice, but nursing-relevant content can be found. It can be linked to the electronic health record and can be used with a portable digital assistant.
- http://www.uptodate.com/index—Like Dynamed, UpToDate is aimed primarily at medical practice. Its methods are somewhat transparent but not easily found. It can be used with a personal digital assistant, contains brief summaries of many types of evidence, and is updated regularly.

You have seen the word *transparent* several times in this chapter as well as in others. This is a key concept to quality evidence. When an evidence source is **transparent**, the authors provide details about its purpose and methods. For example, they need to specify the goals of the guideline, synthesis, synopsis, or summary in the form of a statement or question. They need to explain their search process including where they searched (e.g., databases, organizations) and how they searched. The following statement is an example of good transparency of the search strategies and inclusion criteria used for one summary of a systematic review in the Cochrane Library:

> *In June 2015 we searched: The Cochrane Wounds Specialized Registry, The Cochrane Central Register of Controlled Trials (CENTRAL), The Cochrane Library, Ovid MEDLINE, Ovid MEDLINE (In Process & Other Non-Indexed Citations), Ovid EMBASE and EBSCO CINAHL. We also searched clinical trials registries for registered trials. There were no restrictions with respect to language, date of publication or study setting (Gavin, Webster, Chan & Rickard, 2016, Abstract, para. 3)*

This is typical of a systematic review. Other sources may only discuss the overall methods for a resource somewhere on their Web site or in upfront materials. This makes the source less transparent and more difficult to judge when you must hunt for the methods. You should use caution if a source lacks any description of the method of the search, how exhaustive the search was (i.e., the breadth and number of databases), and what criteria were used to include studies or information in a source.

In addition to transparent methods, look for how the authors ensured **rigor,** meaning the way in which the authors appraise the evidence (look for appraisal checklists and levels of evidence or grades of recommendations) and if more than one person validates the appraisal (if it is a clinical practice guideline or systematic review). For example, in the same systematic review from the Cochrane Library above, Gavin et al (2016) wrote, "Two review authors independently assessed studies for inclusion, performed risk of bias assessment and data extraction" (Abstract, para. 5). Generally, you will see this degree of transparency and rigor only with syntheses, such as systematic reviews.

Defending Your Evidence-Based Position

Once you have selected the best pre-appraised evidence from a synthesized or other digested source, you need to be ready to defend your choice. Not all health-care workers will be familiar with evidence hierarchies, and they may even be skeptical of evidence-based practice itself. You may need to go beyond a plain, uninformative statement such as "My information and reasons are evidence based." Instead, be ready to briefly discuss where your evidence came from and its quality and to provide a quick summary of the results.

In the clinical story, Jacob discovers the physician is reluctant to wait for a full drape to cover the patient and an ultrasound machine that would help the physician know if a vein was patent (i.e., had good circulation and blood flow). Jacob is ready to support his stance. He explains to the physician that the reason he asks her to stop the procedure is that strong evidence from systematic reviews supports full barrier precautions and ultrasound guidance. He says that he used the JBI evidence summaries, which are based on Cochrane Library systematic reviews. In addition, he mentions that he understands her urgency, but the unit standard of practice is consistent with this evidence, and he must stop the procedure to ensure the patient's safety. Once Jacob is able to find the correct equipment, he and the physician start the procedure again.

Increasingly, nursing staff members are empowered to interrupt medical procedures when those involved deviate from the recommended practices (Institute for Healthcare Improvement, 2019). Jacob is confident in his decision to interrupt the procedure because of the high-quality evidence. Having the evidence in hand enhances the nurse's position, even in a situation of conflict with the physician.

■ Summary

In this chapter, you learned about the value of pre-appraised and summarized evidence. In the clinical story, Jacob was able to quickly locate a pre-appraised evidence summary that provided him with important knowledge to maintain the patient's safety. Busy clinicians need systems of evidence they can trust and access quickly at the point of care. You need to understand evidence hierarchies and what they mean in terms of your confidence in the evidence. To this end, evidence ratings can help you quickly assess the trustworthiness of any source and help you defend your clinical decisions. As with any evidence source, pre-appraised sources must be evaluated for their transparency and rigor, but they can be a valuable asset in a busy health-care environment.

CHAPTER QUESTIONS

1. In this chapter's clinical story, what type of evidence source did Jacob rely on? What did it mean that some recommendations were level A and other pieces of evidence were level 2? What is the difference between the level of evidence and level or grade of recommendation?

2. What factors contribute to the rigor of the evidence? What is meant by *transparency*?

3. What are the main similarities and differences among the GRADE Working Group, JBI, and the 6S approaches to ranking evidence?

4. What is a meta-analysis? Is it considered a type of systematic review?

5. Why do most hierarchies rank systematic reviews and meta-analyses as the most ideal evidence?

6. Why does random assignment and concealment of group assignment strengthen a study?

7. How do cohort control, case controlled, and observational study designs compare? Provide an example of each. How do they compare in their ability to control the research conditions?

8. Consider this chapter's clinical story. Was it right for Jacob to stop the procedure? How would you approach a similar situation?

References

Codgill, K. W. (2003). Information needs and information seeking in primary care: A study of nurse practitioners. *Journal of the Medical Library Association, 9,* 203–215.

Coiera, E., Westbrook, J. I., & Rogers, K. (2008). Clinical decision velocity is increased when meta-search filters enhance an evidence retrieval system. *Journal of the American Medical Informatics Association, 15,* 638–646. doi:10.1197/jamia.M2765

DiCenso, A., Bayley, L., & Haynes, R. B. (2009). Accessing pre-appraised evidence: Fine-tuning the 5S model into a 6S model [Editorial]. *Evidence-based nursing, 12*(4), 99–101. doi:10.1136/ebn.12.4.99-b

DiCenso, A., Guyatt, G., & Ciliska, D. (2005). *Evidence-based nursing: A guide to clinical practice.* St. Louis, MO: Elsevier Mosby.

Gavin, N. C., Webster, J., Chan, R. J., et al. (2016). Frequency of dressing changes for central venous access devices on catheter-related infections. *Cochrane Database of Systematic Reviews, 2016*(2). doi:10.1002/14651858.CD009213.pub2

GRADE Working Group. (2019). Organizations that have endorsed or that are using GRADE. Retrieved from https://www.gradeworkinggroup.org

Guyatt, G. H., Oxman, A. D., Vist, G. E., et al. (2008). GRADE: An emerging consensus on rating quality of evidence and strength of recommendations. *British Medical Journal, 336,* 924–926.

Institute for Healthcare Improvement. (2019). Central line insertion checklist. Retrieved from http://www.ihi.org/resources/Pages/Tools/CentralLineInsertionCareTeamChecklist.aspx

Joanna Briggs Institute. (2008). *Joanna Briggs Institute reviewer's manual 2008 edition.* Retrieved from http://www.joannabriggs.edu.au/Documents/JBIReviewManual_CiP11449.pdf

Joanna Briggs Institute (2013a). Grades of recommendation. Retrieved from https://joannabriggs.org/sites/default/files/2019-05/JBI-grades-of-recommendation_2014.pdf

Joanna Briggs Institute. (2013b). Levels of evidence. Retrieved from https://joannabriggs.org/jbi-approach.html

Jordan, Z., Lockwood, C., Munn, Z., et al. (2018). Redeveloping the JBI model of evidence-based healthcare. *International Journal of Evidence-Based Healthcare, 16,* 227–241.

McCaughan, D., Thompson, C., Cullum, N., et al. (2005). Nurse practitioner and practice nurses' use of research information in clinical decision making: Findings from an exploratory study. *Family Practice, 22,* 490–497. doi:10.1093/fampra/cmi042

Melnyk, B. M., Fineout-Overholt, E., Gallagher-Ford, L. et al. (2012). The state of evidence-based practice in US nurses: Implications for nurse leaders and educators. *Journal of Nursing Administration, 42*(9), 410–417.

Pravikoff, D. S., Tanner, A., & Pierce, S. T. (2005). Readiness of U.S. nurses for evidence-based practice. *American Journal of Nursing, 105*(9), 40–51.

Ramos, K., Linscheid, R., & Schafer, S. (2003). Real-time information-seeking behavior of residency physicians. *Family Medicine, 35,* 257–260.

Registered Nurses' Association of Ontario (2005, 2011). Risk assessment & prevention of pressure ulcers. Retrieved from https://rnao.ca/sites/rnao-ca/files/Risk_Assessment_and_Prevention_of_Pressure_Ulcers.pdf

Sivapuram, M. S. (2019. Evidence summary: Central venous access device (CVAD) insertion. *Joanna Briggs Institute EBP Database,* JBI@Ovid, JBI14272.

CHAPTER 12

Apply and Implement I

Decision Making and Integrating Preference and Clinical Expertise

Leslie Rittenmeyer

- Discuss the concept of patient-preference and its relationship to evidence-based practice.
- Explain shared decision making (SDM).
- Summarize the responsibilities of the clinician in SDM.
- Discuss the role of clinical expertise in clinical decision making.

Clinical decision making   **Meaning**
Clinical expertise   **Patient preference**
Local context   **Shared decision making (SDM)**

Clinical Story

Jen, a newly graduated nurse practitioner, is working at a clinic in a rural farming community. The people who work and live in this community are known for their independent thinking and willingness to communicate their ideas and opinions. Jen views these traits as positive, generally leading to an effective, joint decision-making process between patient and clinician, one that moves beyond the research evidence to include patient preferences, values, and clinical expertise. She knows this is the most desirable model for evidence-based practice clinical decision making but admits to her evidence-based practice mentor that it is difficult for her when patients express a preference that she disagrees with. Jen provides an example from her current caseload: a patient who refuses prescribed antihypertensive medication for his high blood pressure. The patient, a 55-year-old farmer who works extremely hard and is exposed to the daily stressors common to the occupation of farming, communicates that the last time he was on this type of medication, his sexual functioning was affected to the point that he prefers not to take them again. At this point, he seems adamant about his decision. Jen wonders what should drive her next actions.

Think Before You Read

- How do you go about engaging patients in decision making about their health?
- Do people vary in what they want to know and how much responsibility they want in making decisions for their health?
- Are there tools that could help patients understand how to work with health-care providers when they share in decision making?
- What factors should be considered in authentic evidence-based decision making?

Introduction

It has often been said that knowledge is power. In nursing, knowledge is derived from many sources, such as systematic reviews, primary research, pre-appraised sources, clinical guidelines, and expert opinion. However, Pravikoff, Tanner, and Pierce (2005) surveyed 3,000 nurses across the United States and found that although nurses needed information to make clinical decisions, they often relied more on peers, colleagues, and the Internet than they did on bibliographic databases, such as the Cumulative Index to Nursing and Allied Health Literature (CINAHL) and PubMed, to obtain it. The study results showed there was more of a reliance on human sources of knowledge, and the study participants felt generally unprepared to do the things necessary to practice evidence-based nursing. Muntean (2012), however, suggests novice nurses regularly encounter new situations, and although there is often more expert advice available to them, the extent to which they communicate a need for assistance seems to be variable. In another study, Hedberg and Larsson (2003) observed experienced nurses and found that communicating and sharing information with colleagues was a large component of the decision-making process, and, through this process of collaboration, the nurses in the study felt it reduced the risk of making errors. Benner (1984) in her seminal book theorized how nurses become expert clinical decision makers. She saw it as happening over time. Research on the clinical decision-making skills of nurses is complex because it involves multiple factors, some that are hard to measure.

In evidence-based practice, knowledge holds a prominent place because its purpose is to inform clinical decision making with the best available evidence. As a nurse, you need to understand how to access knowledge and use it to inform your clinical decisions but at the same time be aware of what may affect your ability to make good clinical decisions, such as the environmental factors, for example, of time pressure and workplace complexity.

However, this is not the complete story. In clinical decision making, the research evidence alone is not necessarily justification for action. There are other considerations such as **patient preference, clinical expertise,** and **local context.**

- Patient preference is the right of an individual to be involved in the planning of his or her own care and ultimately having the final say about which interventions he or she chooses to accept or not accept.
- Clinical expertise is the accumulated knowledge of the professional and how it influences clinical decisions.
- Local context is the circumstances particular to a situation.

All of these considerations together give you the ability to make clinical decisions more clear or, conversely, muddy them. This chapter will address the issues relevant to evidence-based clinical decision making.

Evidence-Based Clinical Decision Making

Haynes, Devereaux, and Guyatt (2002) define evidence-based decision making as the integration of the best available research evidence with clinical expertise and patient values. Clinical decisions are made by balancing four equally important constructs: the clinical circumstance, patient preferences, research evidence, and clinical expertise. Pearson, Wiechula, Court, et al (2005) describe **clinical decision making** within the perspective of giving equal weight to the best available evidence, the context in which the care is given, client preference, and the professional judgment of the health-care professional. The equal weighting of these factors means that research evidence cannot eliminate the wishes of the patient or the clinical expertise of the professional. This fact dispels the belief that evidence-based practice is "cookbook" nursing, making nursing care too prescriptive and removing all creativity. This would be true if clinical decisions were based solely on the research evidence, but that is not the case in actual evidence-based practice (see Chapter 4). When the research evidence, preferences and values of the patient, and the clinical expertise of the professional are in agreement, and there are no contextual issues, the course of action is clear. However, the process gets murky when the research evidence points to one intervention, and the preference of the patient is for another intervention or even in opposition to the evidence. When this happens, it is often the expertise of the clinician that influences the situation.

Jen, the nurse in this chapter's clinical story, understands what should influence clinical decision making but has a hard time accepting patient preference when she feels it is counter to what is medically sound practice. The evidence and her clinical expertise are in accord, but the preference of her patient is not. She asks herself what she should do and what her responsibility is. The answers to these questions should become clear as this chapter progresses.

What Does Patient Preference Really Mean?

There are two ways in which patients and their values and preferences are considered in evidence-based practice. The first is to what extent patients are involved in shared decision making, and the second is the right of patients to choose or reject an intervention. Melnyk and Fine-Overholt (2015) define patient preferences as the "values the patient holds, concerns the patient has regarding the clinical decision/treatments/situations and choices the patient has/prefers regarding the clinical decision/treatment/situation" (p.609). Brennan and Stromborn (1998) state that "patient preferences result from cognition, experience and reflection and exist as the relatively enduring consequence of values. . . . Patient preferences are statements made by individuals regarding the relative desirability of a range of health experiences, treatment options or health states" (pp. 258–259).

Shared Decision Making

Shared decision making (SDM) is a key part of evidence-based practice because it brings together clinical expertise and patient preference. In reviewing the literature, Makoul and Clayman (2006) found that there is great variation in the definitions of shared decision making. The two ideas that appeared most often in the literature were "patient preferences" and "options." Legare, Elwyn, Fishbein, et al. (2008) define SDM as the decision-making process jointly shared by patients and their health-care provider, whereas Thistlewaite, Evans, Tie, et al (2006) describe SDM as a patient-centered consultation in which the patient and clinician discuss disease management and come to mutual decisions. In addition, Towle and Goldolphin (1999) explain that SDM is based on the best evidence of the risks and benefits of all the alternatives. This means that for any clinical decision there are alternatives; you and your patient must weigh the potential harm and potential benefit of any intervention.

Silow-Carroll, Alteras, and Stepnick (2006) state that "the U.S. health care system is experiencing a slow and subtle shift from a professionally driven approach toward one that is 'patient centered' or 'consumer centered.' This stems from a growing recognition that incorporating an individual patient's perspective and greater involvement in his/her care result in better health outcomes and satisfaction" (p. 4). Using an iterative process of reviewing the existing literature and research, the authors identified the following eight core components as a comprehensive patient-centered care approach, especially when caring for vulnerable populations:

1. Welcoming environment
2. Respect for patients' values and expressed needs
3. Patient empowerment and activation
4. Sociocultural competence
5. Coordination and integration of care
6. Comfort and support
7. Access and navigation skills
8. Community outreach

Jen is proud of the fact that her clinic embraces the patient-centered approach to care. She and her colleagues place value on treating their patents within a holistic perspective. She feels that this approach is vital to setting the stage for SDM. Davis, Schoenbaum, and Audet (2005) refer to patient-centered primary care as a system that allows individuals access to a form of health care that works for them, and the Institute of Medicine (IOM) (now called the National Academy of Medicine) identified patient-centered care as one of its six aims of quality. This position illustrates an obvious trend away from the paternalistic view that "the health care provider knows best." Nonetheless, Legare et al (2008) contend that data exist that suggest that SDM has not been broadly adopted in reality. Despite those claims, Clark, Nelson, Valero, et al (2009) cite a large amount of existing literature that suggests SDM is at least being widely discussed in health care.

SDM is not without it controversies. Studies indicate that many patients wish to have active participation in their care (Deber, Kraetschmer, Urowitz, et al, 2007; Funk, 2004; Gilbar & Gilbar, 2007; Heesen, Segal, Kopke, et al, 2004). Conversely, some patients prefer that their health-care provider make decisions for them. Vogel, Bengel, and Helmes (2008) found that 40.2% of the breast cancer patients in their study preferred that their physician make decisions for them. In another study that examined decision-making preferences of 150 women with breast cancer (Beaver, Luker, Owens, et al, 1996), researchers found that 20% of the study participants wanted an active role in decision making, 28% wanted to make a joint decision, and 52% wanted their surgeon to decide for them. In a related follow-up study (Beaver, Bogg, & Luker, 1999), researchers compared the preferences of breast cancer patients (n = 150) against patients with colorectal cancer (n = 48). Results showed that 78% of the colorectal cancer patients preferred to play a passive role in decision making in contrast to 52% of the breast cancer patients.

What does this confusing and sometimes contradictory evidence mean? The answer is not easy, because you cannot assume that you and your patients have the same values. Patient values are as diverse as patients themselves. The important lesson is always to be aware of the differing preferences and values and to communicate respect for your patients. After an exhaustive search of the literature, Clark et al (2009) concluded that preferences for SDM might be age related and possibly a generational phenomenon. The authors posited that younger patients seem to have a preference for patient–provider interaction in health care, possibly because of higher expectations for participation and communication, whereas older individuals seem to be more comfortable with leaving the health-care decisions in the hands of the provider. It is up to the clinician to explore how much or how little involvement the patient wants. If providers make assumptions about their patients' preferences, this is not conducive to a shared decision-making model.

Legare, Bekker, and Desroches (2010) studied the importance of shared decision making in primary care while acknowledging that a great deal of continuing professional development is needed to achieve this goal. Additionally, in recent years, there has been an interest in inter-professional models of shared decision-making. Legare, Stacy, Gagnon et al (2011) developed a conceptual model for an inter-professional approach. This model stresses the importance of facilitating communication between all those that would have responsibility in different stages of the decision-making process. They emphasize that those involved must share knowledge to develop a common understanding of the issues. In this model, the patient and family members (including significant others) are very much part of the shared decision-making team.

Strategies to Encourage SDM

Ford, Schofield, and Hope (2003) investigated the characteristics of a successful evidence-based patient choice consultation. Interviews were done with general practitioners, hospital doctors, practice nurses, academics, and lay people. Six themes emerged from the data:

1. Research evidence/medical information
2. The practitioner–patient relationship
3. Patient perspective
4. Decision-making processes
5. Time issues
6. Establishing the patient problem

Box 12■1 summarizes some of their findings into practical information. Fraenkel and McGraw (2007) also looked at the essential elements to enable participation in medical decision making. They identified five key elements. Box 12■2 summarizes these elements.

It should be clear from the research evidence that SDM does not happen spontaneously. Implementation of an SDM process is a must for patient-centered environments. The health-care system must invest in the ideas and tools, and staff must accept it as part of their obligation to their patients. Elwyn, Laitner, Coulter, et al (2010) identified three major forces that must be present to make SDM part of mainstream clinical practice: (1) access to evidence-based knowledge about treatment options, (2) help in weighing the pros and cons of the various options, and (3) a culture that facilitates patient engagement.

BOX 12■1   **Skills Required for Evidence-Based SDM**

- Communicating complex information using nontechnical language
- Tailoring the amount and pace of the information to the patient needs/preferences
- Drawing diagrams to aid patient comprehension
- Checking patient understanding
- Weighing medical evidence about treatment options while considering patient values
- Conveying objective, nondirective information regarding possible options
- Explaining probability of harm and risk for each option
- Using facilitative skills to encourage patient involvement
- Evaluating Internet information that patients might bring with them
- Creating an environment in which patients feel able to ask questions
- Negotiating skills

Summarized from Ford, S., Schofield, T., & Hope, T. (2003). What are the ingredients for a successful evidence-based patient choice consultation? A qualitative study. *Social Science & Medicine, 56,* 589–602.

BOX 12■2   **Elements That Enable Patient Participation in Medical Decision Making**

- Patient knowledge: Patients being adequately informed is absolutely essential for them to participate in the decision-making process.
- Explicit encouragement of patient participation: Aside from clarifying information, clinicians should facilitate patient participation in decision making by encouraging patients to ask questions.
- Appreciation of the patient's responsibility/rights to play an active role in decision making: Patients should feel that they have a reasonability to actively participate in decisions involving their care.
- Awareness of choice: To participate in decision making, patients must first be aware of the uncertainty in medicine. Patients should realize the importance of participation, particularly when decisions are value based.
- Time: The lack of time spent with patients has been identified as a barrier. Limited time has been seen as a barrier to becoming informed.

Summarized from Fraenkel, L., & McGraw, S. (2007). What are the essential elements to enable patient participation in medical decision-making? *Journal of General Internal Medicine, 22*(5), 614–619.

Patient Choice

As previously discussed, patients come to the health-care setting with many different perspectives and values. As Hope (1996) observed, patients differ both in what they value and their tendency to accept risk. In this chapter's clinical story, Jen's patient is choosing to reject the treatment recommendation. She acknowledges his right to do so but admits it upsets her that he is making that decision. In this case, the patient seems to value his sexual function more than he values treating his hypertension.

The right of a patient to choose health-care options has existed for some time. When talking and writing about patient-centered care, nurses have long recognized patient autonomy. Ford et al (2003) describe patient choice as originating from the doctrine of informed consent. They state that in English and U.S. law, a competent individual has a legal right to refuse even lifesaving treatment. Patient choice from an evidence-based practice context goes beyond just informed consent; it actively involves the patient in the decision-making process. Knowledge is given to patients with the explicit purpose of giving them choice. This is more than respect for patient autonomy; there is full recognition of individual preferences (Hope, 1996).

In the clinical story, Jen might speculate about why her patient values his sexual function more than he values his health, but in trying to understand his decision she should consider the **meaning** both have for him. Until she is able to discover this information, she will probably have difficulty engaging in SDM with him. *Meaning* is the subjective interpretation an individual places on something. To glean the meaning of something, you have to attempt to understand your patient's story. Nurses should ask, "Help me understand how you came to this decision," so the patient can provide insight into his or her decision-making process. Although it is sometimes difficult, it is always better to bring a nonjudgmental attitude to the nurse–patient relationship. If you are to be given the privilege of hearing the patient's story, then the patient has to feel comfortable sharing it with you.

Another way in which you might get in touch with the meaning of particular phenomena is by searching for research evidence or synthesized evidence that will give you more information. For example, Jen decides to explore the evidence for anything that will provide her with a greater understanding of her patient's decision. Realizing that systematic reviews are a higher level of evidence, she first goes to the CINAHL and MEDLINE databases and searches for any systematic reviews (in the form of a meta-synthesis or meta-aggregation) on the meaning of "sexual dysfunction as a result of taking hypertensive medication." She does not find a systematic review but is excited to find a primary qualitative research study in which Volis, Sandelowski, Dahm, et al (2008) explored the adherence to antihypertensive medications as a patient-driven means to preserving sexual potency. Jen first critically appraises the study and determines that it is of high quality. After reading this study, she thinks she better understands her patient's decision. Box 12■3 summarizes what she learned from this study that helped her to better understand the context of her patient's preferences.

After reading this meaningfulness study, Jen believes she has a better understanding of the factors that are influencing her patient's decision. Next, she needs to search for the best available evidence that will assist her in identifying alternative forms of hypertensive treatment that might target the diagnosis but not have the same side effects. Armed with some new insights and information, Jen now plans to engage her patient during the next office visit to further explore his perspective. She wishes to discuss if he has considered how this decision will affect his

BOX 12■3 **Findings on Preserving Sexual Potency While on Hypertensive Medication**

- The male patients felt that sexual activity reduced stress caused by high blood pressure.
- The male patients felt that sex lowers your blood pressure and the lack of it is unnatural.
- "Sexual intercourse is part of your makeup. Part of your spiritual makeup, part of your mental makeup and you need to get some."
- Patients felt the antihypertensive medications interfered with their desire and ability to have sexual intercourse, causing them to pursue strategies to preserve sexual function.
- Some reported selecting/adhering to the medication, stopping when a romantic time was planned.
- Spouses thought the sexual dysfunction took low priority to health.

Source: Volis, C., Sandelowski, M., Dahm, P., et al. (2008). Selective adherence to antihypertensive medications as a patient-driven means to preserving sexual potency. *Patient Preference and Adherence, 2,* 201–206.

relationships with significant others and if he has shared his preference with significant others. If he is firm in his decision, then she wants to discuss potential risks and offer him some alternative treatment options.

Whatever the patient's final decision, Jen has researched and answered her own questions about her responsibility when a patient's preference is different from the evidence-based recommended intervention. She realizes she must (1) struggle to understand the meaning of the patient's decision; (2) search for the best available evidence of alternative treatments that will minimize the patient's perception of risk but still target the diagnosis; (3) empower the patient with the necessary knowledge to make the decision; (4) enter into a shared decision-making dialogue; and (5) ultimately accept the patient preference.

Patient Decision Aids

Patient decision aids are tools to support patients during decision making. They are evidence based and are part of a shared decision-making process. These tools are meant to supplement the practitioner–patient relationship, not replace it. O'Connor, Llewellyn-Thomas, and Flood (2004) identified that these tools can come in many forms such as print, video, audio, and Internet-based delivery systems. They can be self- or practitioner administered. They usually provide high-quality, up-to-date information on a particular clinical condition, a section where values are clarified and explored, and opportunities for guidance and coaching. The International Cochrane Collaboration Review Group on Decision Aids (2004) found that when patient decision aids are used, they are more effective than just usual factors on decision quality, understanding of options, and cost-effectiveness (O'Connor et al, 2004).

BOX 12■4   **Examples of Shared Decision-Making Tools**

■ Ottawa Hospital Research Institute, Patient Decision Aids (https://
   decisionaid.ohri.ca)
■ Dartmouth-Hitchcock Center for Shared Decision-Making Center (https://
   med.dartmouth-hitchcock.org/csdm_toolkits.html)
■ Decision Support Toolkit for Primary Care Center for Shared Decision
   Making (https://med.dartmouth-hitchcock.org/csdm_toolkits/primary_care_
   toolkit.html)
■ Substance Abuse and Mental Health Services Administration Shared
   Decision Making Tools (https://www.samhsa.gov/brss-tacs/recovery-
   support-tools/shared-decision-making)

Decision-making aids are readily available by searching on the Web with the keywords "decision making tool kits." Please see Box 12■4 for an array of Web sites that will provide you with portals to decision-making tools. Remember, though, decision aids are meant to be used in conjunction with a shared decision model, implemented in a patient-centered environment.

Role of Clinical Expertise

What is the role of clinical expertise in evidence-based health care? Does clinical expertise hold more weight than other factors, such as research evidence or patient preference? As previously mentioned in this chapter, clinical expertise should be weighed equally with research evidence and patient preference. Although the research evidence is of utmost importance as a starting place, an expert clinician will address an array of other considerations such as sociocultural factors, access to transportation, insurance coverage, and ethical concerns before making decisions. Jen, the nurse in our clinical story, used her expertise to diagnose her patient's hypertension and suggest evidence-based treatment. When her patient declined the treatment, she then used her expertise to better understand his decision and to look for alternatives that would decrease his perception of risk.

Within the evidence-based practice movement, it is expected that expert clinicians will inform their practice with the best available evidence. As Haynes et al (2002) state, "Application of current best evidence from healthcare research is now an expected adjunct to clinical acumen" (p. 36). In that context, clinical expertise is a union of knowledge of the best available evidence, competent clinical skills, and clinical experience (Boxes 12■5 and 12■6). In an evidence-based practice setting, the clinician will use his or her clinical expertise to balance relevant research evidence, the patient's clinical state and circumstances, and the patient's preference and values before determining action. It is through this expertise that the intricacies of good clinical decision making take into account preferences of the patient and the context in which the care is delivered.

BOX 12■5 **Interdisciplinary Rounds**

You would like to find out how experienced clinicians implement a shared decision-making model in their evidence-based practice. You talk to some colleagues from different disciplines and organize a brown bag lunch once a month to discuss their perspectives on patient preference and shared decision making.

BOX 12■6 **Tools for Learning and Practice**

■ Read Haynes, R. B., Devereaux, P. J., and Guyatt, G. H. (2002). Clinical expertise in the era of evidence-based medicine and patient choice. *Evidence-Based Medicine, 7,* 36–38, and summarize the article's six most salient points.
■ Ask three people in your family how involved they would like to be in making clinical decisions in conjunction with their health-care practitioner.
■ Conduct an Internet search for the term "patient-centered care" and compare the characteristics with evidence-based clinical decision making.

■ Summary

Clinical decision making is a process that includes more than the application of the best available research evidence to a clinical situation. This alone is not sufficient to justify any action on the part of the health-care provider. Consideration of other factors such as preferences and values of patients, the context or circumstances that influence the situation, and the available resources is warranted. Patient preference is valued through shared decision-making models and respect for patients' autonomy in accepting or refusing a treatment.

Clinical decision making is not always an unambiguous process because patients sometimes choose not to accept a suggested treatment. It is during this time that clinicians need to explore the meaning of the patient's decision to better understand it and to search for acceptable alternatives. The expertise of the clinician is what drives this process. Combining knowledge of the best available research evidence with competent clinical skills and clinical experiences while respecting the preferences and values of patients within the context or circumstance of the situation influence the achievement of good clinical outcomes. Including patient preference and clinical expertise in the clinical decision-making process is essential for maintaining the theoretical underpinning of holistic nursing practice.

CHAPTER QUESTIONS

1. Why do you think Jen, the nurse in the clinical story, felt concerned about her patient's decision?

2. What steps would you take if this happened to you?

3. How much weight do you feel should be given to patient preferences?

4. What role does meaning have when considering patient preferences?

5. What are the most important elements to consider in SDM?

6. Explain the role of clinical expertise in clinical decision making.

References

Beaver, K., Bogg, J., & Luker, K. A. (1999). Decision making role preferences and information needs: A comparison of colorectal and breast cancer. *Health Expectations 2*, 266–268.

Beaver, K., Luker, K. A., Owens, R. G., et al. (1996). Treatment decision making in women newly diagnosed with breast cancer. *Cancer Nursing, 19*(1), 8–19.

Benner, P. (1984). *From novice to expert: Excellence and power in clinical nursing practice*. Menlo Park, CA: Addison-Wesley.

Brennan, P., & Stromborn, I. (1998). Improving health care by understanding patient preferences. *Journal of the American Medical Informatics Association, 5*(3), 257–262.

Clark, N. M., Nelson, B. W., Valero, M. A., et al. (2009). Consideration of shared decision making in nursing: A review of clinician's perceptions and interventions. *The Open Journal of Nursing, 3*, 65–75. doi:10.2174/1874434600903010065

Davis, K., Schoenbaum, C., & Audet, J. (2005). A 2020 vision of patient-centered primary care. *Journal of Internal General Medicine, 2*(10), 953–957.

Deber, R. B., Kraetschmer, N., Urowitz, S., et al. (2007). Do people want to be autonomous patients? Preferred roles in treatment decision making in several patient populations. *Journal of Public Participation in Health Care and Health Policy, 10*(3), 248–258.

Elyn, G., Laitner, S., Coulter, A., et al. (2010). Implementing shared decision making in the NHS. *BMJ: British Medical Association, 341*, c5146.

Ford, S., Schofield, T., & Hope, T. (2003). What are the ingredients for a successful evidence-based patient choice consultation? A qualitative study. *Social Science & Medicine, 56*, 589–602.

Fraenkel, L., & McGraw, S. (2007). What are the essential elements to enable patient participation in medical decision-making? *Journal of General Internal Medicine, 22*(5), 614–619.

Funk, L. M. (2004). Who wants to be involved? Decision making preferences among residents of long-term care facilities. *Canadian Journal of Aging, 23*(1), 47–58.

Gilbar, R., & Gilbar, O. (2007). The medical decision making process and the family: The case of breast cancer patients and their husbands. *Bioethics, 23*(3), 183–192.

Haynes, R. B., Devereaux, P. J., & Guyatt, G. H. (2002). Clinical expertise in the era of evidence-based medicine and patient choice. *Evidence-Based Medicine, 7*, 36–38.

Hedberg, B., & Larsson, U. (2003). Observations, confirmations, and strategies—useful tools in decision-making process in nursing practice? *Journal of Clinical Nursing, 12*, 215–222.

Heesen, C., Segal, J., Kopke, S., et al. (2004). Decisional roles preference, risk knowledge, and information interests in patients with multiple sclerosis. *Multiple Sclerosis, 10*(6), 643–650.

Hope, T. (1996). *Evidence based patient choice*. London, United Kingdom: Kings Fund.

Legare, F., Bekker, H., & Desroches, S. (2010). Effective continuing professional development for translating shared decision making in primary care: A study protocol. *Implementation Science, 5*, 83. doi:10.1186/1748-5908-5-83

Legare, F., Elwyn, G., Fishbein, M., et al. (2008). Translating decision-making into healthcare clinical practices: Proof of concepts. *Implementation Science, 3*(2). doi:10.11866/1748-5908-3-2

Legare, F., Stacey, D., Gagnon, S., et al. (2011). Validating a conceptual model for an inter-professional approach to shared decision-making: A mixed method study. *Journal of Evaluation in Clinical Practice, 17*(4). doi:10.1111/j.1365-2753.2010.01515.x

Makoul, G., & Clayman, M. L. (2006). An integrative model of shared decision making in medical encounters. *Patient Education and Counseling, 60*(3), 301–312.

Melnyk, B., & Fineout-Overholt, E. (2015). *Evidence-based practice in nursing and healthcare. A guide to best practice.* (3rd ed.). Philadelphia, PA: Wolters Kluwer.

Muntean, W. (2012). Nursing clinical decision-making: A literature review. Paper commissioned by the National Council of State Boards of Nursing.

O'Connor, A. M., Llewellyn-Thomas, H. A., & Flood, A. B. (2004). Modifying unwarranted variations in health care: Shared decision-making using patient decision aids. *Health Affairs, 23*(Suppl. 2). https://doi.org/10.1377/hlthaff.var.63

Pearson, A., Wiechula, R., Court, A., et al. (2005). The JBI model of evidence-based healthcare. *International Journal of Evidence-Based Healthcare, 3,* 207–215.

Pravikoff, D. S., Tanner, A. B., & Pierce, S. T. (2005). Readiness of U.S. nurses for evidence-based practice. *American Journal of Nursing, 105,* 40–45.

Silow-Carrol, S., Alteras, T., & Stepnick, L. (2006). *Patient-centered care for underserved populations: Definition and best practices.* Washington, DC: Economic and Social Research Institute.

Thistlewaite, J., Evans, R., Tie, R., et al. (2006). Shared decision making and decision aids—a literature review. *Australian Family Physician, 35*(7), 537–540.

Towle, A., & Goldolphin, W. (1999). Framework for teaching and learning informed shared decision making. *British Medical Journal, 319,* 766–771.

Vogel, B. A., Bengel, J., & Helmes, A. W. (2008). Information and decision making: Patients needs and experiences in the course of breast cancer treatment. *Patient Education and Counseling, 71*(1), 79–85.

Volis, C., Sandelowski, M., Dahm, P., et al. (2008). Selective adherence to antihypertensive medications as a patient-driven means to preserving sexual potency. *Patient Preference and Adherence, 2,* 201–206.

CHAPTER **13**

Apply and Implement II
Individual Nurse Implementation

Lisa Hopp

LEARNING OBJECTIVES

- Given a clinical scenario, identify the problem that is amenable to using evidence to inform an individual nurse's decision to intervene.

- Discuss common barriers and nurses' characteristics that relate to their use of research.

- Explore the concept of knowledge translation and how it relates to using evidence in nursing practice.

- Considering common barriers and facilitators for using evidence in individual nurse's daily practice, develop a plan to overcome these barriers.

- List evidence-based strategies related to improving how nurses implement evidence.

KEY WORDS

Academic detailing
Audit and feedback
Conceptual research utilization
Context
Implementation science
Instrumental research
  utilization

Knowledge translation (KT)
Opinion leaders
Patient-mediated strategies
Persuasive research utilization
Reminders

Clinical Story

The first sign of trouble in Ms. B's breathing is the telltale wheeze that Rory could hear without a stethoscope. When she sees Ms. B. in the emergency department's (ED) triage area at 3 a.m., Rory knows that she needs to move the patient to the back for treatment immediately. Ms. B. is 20 years old and her family physician diagnosed her asthma just a few days prior to her visit to the ED. When she arrives, Ms. B. has a difficult time speaking because of her shortness of breath. Her respiratory rate is 22 breaths per minute. She is sitting upright and working hard to breath. Rory listens to her chest and hears distant breath sounds and expiratory wheezes. The ED physician immediately orders a nebulizer treatment with a fast-acting bronchodilator. Within about 15 minutes of the treatment, Ms. B. begins to feel better; her respiratory rate decreases and she can talk more easily. She tells Rory she has been taking inhaled medicines since her physician prescribed them, but she wasn't sure if she was using the inhaler correctly. She says she recognized her symptoms but then began to panic as her wheezing and chest tightness seemed to worsen. She tells Rory she just didn't know what to do.

In her years as a nurse, Rory has seen many patients in the ED who cannot recognize and care for their early asthma symptoms. She knows that a patient needs to use the right technique for the inhaled medications to reach the bronchioles. She also knows that if patients wait until they have audible wheezing and chest tightness, they may have waited too long for the rescue inhaler to work. Rory wants to use the best evidence to teach her young patient how to control her asthma as much as possible to avoid future hospital visits and the fear associated with severe shortness of breath. Ms. B. will be discharged from the ED in about an hour, so Rory needs to find the best evidence and tools for teaching quickly.

To start her search, Rory thinks about the issues facing Ms. B. that she can feasibly address, and she prioritizes these issues. Rory is highly motivated to find the right answers to help Ms. B. because she has seen patients newly diagnosed with asthma return to the emergency room in distress many times. Even though she has only a short amount of time to work with patients once their attack is controlled, she knows can make an impact when they have recovered from the severe symptoms but she must focus on some "just-in-time" teaching. To help Ms. B. and future patients, Rory wants to provide the best resources and information that she can.

Think Before You Read

- What are barriers to using evidence to support everyday decision making in nursing practice?
- How does the context of care potentially shape how you might use evidence in your decision making?

- What would be the best tools to help Rory translate what the evidence suggests as the right way(s) to intervene?
- What strategies might be important to influence other nurses to use evidence in their decision making?

Introduction

Clinical reasoning and decision making are at the center of nursing care. Individual nurses decide how and when to assess patients; they identify problems and make diagnoses; they select, implement, and evaluate their interventions. At each step, they need to use information to make the best decisions. The evidence-based practice movement calls for this information to be based on the best available evidence from research. In the previous chapters, you learned that evidence is rarely the only factor to consider. Patient preferences, clinician expertise, and available resources also play roles in the decision-making process. In addition to using evidence to inform their decisions, nurses do not make decisions in a vacuum. They are part of the clinician–patient/family relationship and members of a patient care unit, a multidisciplinary team, a health-care organization, and a public health context. In this chapter, you will learn how to use evidence in your everyday decision making as an individual practitioner. Although you make autonomous decisions for which you are accountable, you make these decisions in the midst of many influences in your practice setting (Box 13■1).

BOX 13■1 Significance of Individual Implementation of Evidence in Nursing Practice

---

- When nurses do not use the evidence from research and other sources, uptake is slow and patient outcomes may be affected.
- Research use may take the form of influencing others, changing thinking or actual practices.
- The characteristics of the evidence, setting, and nurse affect how individual nurses use evidence.
- Clinical context including organizational culture, leadership, and evaluation practices can positively and negatively affect how bedside nurses use evidence.
- Individual characteristics that are more likely associated with research utilization are holding an advanced practice degree, being in a leadership role, practicing in a specialty area (e.g., critical care, diabetes care), and being satisfied in the job.

Nurses and Research Utilization

Research utilization is one aspect of the evidence-based practice process. For several decades, nurse researchers have studied how nurses use research, yet a research–practice gap remains. Uptake of research is not fast or consistent enough, so patients do not consistently benefit from the investment in research and may even be harmed because of slow uptake (Squires, Estabrooks, Gustavsson, et al, 2011). A number of researchers have studied how nurses perceive how they use research. Squires, Hutchinson, Bostrom, et al (2011) conducted a systematic review to identify and analyze how nurses use evidence in their practice. They searched the international literature, including in both English and Scandinavian languages. They retrieved 133 articles from an initial list of 12,418 titles, with the most recent titles published in March 2008. After using standard tools to appraise all of the articles they retrieved, they ultimately included 55 studies of varying research designs. They found researchers used several different tools to measure nurses' research use, and they summarized the level of research use with a simple "low to high" research use scale. The studies represented nurses from North America (71%), Europe (22%), Asia (5%), and Oceania (2%). The trend showed more studies were conducted after 1995, and nurses reported increasingly higher levels of research use since 1995. Overall, nurses classified their research use in the moderate-high level (the second highest level) (Squires, Hutchison, et al, 2011). The authors of this systematic review are cautious about the validity of the research and recommended further research to measure research use more directly.

The manner in which nurses use research is important and varies, depending on the person, the evidence, and the situation. Some researchers differentiate instrumental, conceptual, and persuasive ways of using research. In **instrumental research utilization,** you apply the research in some concrete way. For example, if a systematic review indicates a pressure-reducing bed surface is best for preventing pressure ulcers in at-risk adults and this causes nurses to change from a standard mattress to a specialized bed surface for certain patients, then they would be using research in an instrumental manner. In **conceptual research utilization,** you think differently after understanding research but do not change your behavior. Consider the following example: Nurses read about pregnant women's experience of being confined to bed because of the threat of premature labor, and they consider this research the next time they work with a pregnant woman who has been put on bedrest. However, they ultimately do not use the evidence to make a decision about counseling the patient on her activity. In **persuasive research utilization,** you use research to influence the others. For example, nurses might use evidence related to the effectiveness of bedrest in premature labor to persuade midwives when they make recommendations (Squires, Hutchinson, et al, 2011).

The evidence-based practice movement has changed the way nurses think about using research. Now, they focus on finding the best available evidence instead of just any piece of research. The goal is to use evidence in concrete, instrumental ways to improve patient outcomes. Moreover, the definition of evidence-based practice includes clinical expertise and patient preferences in the decision-making process.

Barriers to Evidence Utilization

Moving evidence into practice is the responsibility of both individual nurses and the organizational context in which they work. This means you, as an individual nurse, are accountable for using the best available evidence. However, you work within an organization, whether it is an acute care hospital, a community health agency, a long-term care setting, or some other type of health-care facility. Organizations, their leaders, and systems of care greatly affect how individual nurses use evidence; they share the responsibility for providing nursing care based on the best available evidence. Any individual nurse will find it difficult to use evidence if elements of the organization pose too many barriers. Similarly, organizations can create a positive context, making it easier for individual nurses to act and advance evidence uptake (Estabrooks, Scott, Squires, et al, 2008; McCormack, Kitson, Harvey, et al, 2002).

A great deal of literature exists related to barriers to evidence implementation. You need to be aware of these barriers so that you are able to anticipate common challenges you may face and to understand the complex process of moving evidence into practice. Barriers tend to cluster around the following themes: the nature of the evidence (e.g., amount, novelty, presentation of evidence, quality, accessibility), the setting (e.g., time, resources, support, leadership), and characteristics of the individual nurse (e.g., knowledge, time, attitude) (Jun, Kovner, & Stimpfel, 2016; Kajermo, Bostrom, Thompson, et al, 2010; Kent, Hutchinson, & Fineout-Overholt, 2009).

In the next chapter, you will learn more about these barriers and how important the organizational culture and systems are to the success of evidence implementation. This chapter explores what individual nurse characteristics are most important to successful implementation of evidence.

Individual Nurse Characteristics That Pose Barriers to or Aid Evidence Implementation

In a systematic review of barriers related to nurse characteristics, Kajermo et al (2010) found the top three hurdles to using research in practice were (1) nurses being unaware of research, (2) nurses not feeling capable of evaluating the quality of research, and (3) nurses being isolated from knowledgeable colleagues with whom they could discuss research. Closely related to these nurse characteristics were barriers related to organizational setting: insufficient time on the job to implement new ideas, insufficient time to read research, lack of authority for patient care procedures, unsupportive staff, and uncooperative physicians.

Pravikoff, Tanner, and Pierce (2005) surveyed a broad spectrum of practicing nurses in the United States. They found the most frequent individual barriers to using research in practice were the following: lack of time, lack of value for research in practice, lack of skills for using or accessing electronic information and databases, and difficulty understanding research. Subsequent research supports Pravikoff and colleagues' initial work and time. Lack of leadership support continues to be a barrier to individual uptake of evidence (McKinney, DelloStritto, & Branham, 2019).

Individual attributes can change if nurses are willing to learn information management skills, are open to using evidence, and are willing to learn more about judging the quality of evidence. Appraisal checklists that are brief and include hints about what to look for in the research are very helpful for the novice as well as the experienced appraiser (see Chapter 10). Nurses can build confidence in their appraisal skills by joining a journal club on their unit. In addition, clinical and academic educators can provide opportunities for nurses to acquire the appropriate skills and knowledge. Researchers have studied what conditions aid or slow the use of evidence in nursing practice. In a recent systematic review, Squires, Estabrooks, et al (2011) found the following individual nurse characteristics were more commonly associated with the use of research-based evidence:

- Having a positive attitude toward research
- Being engaged in research activities
- Having a greater tendency to seek information
- Holding a graduate degree
- Having certain professional characteristics

According to the review, nurses were more likely to use evidence if they held advanced practice degrees or leadership roles, practiced in a specialty area (e.g., critical care or diabetes care), or were satisfied in their jobs. Years of experience did not relate to evidence use (Squires, Estabrooks, et al, 2011). This evidence reinforces the need to remain curious, inquisitive, and interested in continuously searching for evidence that helps you provide the right intervention to the right patients in the right way at the right time.

Knowledge Translation—Part of the Implementation Puzzle

Although individual nurses are responsible and accountable for using the best available evidence to make clinical decisions, you still need to learn how to accomplish that goal. The next phase in the evidence-based practice movement begins with investigators focusing on how best to translate knowledge from research and other sources into everyday practice. Some refer to this process as **knowledge translation (KT).** Many countries, including Canada, the United States, the United Kingdom, and Australia, have developed programs to enhance the uptake of evidence. For example, the Canadian Institutes of Health Research (CIHR) has committed to integrating knowledge translation into its core mission. CIHR defines KT as "a dynamic and iterative process that includes synthesis, dissemination, exchange and ethically sound application of knowledge to improve the health of Canadians, provide more effective health services and products and strengthen the health care system" (Canadian Institutes of Health Research, 2016, Knowledge Translation—Definition, para. 1). This means that moving knowledge from research to practice does not happen in a linear fashion via a lone practitioner; it is not context free and may occur at the end or may be integrated throughout the research process. The implementation process requires the knowledge creators and the users to interact, reflect, revise, and reflect again on practice changes within their own environments. The tools and mechanisms of KT involve synthesizing multiple sources of knowledge (i.e., more than one study as well as other sources of knowledge such as local data, patient experiences, and clinician expertise) and novel, innovative ways of getting the information to the knowledge users (clinicians and patients).

Exchange is another important characteristic of effective KT. This step may be as simple as engaging patients and their families in the discussion and shared decision-making process about their care. It can be as complex as national and international networks of patients, researchers, and clinicians working together for evidence-based solutions.

You can become a part of future KT efforts by volunteering to take part in research or evidence-implementation projects. Some KT models indicate that you could be involved from the very inception of the research project by helping researchers identify important questions to your nursing practice and the health needs of your patients. If you become a part of the research process itself, you can help ensure the relevance of the findings and use the evidence in your practice to contribute to the advancement of the profession.

Context of Care

Although this chapter focuses on what the individual nurse can do to implement evidence in practice, it is important to recognize that this always occurs within a context that influences how and if change can happen. Context is a very broad concept with many definitions. Two groups have used a concept analysis approach to help clarify what context is and isn't. McCormack, Kitson, Harvey, et al (2002) defined **context** as "the environment or setting in which the proposed change is to be implemented" (McCormack et al, 2002, p. 96). According to the Promoting Action on Research Implementation in Health Services (PARIHS) framework (see Chapter 5 for more detail), context includes the subelements of organizational culture (e.g., values, beliefs, regard for individuals, how learning happens, teamwork), leadership (e.g., style, structures, roles, methods of teaching), and evaluation (e.g., feedback mechanisms, sources and methods of measurement) (McCormack et al, 2002). Squires, Graham, Bashir, et al (2019) expanded on this greatly by reviewing a wide range of literature in a very systematic manner. They identified 6 domains, 21 attributes, and 89 shared features organized in a hierarchical but interconnected manner that illustrates the complexity of context (Squires et al, 2019).

Many evidence-based practice models (see Chapter 5) take context into consideration in some manner. However, although there is broad recognition that context and organizational cultures affect the implementation of evidence, a systematic review of strategies for change in organizational culture indicates evidence is lacking about how to effectively change cultures (Parmelli, Flodgren, Beyer, et al, 2011).

Kent and McCormack (2010) note that the emphasis on quality, safety, and effectiveness in health care has caused organizational cultures to shift away from paternalistic, provider-centered care toward more patient-centered care. To work in this culture, practitioners need to change how they approach care, and nurses need to be reflective, critical-thinking, "knowledge-based doers" (p. 11).

In this chapter's clinical story, Rory is always pressed for time in the busy emergency department. Despite the rapidly changing conditions of the environment, she is open to using evidence to make a difference in the many patients she sees with acute exacerbations of asthma, but she must be able to trust the information she uses to advise her patients. She needs the skills to find the information quickly, to judge the quality of the information rapidly, and to use the tools to intervene within a short window of opportunity with her patient. Rory values the evidence from research, and she has good searching skills so she can quickly find evidence from the databases immediately available on the computers in the patient care bays and at the nurse's station. She must also understand she has the authority to make these decisions about using evidence in patient care; her manager and the organizational leaders not only support her but expect that she will use the evidence in collaboration with her patient.

Not all nurses in the United States and in other countries experience these ideal conditions. In this chapter's clinical story, Rory has an inquisitive mind, knowledge, and resources, which lead to her use of evidence. She did not have to overcome barriers such as no access to electronic databases, lack of skill or confidence to search and evaluate the evidence, or inadequate autonomy to pursue the issue. If she had to face these barriers, she may have discharged the patient without an evidence-based solution to address the patient's need to understand and manage her asthma symptoms.

From Question to Evidence

In previous chapters, you studied how to ask, acquire, and appraise the evidence to decide how to apply the evidence in a particular context while also considering the patient's values and preferences. Just as Rory did when she first assessed Ms. B., you can form a mental checklist to help you quickly move from messy, poorly structured problems to focused questions that will lead to the right evidence. For example, ask: What is at the center of the patient's condition that you can change? What are the nursing interventions that relate to the patient problem? If you keep the focus on the patient's needs, you will stay centered on the higher priority questions.

In the clinical story, Rory identifies that the patient needs to understand how to self-manage her asthma. This problem could generate many questions such as: What is the effectiveness of asthma self-care action plans (intervention) versus brief oral instruction (comparison) on frequency of asthma exacerbations (outcome) in newly diagnosed adult asthma patients (population)? Rory is time pressured and needs to find a brief summary of the evidence to help her counsel the patient. She searches "asthma self-care" in the JBI evidence database, which is available in the emergency room. She immediately finds two evidence summaries that fit the patient's problem—one on self-management and another on effective inhaler techniques. This type of evidence is ideal for point-of-care use. The summaries are short yet transparent, meaning Rory can immediately determine the level of evidence supporting each recommendation. In fact, she can see the original sources cited along with a summary of the type of evidence underpinning the recommendations (James, 2019).

If Rory did not have access to this type of evidence source, she could have generated several questions (see Chapter 8 for more information on questioning) from her mental checklist such as the following:

- What is the effect of a written self-management action plan that includes self-adjusting medications versus regular visits with a primary care provider on the number of return emergency room visits for acute exacerbations in patients with new diagnosis of asthma?
- What is the effect of regularly using a peak-flow meter (a handheld device that measures airflow) versus no self-monitoring to identify worsening symptoms in patients with asthma?
- What is the effect of time of day on the occurrence of wheezing, chest tightness, and cough in patients with asthma?
- What are effective ways to manage allergy-related triggers of bronchospasm and an asthma attack?

The experience of an acute exacerbation merits exploration as well. Rory could ask the following meaningfulness questions:

- What is the experience of dyspnea (shortness of breath) in patients in the midst of an acute exacerbation?
- What is the meaning of receiving a diagnosis of asthma?
- What is the meaning of avoiding allergic triggers and its impact on quality of life for people with asthma?

Implementing the Evidence

You have read about several conceptual frameworks and models to guide the evidence-based practice process. Once you have worked through the question, evidence search, and appraisal process, the next step is to apply the evidence. The model or framework that you choose will influence how you apply the evidence. In addition to theory, there is a growing body of research that supports how to improve the uptake or application of evidence. This evidence comes from KT and implementation science work. **Implementation science** means the "scientific study of methods to promote the systematic uptake of clinical research findings and other evidence-based practices into routine practice, and hence to improve the quality and effectiveness of health care. It includes the study of influences on healthcare professional and organizational behavior" (Eccles & Mittman, 2006, para. 2). Just as you use the evidence to determine the right intervention, you need to consider what works to apply evidence.

Several systematic reviews of implementation methods have already been conducted, but they reveal this is an emerging science and much remains to be learned. In addition, most of the completed studies relate to physician uptake of evidence-based guidelines (Table 13■1). Thompson, Estabrooks, Scott-Findley, et al (2007) reviewed the evidence related to enhancing research use in nursing practice. Despite screening over 8,000 titles in their initial search of multiple databases, only 4 studies met their quality criteria. The most frequent intervention to enhance research uptake was an educational meeting of some sort, but no study showed an increase in evidence uptake. Educational meetings with local opinion leaders and multidisciplinary committees showed more promise, but the authors concluded that current evidence has not produced much guidance on effective strategies (Box 13■2). In 2015, Yost, Ganann, Thompson, et al conducted the most comprehensive systematic review of strategies specifically aimed at nurses using evidence in their clinical decision making. Based on their analysis of 30 citations, there was too much variation among the studies and systematic reviews to make definitive recommendations. However, the authors concluded that there is value in educational efforts, the involvement of leadership is important to the success of implementation of evidence, and dyads (staff and leaders) working in tandem may improve the translation of evidence into practice (Gifford, Squires, Angus, et al, 2018; Yost et al, 2015).

In the clinical story, Rory is ready to use the evidence in the short time she has to work with Ms. B. Although she recognizes that asthma self-management can

TABLE 13■1 Strategies and Examples That May Promote Evidence Uptake

Strategy	Potential Application
[1]Audit and feedback	Observations and chart review to monitor adherence to evidence-based interventions for central-line infections with monthly feedback to the nursing care unit
[2]Reminders	Colored patient wrist bands indicating allergies and risks for falls or pressure ulcers
[3]Opinion leaders	Well-respected staff nurses give a demonstration of an evidence-based procedure and work one-to-one with other nurses to coach them through the procedure
[4]Patient-mediated interventions	When orienting patients and families to the hospital, inform them that everyone who enters the room should wash their hands or use the alcohol scrub before working with the patient
[5]Academic detailing	A nursing instructor from the local university works with the nursing staff to develop evidence-based interventions

[1]Jamtvedt, Young, Kristoffersen, et al, 2006; [2]Shojania, Jennings, Mayhew, et al, 2009; [3]Flodgren, Parmelli, Doumit, et al, 2007; [4]Fraenkel & McGraw, 2007; [5]O'Brien, Rogers, Jamtvedt, et al., 2006.

BOX 13 ▪ 2 **Interdisciplinary Rounds**

- Consider evidence from multiple disciplines when searching for the best evidence to make well-informed decisions.
- Join an interdisciplinary journal club to review research related to a topic of common interest.
- More systematic reviews of research exist related to strategies to promote individual physician adoption of evidence-based decisions. Brainstorm with other nurses how this research does or does not translate to nurse behaviors.
- Collaborate with other disciplines to build consensus around evidence-based patient care to increase the chance that practitioners use evidence.
- With physicians, physiotherapists, occupational therapists, and other professionals, discuss the use of patient-mediated interventions that result in empowering patients to urge their health-care providers to use evidence. What are their concerns and ideas about this strategy?
- Become a part of an interdisciplinary team to improve a patient outcome through the implementation of an evidence-based practice. How might you use audit and feedback, reminders, and prompts? For each discipline involved in the project, consider who would be the most effective opinion leader. Would an outside expert influence the adoption of the evidence?

---

be complicated for patients, she has just a brief opportunity to intervene and that shapes how she uses the evidence (Box 13▪3). After reading the one-page summary on asthma self-care, she focuses on three key goals for her intervention:

1. The patient will be able to demonstrate how to use a peak expiratory flow meter and record her measurement in a diary.
2. The patient will be able to demonstrate how to use a rescue inhaler.
3. The patient will be able to state what to ask her primary care provider to help her manage her asthma.

The evidence related to strategies to achieve these outcomes is ranked level I, the most trustworthy type, which is based on systematic reviews of randomized controlled trials, with grade A recommendations (strong support for application) (James, 2019). Rory gathers the equipment she needs (a peak expiratory flow meter and diary to record the reading, date, and time that accompanies the meter), a metered-dose inhaler with the appropriate medication (a handheld "puffer" device and short-acting bronchodilator to relax the airways), and a simple patient instruction pamphlet with brief directions on the use of the meter and inhaler as well as a reminder to schedule a visit with her primary care provider and a prompt for questions to ask her provider.

BOX 13■3 **Tools for Learning and Practice**

- Use brief, trustworthy pre-appraised evidence summaries when making individual decisions on the fly.
- Checklists, prompts, and reminders can be good memory aids and help all bedside practitioners use evidence in their everyday practice.
- Seek feedback from clinical audits to check your own adherence to evidence-based practices.
- Work with advanced practice nurses to uncover the best available evidence to create pre-appraised evidence sources about the high-frequency, high-impact nursing care interventions if no existing summaries are available.
- Provide patients and their families with information and resources that help them ask the right questions and engage in shared decision making, including the following:
  - Joint Commission Speak Up Program (http://www.jointcommission.org/speakup.aspx)
  - Agency for Healthcare Quality and Research consumer and patient information (http://www.ahrq.gov/consumer/)
  - Agency for Healthcare Quality and Research Health Tips (http://healthcare411.ahrq.gov/)
  - United Kingdom National Health Services Choices for consumers (http://www.nhs.uk/Pages/HomePage.aspx)
  - Explore Canadian Institutes of Health Research's Café Scientifique idea for developing a local consumer discussion or to take part in an online discussion (https://cihr-irsc.gc.ca/e/41750.html)

Engaging Patients in the Evidence That Affects Their Care

Nurses have long valued the idea that patients should be partners in their care. Recall that the definition of evidence-based practice includes patient preferences and values. But evidence related to the role of patients in shared evidence-based decision making is still emerging. In the previous chapter, you learned about the evidence that currently exists. Some of the key recommendations from this work (Buzza, Williams, Vander Weg, et al, 2010; Ford, Schofield, & Hope, 2002; Fraenkel & McGraw, 2007) include the following:

- Use plain language for explanations to ensure that patients understand their options.
- Explicitly encourage their participation.
- Provide an unhurried atmosphere of listening.

- Encourage patients to ask about the evidence-based approaches to care (activating the patient to encourage their providers to use evidence-based strategies).
- Use decision aids to help patients understand their alternatives.

In the clinical story, Rory closes the drapes so she can remain focused on what the patient says. Rory then sits down so she can maintain level eye contact, and she listens to her patient's main concerns about being able to manage her asthma. Ms. B. says she was very frightened by her attack, and she worries that it will happen again. She states she wants to take care of herself. Rory focuses her interventions on these issues. Rory tells Ms. B. there is good evidence that patients can manage their asthma with the help of a written action plan (James, 2019) and by working with their primary care provider. In addition, by using a peak flow meter, patients can better detect when their asthma is flaring so they can give themselves the right medicine to prevent worsening symptoms. Ms. B. is relieved and asks for more information. Rory teaches her how to perform a good measurement with the peak expiratory flow meter by blowing out as hard and fast as she can through the mouthpiece. In just a few tries, Ms. B. is able to reproduce her best measurement. Because her medicine has not completely opened her airway yet, the meter registers a decreased measurement. Rory discusses the result with Ms. B. and asks her to record the measurement, her current shortness of breath, and the time of day in the diary (4 a.m.). Rory emphasizes that patients often experience more bronchospasm and coughing during the nighttime than during the daytime. Next, Rory shows Ms. B. how to use the inhaler, emphasizing the need to coordinate activation of the inhaler by taking a deep breath in and then holding it as long as she can. Ms. B. practices first without activating the medicine and then demonstrates the technique with the medication as she still has some airflow limitation (the key breathing problem in asthma). Rory congratulates her on her good technique and again encourages her to record taking the medication in the diary.

After about 15 minutes, Rory returns to Ms. B. and asks her to repeat her peak flow measurement and to write it down. They are both happy to see that the measurement has improved. Rory assesses Ms. B.'s chest sounds one last time and is pleased to hear very few wheezes. Finally, Rory provides Ms. B. with the printed pamphlet of the techniques they discussed and asks Ms. B. to make sure she contacts her primary care provider the next day to schedule a return visit. Rory sits with her for 5 more minutes to generate the following questions that Ms. B writes down to ask her primary provider:

1. How often and when shall I measure my expiratory peak flow?
2. What medicine should I use and in what sequence should I use them when my expiratory flow decreases?
3. What is the written plan that I will use to take care of my asthma?
4. When should I call my primary care physician?
5. Under what circumstances should I go to the emergency room?

These are the top five questions based on Rory and Ms. B.'s shared concerns about Ms. B.'s condition and ability to manage her asthma. Ms. B. leaves the ED breathing better and armed with the information that Rory is confident reflects the best available evidence, represents the desires and preferences of the patient, and will help Ms. B. manage her asthma.

■ Summary

Bedside clinicians rarely make decisions in isolation or out of context. Rather, they are part of a larger system and environment that influence how they use evidence and make decisions. Barriers and facilitators of knowledge translation can arise from the individual practitioner, the evidence itself, or the context of the evidence implementation. Strategies to help individuals translate knowledge into practice include **audit and feedback, reminders, opinion leaders, patient-mediated interventions, academic detailing,** and combinations of these strategies (Box 13■1). When nurses engage patients in the process of knowledge translation, the patient preferences are honored, and the gap between research and practice narrows.

CHAPTER QUESTIONS

1. Think about a time when you were unsure about what to do in a certain clinical situation. What could be on your mental checklist to help you formulate a question that enables to you isolate the main questions and locate evidence?

2. Consider this scenario: You are searching for new employment as a bedside nurse. You are passionate about using evidence in your nursing practice. You want to determine whether the organization is an environment that would enable you to use evidence in your everyday practice. What are some questions that you would ask during your interview with the human resources representative, the nursing leader of the unit you are considering, and a staff nurse who currently works on the unit?

3. What are common individual barriers to using evidence that nurses commonly identify? How might you overcome those barriers to enhance how you and your colleagues use evidence?

4. Using a common search engine such as Google, search the term "knowledge translation." How are different organizations and national groups defining "knowledge translation" and supporting knowledge translation efforts? Do you think that knowledge translation is important to everyday nursing practice?

(continues on page 200)

CHAPTER QUESTIONS (continued)

5. Think about a routine nursing practice. How do you know that the practice is right? Have you questioned a nursing procedure or intervention in the past? Have you noticed any clinical reminders, prompts, or cues in your practice setting? How well have they worked? Did they represent an evidence-based practice? Does the effect of these strategies change over time?

6. Consider this situation: You are a staff nurse caring for a patient in a critical care unit. The unit policy limits visitors to 10 minutes on the even hours. You find yourself needing to frequently bend the rules because some families and their critically ill loved ones want to spend more time together and they want more flexibility to visit. How might you investigate whether this practice reflects the best available evidence? How might patients' and families' wishes be better incorporated to change the practice?

References

Buzza, C. D., Williams, M. B., Vander Weg, M. W., et al. (2010). Part II, provider perspectives: Should patients be activated to request evidence-based medicine? A qualitative study of the VA project to implement diuretics (VAPID). *Implementation Science, 5*(24). doi:10.1186/1748-5908-5-24

Canadian Institutes of Health Research. (2016). More about knowledge translation at CIHR. Retrieved from http://www.cihr-irsc.gc.ca/e/29418.html

Eccles, M. P., & Mittman, B. S. (2006). Welcome to *Implementation Science. Implementation Science, 1*(1). doi:10.1186/1748-5908-1-1

Estabrooks, C. A., Scott, S., Squires, J. E., et al. (2008). Patterns of research utilization on patient care units. *Implementation Science, 3*(31). doi:10.1186/1748-5908-3-31

Flodgren, G., Parmelli, E., Doumit, G., et al. (2007). Local opinion leaders: Effects on professional practice and health care outcomes. *Cochrane Database of Systematic Reviews, 2007*(1). doi:10.1002/14651858.CD000125.pub3

Ford, S., Schofield, T., & Hope, T. (2002). Barriers to the evidence-based patient choice (EBPC) consultation. *Patient Education and Counseling, 47*, 179–185.

Fraenkel, L., & McGraw, S. (2007). What are the essential elements to enable patient participation in medical decision making? *Journal of Internal Medicine, 22*, 6114–6119.

Gifford, W. A., Squires, J. E., Angus, D. E., et al. (2018). Managerial leadership for research using in nursing and allied health care professions: A systematic review. *Implementation Science, 13*, 127. doi:10.1186/s13012-018-0817-7

James, A. H. (2019). Evidence summary: Asthma educational interventions delivered to adults in the emergency department. The Joanna Briggs Institute EBP Database, JBI@Ovid, JBI7779.

Jamtvedt, G., Young, J. M., Kristoffersen, D. T., et al. (2006). Audit and feedback: Effects on professional practice and health care outcomes. *Cochrane Database of Systematic Reviews, 2006*(2). doi:10.1002/14651858.CD000259.pub2

Jun, J., Kovner, C. T. & Stimpfel, A. W. (2016). Barriers and facilitators of nurses' use of clinical practice guidelines: An integrative review. *International Journal of Nursing Studies, 60*, 54–68. https://doi.org/10.1016/j.ijnurstu.2016.03.006

Kajermo, K. N., Bostrom, A. M., Thompson, D. S., et al. (2010). The BARRIERS scale—the barriers to research utilization scale: A systematic review. *Implementation Science, 5*(32). doi:10.1186/1748-5908-5-32

Kent, B., Hutchinson, A. M., & Fineout-Overholt, E. (2009). Getting evidence into practice—understanding knowledge translation to achieve practice change. *Worldviews on Evidence-Based Nursing, 6*, 183–185. doi:10.1111/j.1741-6787.2009.00165.x

Kent, B., & McCormack, B. (2010). Context: Overview and application. In B. Kent & B. McCormack (Eds.), *Clinical context for evidence-based nursing practice*. West Sussex, United Kingdom: Wiley-Blackwell.

McCormack, B., Kitson, A., Harvey, G., et al. (2002). Getting evidence into practice: The meaning of "context." *Journal of Advanced Nursing, 38*(1), 94–104.

McKinney, I., DelloStritto, R. A., Branham, S. (2019). Nurses' use of evidence-based practice at point of care: A literature review. *Critical Care Nursing Quarterly, 42*, 256–264. doi:10.1097/CNQ.0000000000000266

O'Brien, M. A., Rogers, S., Jamtvedt, G., et al. (2007). Educational outreach visits: Effects on professional practice and health care outcomes. *Cochrane Database of Systematic Reviews, 2007*(4). doi:10.1002/14651858.CD000409.pub2

Parmelli, E., Flodgren, G., Beyer, F., et al. (2011). The effectiveness of strategies to change organisational culture to improve healthcare performance: A systematic review. *Implementation Science, 6*(33). doi:10.1186/1748-5908-6-33

Pravikoff, D. S., Tanner, A. B., & Pierce, S. T. (2005). Readiness of U.S. nurses for evidence-based practice. *The American Journal of Nursing, 105*(9), 40–51.

Shojania, K. G., Jennings, A., Mayhew, A., et al. (2009). The effects of on-screen, point of care computer reminders on processes and outcomes of care. *Cochrane Database of Systematic Reviews, 2009*(3). doi: 10.1002/14651858.CD001096.pub2

Squires, J. E., Graham, I., Bashir, K., et al. (2019). Understanding context: A concept analysis. *Journal of Advanced Nursing, 75*, 3448–3470. doi:10.1111/jan.14165

Squires, J. E., Estabrooks, C. A., Gustavsson, P., et al. (2011). Individual determinants of research utilization by nurses: A systematic review update. *Implementation Science, 6*(1). doi:10.1186/1748-5908-6-1

Squires, J. E., Hutchinson, A. M., Bostrom, A-M, et al. (2011). To what extent do nurses use research in clinical practice? A systematic review. *Implementation Science, 6*(21). doi:10.1186/1748-5908-6-21

Thompson, D. S., Estabrooks, C. A., Scott-Findlay, S., et al. (2007). Interventions aimed at increasing research use in nursing: A systematic review. *Implementation Science, 2*(15). doi:10.1186/1748-5908-2-15

Yost, J., Ganann, R., Thompson, D., et al. (2015). The effectiveness of knowledge translation interventions for promoting evidence-informed decision-making in tertiary care: A systematic review and meta-analysis. *Implementation Science, 10*(1), 1–15. doi:10.1186/s13012-015-0286-1

CHAPTER **14**

Apply and Implement III

Nursing Systems of Evidence Implementation

Beth Vottero

 LEARNING OBJECTIVES

- Distinguish among organizational, setting, and individual barriers to evidence implementation.
- Describe how the organizational culture affects evidence implementation.
- Explain how knowledge of system barriers can facilitate evidence implementation.
- Develop a planning process to minimize system barriers while maximizing system facilitators.
- Examine your own individual barriers and facilitators for evidence implementation.
- Identify potential implementation strategies.

 KEY TERMS

Accountability
Ad hoc committees
ANCC Magnet Recognition
  Program®
Authority to change practice
Barriers

Chief nursing officer/chief
  nursing executive
Embedded evidence
Empirical quality outcome
Enculturation
Facilitators

202

KEY TERMS (continued)

Forces of magnetism	**Organizational culture**
Implementation science	**Shared governance**
Journal clubs	**Structural supports**
Levels of administration	**Unit practice councils**
Magnet model	

Clinical Story

Ann is the quality representative on a critical care unit. As part of her responsibilities, she monitors data from catheter-associated urinary tract infections (CAUTI). Over the past two quarters she notices an increase in the number of CAUTIs on her unit. As a nurse-sensitive indicator, CAUTIs reflect the quality of care provided for catheterized patients. Ann is determined to make a change. Ann begins by reviewing the current evidence on care of patients with an indwelling urinary catheter. She then examines the organization's policies and protocols on the care of patients with an indwelling catheter to see if she can find discrepancies between the evidence and the policies. Finally, Ann looks at the current protocols. Ann believes that she could make a change but is unsure about how to go about it.

Think Before You Read

- What role do you think evidence should play in systems that are aimed at improving the quality of patient outcomes?
- What barriers might systems of care (e.g., the way that hospitals design and distribute policies) pose for individual nurses trying to use evidence-based practice in their everyday nursing practice?
- How does the organizational culture influence how nurses can use evidence to make clinical decisions?
- How might a nursing leader influence the success or failure of making an evidence-based change in nursing practice?

Introduction

The success of any evidence implementation project is directly associated with **organizational culture** (Squires, Aloisio, Grimshaw, et al, 2019). The culture of an organization is the bedrock for germinating new ideas and innovations. Why is organizational culture important? Similar to creating a garden, where starting with the right soil mix and fertilizer ensures healthier plants, organizational culture can foster opportunities and sustain integration of evidence implementation. The culture reflects the values of the organization, from the bedside nurse to the highest levels of administration.

You may have noticed that different organizations have different cultures, manifested in part through nurse-sensitive outcomes and nurse satisfaction, autonomy, and accountability over nursing practice as well as patient outcomes. Health-care organizations that nurture a culture of evidence demonstrate higher nursing satisfaction and lower turnover rates while maintaining positive patient outcomes (Mannion & Davies, 2018). However, the creation of such a culture is a multifaceted and complex endeavor, requiring the inclusion of nurses from the bedside to the boardroom. This leads us to the question, What are the **barriers** and **facilitators** to creating an effective culture for evidence implementation?

To understand barriers and facilitators, it helps to organize them in terms of organizational, setting, and individual. Organizational barriers and facilitators consist of management/administration priorities involving evidence-based practice processes, communication channels, organizational culture, and resources for skill development. Examples of setting barriers and facilitators include policies and procedures, design and type of unit, and the workload constraints that affect implementation of evidence-based practice. Finally, individual barriers and facilitators consist of nurse competence in evidence-based practice procedures, presence or lack of skills, and ability to apply research to practice.

Organizational Barriers and Facilitators

In the clinical story, Ann is positioned to affect a change in practice. As a first step, Ann approaches her director about her analysis of the data and redesigning care related to indwelling catheters. She believes that the current protocols should be reviewed against the best available evidence to support care, but is unsure about how to begin. The director recognizes an opportunity to meet the organizational goals of providing evidence-based care as well as aligning the **chief nursing officer**'s (CNO) or **chief nursing executive**'s (CNE) vision with nursing practice on the unit level. The CNO or CNE is the most senior nursing leader in the organization who is administratively responsible for all aspects of the nursing care such as budget, patient care services, and patient care outcomes. Sometimes the CNO or CNE carries the title of vice-president. The director encourages Ann to enlist other nurses' involvement during the next unit meeting.

Organizational Priorities

Although much of the duty for evidence-based practice falls on clinical nurses, the actuality is that evidence-based practice is a complicated undertaking requiring organizational dedication to embrace an evidence-based practice culture (Box 14■1). Organizational barriers strongly affect the ability of nurses to implement evidence. In the overall leadership structure, it is essential to have a CNO or CNE with a voice and vote to represent nursing and evidence-based practice at the organization's highest **levels of administration.** The administration includes all of the executive leaders in the organization who make critical financial, strategic, and patient care

> **BOX 14■1 Significance of Nursing Systems in Implementing Evidence**
>
> ■ Organizations that foster a culture of evidence have higher nurse satisfaction and a more stable workforce, and demonstrate positive patient outcomes (Mannion & Davies, 2018).
> ■ Leaders set the tone and expectations for the members of the organization.
> ■ Systems that enhance evidence uptake include effective communication channels; shared, decentralized governance structures; resource allocation; access to evidence; coaches; and mentors.
> ■ Evaluation systems that enhance evidence uptake provide meaningful, accessible data and feedback mechanisms that are timely, individualized, and focused.

decisions on behalf of all aspects of the agency. Embedding a value for evidence-based practice at the administrative level ensures that leadership of the entire organization shares the same goals. Subsequently, evidence-based practice becomes an essential part of the strategic plan for the organization. To facilitate evidence-based practice, direct care nurses need an advocate at the highest levels to obtain resources in finance, human resource, operations, technology, quality information, and procurement as well as from other departments in the facility. The CNO/CNE is positioned to initiate critical conversations on evidence-based practice with an opportunity to provide a clear vision for the entire organization.

Similarly, the CNO/CNE's ability to understand and support evidence implementation reflects down the hierarchy to middle management's appreciation for evidence-based nursing practice. Unit managers/directors must have explicit expectations to grow a climate that values and supports evidence-based practice. The CNO/CNE functions as a catalyst, bringing together the appropriate high-level administrative entities and the middle management layer to ensure that the direct care nurse has the necessary resources to implement evidence into practice. The ability of middle management to cultivate interest and opportunities for EB initiatives is the beginning of culture development. In the clinical story, the director recognizes how Ann's project is aligned with the organization's values.

Organizational Culture

Enculturation—the process of being socialized to a culture—of evidence-based practice as an organizational value has a strong impact on frontline nursing. To understand the true barriers to evidence-based practice implementation, one must be aware of nurse-identified management issues. Such barriers include a lack of interest, motivation, leadership, vision, strategy, and direction (DiCenso, 2003). To counteract such barriers, organizations have initiated ongoing leadership development, communication training, and education on evidence-based practice and coaching and mentoring skills. Some facilities use outside consultants, whereas others work with professional organizations such as the American Organization for Nursing

Leadership (AONL) or the American Nurses Credentialing Center (ANCC) to offer preparation courses for certification as a nurse executive. The American Nurses Association's (ANA) certification requires that candidates are well versed in the body of knowledge, consisting of leadership and management styles, theoretical underpinnings of management, culture development, and strategic planning. These skills are essential for progressing an organizational culture and philosophy that is founded on evidence-based practice.

The CNO/CNE can instill **accountability** for evidence-based practice implementation into performance evaluations for middle nursing management. This includes setting explicit expectations for developing evidence-based practice opportunities. Middle managers are charged with the task of creating an environment supportive of practice innovations, and assume direct responsibility for setting the stage for evidence-based nursing practice. When looking at the clinical story, it is clear that Ann's manager supported her initiative and promoted involvement of other nurses. Identifying potential facilitators, supporting time to work on the project, bringing key stakeholders to the table, and acquiring access to databases for literature reviews make up some actions that middle management take to support nurse-driven initiatives. Managers also must learn how to gather and watch how data are trending regarding the effectiveness of evidence-based practice initiatives. Supportive documentation exposes the degree of enculturation for evidence implementation projects, including the significance for enhancing patient outcomes.

Adding an evidence-based practice component to the nurse's position description, leveled for educational preparation, can support commitment to evidence-based practice. Clearly detailing expectations for evidence-based practice increases nurse awareness and responsibility for providing evidence-based care. In 2003, the Institute of Medicine (IOM) initiated discussion on the need to include evidence-based practice processes in the education of health-care workers through their publication, *Health Professions Education: A Bridge to Quality*. The IOM proposed that all health-care professionals be educated to deliver patient-centered care as members of an interdisciplinary team, emphasizing evidence-based practice, quality improvement approaches, and informatics (IOM, 2003). For direct care nurses, the expectation could include identifying practice issues, using organizational resources to develop an evidence-based project, creating a PICO question, participating in an evidence-based project, becoming a member of the research committee, or attending educational offerings that increase awareness of research and evidence-based nursing practice. When the position description includes evidence-based practice processes, there must be coexisting structural supports to help nurses achieve expected performance levels.

Communication

A key to successful implementation of evidence-based practice organization-wide is having clear channels of communication. This is important when working on evidence-based practice projects on a unit within a larger organization. Communication allows a sharing of ideas, thoughts, practices, challenges, and promotes collaboration

BOX 14■2 **Interdisciplinary Rounds**

■ All disciplines contribute to the organizational culture, including the chief executives of various disciplines such as nursing, medicine, and information services.
■ Most problems affect other disciplines. For example, preventing CAUTIs requires collaboration and cooperation among nurses, nursing care technicians, physicians, infectious disease professionals, quality and safety officers, purchasing and supply chain managers, clinical educators, advanced practice nurses, finance officers, and risk managers.
■ Some disciplines, like nursing, affect how evidence informs practice directly because they are at the point of care. Other disciplines, such as purchasing and supply chain managers, affect how the organization uses evidence indirectly because they influence the structures important to evidence uptake. For example, those who make decisions about what urinary catheter to buy must understand the evidence related to the effectiveness of one catheter type over another.
■ Magnet-recognized facilities promote interdisciplinary engagement by creating structures for nurses to participate in diverse teams and work groups.
■ Depending on the problem you approach, the departmental leaders can either facilitate or pose barriers to evidence implementation.
■ Effective and respectful interdisciplinary communication helps move evidence into practice and creates a positive organizational culture.

among various units and disciplines (Box 14■2). For example, if another unit revises its CAUTI care practices, the sharing of their experience and knowledge could help Ann with her project. In addition, communication is significant for enhancing collaboration between disciplines (Zwarenstein, Goldman, & Reeves, 2009). An essential piece of any nursing care project is the input from other disciplines. If Ann were to work on her project without the input from other areas such as laboratory personnel, physicians, or infection control staff, she might lose out on some wonderful opportunities to bring in various elements needed for a successful project. Laboratory information affects turnaround time for urinalysis results. Physician collaboration assists by creating orders responsive to the patient's need and nurse's judgment for catheter removal. Infection control's participation includes bringing data from CAUTI rates to the table and determining effective practice changes.

One method for enhancing communication is a functional and ingrained **shared governance** structure. Ideally, when a functional shared governance structure is in place, nurses are given the power, autonomy, and authority to control nursing practice. Porter-O'Grady defined three principles of professional nursing shared governance: it is "grounded in practicing nurse accountability; structures are built around professional accountability and clinical decision-making; and professional

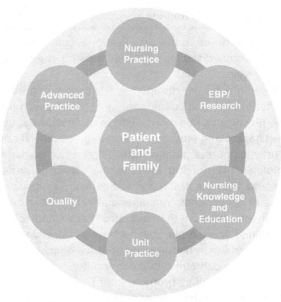

FIGURE 14■1 Example of a shared governance council structure

governance structures reflect distributive decision-making" (2019, p. 37). Organizations with strong shared governance structures are shown to demonstrate sustained evidence-based practice integration (Rycroft-Malone, 2008). One of the **forces of magnetism** (American Nurses Credentialing Center, 2019) is decentralized decision making, whereby nurses throughout an organization are engaged in self-governance and forums to address practice issues (related to Force of Magnetism #2: Organizational Structure). A variety of shared governance structures are found in the literature, the most common being the council format. In this model, councils are created based on functions (quality, research, evidence-based practice, education, advocacy, retention/recruitment, etc.) and include nursing representation (Fig. 14■1). The different councils work toward improving patient care and the patient/family experience. With the patient/family at the center, the model ensures that all issues keep a focus on the patient and family. Unit-based councils focus on specific unit practice issues; they are the only councils that include direct care nurses on each specific unit. All other councils have a representation and a voice to promote communication of issues.

Establishing a formal communication configuration allows the sharing of ideas among all areas. For example, **ad hoc committees** can develop from the original group, allowing key stakeholders to work with nurses to support implementation of evidence-based practice innovations. Ad hoc committees are formed by the owner of the project to address short-term issues. Composition of the committee includes experts in the area, those directly affected by the practice, and both managers and direct care nurses. The committee works solely on the identified issue, then disbands after completion of the project.

In the clinical story at the beginning of the chapter, Ann presented her project at the unit practice council meeting. Two other nurses expressed an interest in working with Ann on the project. Ann also communicated her ideas to the evidence-based practice council as a project proposal. To help Ann and her team, the committee suggested working with a mentor who could help work through the process of an evidence-based practice project with the team. The evidence-based practice council works in concert with the other councils to establish a roster of nurses who possess training and experience in evidence-based practice processes. From this roster, an appropriate mentor is contacted and agrees to work with Ann and her team.

Resources at the Organizational Level

Organizational support for evidence-based practice is critical, especially in organizations where nurses think they lack the authority, autonomy, or power to implement a change in patient care practices (Kueny, Shever, Mackin, et al, 2015). Such barriers relate to the critical need for leadership styles that promote a patient-centered environment in which nurses believe they are valued and incorporate a learning culture that encourages evidence-based practice. To counteract the barriers, some organizations create evidence-based practice councils, teams, mentors, interdisciplinary councils, and evidence-based, practice-focused education, all designed to support nurse participation in evidence-based practice. Such tools and resources can effectively promote evidence-based practice when used in conjunction with leadership empowerment for nurse participation.

A critical need exists for collaboration with physicians on evidence-based practice initiatives from a big picture perspective. Having a physician champion does not mean that nursing initiatives must transform into medical projects. Rather, a physician champion opens doors to medical staff committees that might have a piece of your evidence-based practice puzzle. For instance, in the clinical story, Ann wants to change current practice based on a review of the evidence for CAUTIs. The new protocol may require changes in treatment, including pharmacology management. Having a physician champion on board at the beginning of discussions can minimize problems later during implementation. During the stages of protocol development, the physician champion becomes a communication conduit between the CAUTI committee and physician committees. Issues, problems, concerns, and ideas are discussed during development, minimizing the chance that opposition will arise during implementation.

To appreciate the big picture of potential barriers and **facilitators** from an organizational perspective, it helps to see how the structure and resources can affect evidence integration (Box 14■3). It is clear that consideration of organizational issues affecting evidence integration is widespread and varied. Having a basic understanding of such issues can help you identify your own organization's potential problem areas as well as highlight exemplary processes.

BOX 14■3 **Tools for Learning and Practice**

■ Ask for an organizational chart to understand the reporting structure in your organization.
■ Find out if your organization has an evidence-based practice council and determine whether you are eligible to participate on the council or find out who your representative is.
■ When planning a unit-level or systemwide evidence-based change, use tools to assess the organizational culture, context, and stakeholders:
  ■ Use the Context Assessment Index (related to the i-PARIHS model) to determine the strengths of leadership, evaluation methods, and organizational culture.
  ■ Use the Guideline Implementation Toolbox available from the Registered Nurses' Association of Ontario to analyze a system's readiness for change, stakeholders, and to plan implementation strategies (http://www.rnao.org/Storage/12/668_BPG_Toolkit.pdf)
  ■ Systematically identify barriers and promoters of change.
■ Work with an advanced practice nurse to help you find, appraise, and plan change.
■ Engage your information technology team to create quick links to excellent evidence-based sources available through one-click on your unit's desktops.
■ Support and get involved with policy committees to make evidence transparent and embedded in the policy.
■ Participate in journal clubs and encourage peers to join.

Setting Barriers and Facilitators

Organizations with successful evidence integration have something in common; each embeds evidence into policies, procedures, clinical pathways, standards, protocols, and documentation systems (Zwarenstein et al, 2009). These actions build strong structural supports that externalize the internal cultural value for evidence-based nursing practice. When providing care for a specific patient population and diagnosis, such as asthmatic children or adults with heart failure, pathways or protocols prescribe nursing interventions. When based on evidence, the pathway or protocol can increase the likelihood of achieving desired patient outcomes.

Ann's team has worked diligently for over a month on the new protocol. During one meeting, a team member tells the group that besides her normal 40-hour workweek, she has put in at least 20 hours per week of her own time on the project. The other team members agree that the project is time-consuming, provides no reimbursement, and is beginning to affect their family life. The team members also discuss difficulties accessing databases, not knowing how to search effectively, and needing help to find articles. Ann can feel the group's enthusiasm starting to wane and decides to speak to the director about the new issues.

Time Constraints

Nurses very commonly perceive that insufficient time poses a primary setting barrier to being able to implement new practices (Geerligs, Rankin, Shepherd, et al, 2018). These time constraints include short staffing, lack of time for patient care, too much work, and high patient acuity. In addition, nurses may believe that time constraints extended to personal time (Kueny et al, 2015). All are valid and pertinent points. You may have considered the amount of time needed for developing and instituting an evidence-based practice project and wondered how you will incorporate it into your nursing practice. Strategies to overcome the time barrier require an organizational commitment to evidence-based nursing practice. For example, the CNO/CNE can develop and support a policy allowing paid time off for working on research or evidence-based practice that directly relates to the area of nursing. In addition, the unit director or manager may allow time off to work on initiatives that improve the quality of care. In both cases, the key issue is that nurses need dedicated time away from direct care responsibilities to work on evidence implementation.

Ann speaks to her director about the concerns of the group. The director acknowledges the validity of the concerns and agrees to bring it up to the CNO/CNE. During the meeting, both identify the need to support direct care nurses engaged in evidence-based practice initiatives and brainstorm on creative ways to meet the need for time release. A unique feature of their organization is the presence of a highly functioning and nurse-dedicated foundation. The foundation agrees to fund half a nurse's salary for 1 month while working on an evidence-based practice project and promises to expand the program up to a total of five nurses per year. The program allows Ann's team to split the time off and continue with the project.

Resource Availability

Another organizational characteristic involves resources available to nurses. In the clinical story, Ann's team quickly identified the need to access databases to review the literature on catheterized patients. When you encounter a practice issue, you will need to have accessible and reliable databases for reviewing the literature. Professional literature is essential for developing a change in practice that is consistent with best evidence (Pravikoff, Tanner, & Pierce, 2005). This step requires a dedicated budget for purchasing appropriate library resources. The economics of health care makes it important to have a champion at the administrative level that values knowledge generation and defends the need for budget allocations. Imagine if Ann and her team did not have access to the necessary literature; the entire project would have been compromised.

Having accessible databases demonstrates the dedication of the organization for knowledge growth. In addition, an experienced on-staff librarian can help immensely when locating appropriate and reliable literature. Some smaller organizations employ a librarian for use by both physicians and nurses, whereas others have dedicated staff for each department. The function and title of a hospital-based librarian varies in each facility. Some may combine several duties together, whereas other facilities maintain a pure librarian position. However it is handled in your organization, you should be familiar with the structure and position of the librarian, as he or she will become an invaluable resource to you.

Even with database resources, the logistics of accessing information can still be a barrier. Having Internet access throughout the units with the ability to acquire full-text articles or guidelines on the nursing unit is significant to linking evidence to the point of care. Minimizing the steps nurses must perform to get the evidence into practice facilitates the process. Some of the more technologically advanced health-care organizations have **embedded evidence** into their charting systems by linking policies, protocols, and pathways to specific nursing care instances. For example, while caring for a patient with ventilator-acquired pneumonia (VAP), the nurse is prompted to perform certain care when entering information into the patient's medical record. A link to the protocol allows the nurse to access the evidence-based care interventions at the point of care.

Some organizations, recognizing the need to provide strong **structural supports** for evidence-based practice, have created dedicated nursing education departments. These departments go beyond teaching; they can also include primary responsibility for purchasing and maintaining resources such as databases and memberships for the organization. Education departments identify the learning needs of the organization and develop or bring in experts to meet such needs. The departments also help make connections between those desiring to work on an evidence-based project and those experienced in the processes. For example, Kaiser Permanente, a large health-care organization in California, wanted to expand its nursing workforce's knowledge of research and evidence-based practice. The organization's Nursing Education Department developed a Nursing Pathways Web site devoted to knowledge generation and dissemination (https://www.kpnursing.org/research/index.html). This action allows nurses to expand their understanding of evidence-based practice and share initiatives throughout the organization.

Dedicated mentors, well versed in evidence-based practice processes, can provide a support mechanism for initiating and sustaining evidence-based practice initiatives. Having someone knowledgeable in the process of crafting a question from a practice issue, experienced in searching the literature, and familiar with the organizational policies for putting evidence into practice is vital for constructing an evidence-based practice culture. Some larger organizations employ a dedicated nurse researcher. Smaller organizations may have nurse mentors who are practicing nurses experienced in evidence-based practice processes. Regardless of how the process is handled, having available mentors demonstrates organizational commitment toward initiating and sustaining an environment for evidence-based practice.

Even with available time for evidence-based practice, adequate database resources, a mentor to assist in the process, support from management, and Internet access, other unexpected issues can still arise. The key is that with the aforementioned support mechanisms, most of the other barriers can be overcome or minimized to increase an organization-wide culture for evidence-based practice.

Individual Barriers and Facilitators

Ann's team completes the project and is ready to present their protocol and supportive evidence to the unit's practice council. While preparing for the meeting, Ann begins to think that she might not be able to affect changes in practice, even though she knows that the team developed a valid process and is confident in the project findings.

Individual barriers consist of both intrinsic and extrinsic factors such as lack of knowledge and skills, uncertainty about how to proceed with a project or formulate a question, belief that the goal of implementing evidence-based practice is unattainable, heavy workloads, lack of resources, and minimal support (Geerligs, et al, 2018). Research shows that there are six individual determinants that affect evidence implementation at the individual level; beliefs and attitudes, information seeking, education, professional characteristics, and involvement in research activities (Estabrooks, Floyd, Scott-Findlay, et al, 2003). Education about evidence-based practice processes is fundamental to building the foundation for an evidence-based practice culture but is most effective when lack of knowledge is identified as a primary barrier. A multifaceted approach includes seminars and workshops. The education is most effective when it is highly interactive, the content is highly relevant, and nursing leaders indicate that attendance is important. Education by itself will probably not change complex behaviors (Forsetlund, Bjorndal, Rashidian, et al, 2009). Healthcare opinion leaders providing educational outreach are successful in reducing bias.

Implementation Science

Implementation science is the study of "methods to promote the systematic uptake of research findings and other evidence-based practices into routine practice, and, hence, to improve the quality and effectiveness of health services and care" (Eccles & Mittman, 2006). Implementing a change in practice requires you to attend to how you implement the change. Selecting appropriate implementation strategies can mean the difference between a successful project and one that may fail over time. Selecting appropriate strategies requires attention to the context for which the change is designed and the stakeholders integral to the change. There are four functional groups of implementation strategies: "(1) build health information technology to support data-informed quality improvement (QI); (2) build QI capacity and improve outcomes; (3) enhance clinician and practice member knowledge; (4) build community connections and patient involvement" (Perry, Damschroder, Hemler, et al, 2019). Commonly used implementation strategies can be viewed in Table 14■1.

Beliefs and Attitudes

A frequently cited individual barrier to evidence implementation is the nurses' perception that they did not feel they had the **authority to change practice** (Brown, Wickline, Ecoff, et al, 2009). This brings up an interesting question: If nurses do not have control over their practice, then who does? Contrary to what some nurses

TABLE 14■1 **Common Implementation Strategies**

Implementation Strategy	Definition
Audit and Feedback	Collect data on the change and report back
Educational Outreach	Trained person provides education in the practice setting
Local Opinion Leaders	Train those with influence in the practice setting to adopt change and sway opinion
Early Adopters	Identify early adopters and learn from their experiences with the change
Tailor Strategies	Personalize the implementation strategies to the specific context barriers
Conduct Cyclical Tests of Change	Implement change for a small group and conduct tests to inform modifications

Source: Powell, B. J., Waltz, T. J., Chinman, M. J., et al. (2015). A refined compilation of implementation strategies: results from the Expert Recommendations for Implementing Change (ERIC) project. *Implementation Science, 10*, 21. doi:10.1186/s13012-015-0209-1

may believe, nurses absolutely have authority to change practice and should take control of the process. The bigger issue is the reason that nurses feel this way and what can be done to counteract it. This feeling can be related to the culture of the organization as well as an understanding of the professional nursing concepts of accountability and autonomy.

Continuity of care is another means of supporting nurses in applying evidence-based practice. When nurses have the same assigned patients (i.e., a caseload), they not only develop relationships with their patients, but they also have the opportunity to learn about their patients' preferences. When nurses' patient assignments change each day, they cannot easily identify subtle changes in their patients' status. They will need more time to understand trends, to apply interventions for the specific patient's care needs, and to see outcomes from interventions when the patient load varies.

It helps when there is a structure in place for nurses to bring practice issues forward. **Unit practice councils** or similar formal venues allow nurses to voice their concerns and be involved in making practice changes. Councils, made up of direct care nurses, allow exploration of practice issues and create opportunities for supporting evidence-based practice. Such formats encourage all nurses to take an active role in deciding how nursing care will be provided. Consider in the clinical story how Ann was part of a unit practice council with a direct link to larger, hospital-wide nursing councils. The larger nursing councils also had a direct link to various committees made up of management. How would the progression and sustainability of the initiative change if this chain of support and communication were not present?

Education

Knowledge of research, including how to read, understand, and assimilate findings, can be a barrier to evidence-based initiatives. It is estimated that 37.9% of direct care nurses possess an associate's level degree (HRSA, 2008). Because of this, research knowledge and skills cannot be expected from nurses who have not had formal education on this topic. To counteract this, many facilities have initiated RN-BSN or RN-MSN program affiliations with academic partners. Such partnerships bring a twofold benefit to the organization. First, the partnership supports the continuation of professional development for nurses by encouraging formal education for the nursing staff. Second, it links academic resources to the organization. For some organizations, this partnership has helped to formalize research committees and journal clubs and provided research opportunities for educators.

Other organizations have turned to advanced practice nurses (APNs) to help support evidence-based initiatives. In particular, **clinical nurse specialists** (CNSs) are APNs with master's or doctoral degrees and they are prepared with a specialty focus and are able to lead practice change at multiple levels, including influencing individual nurses, units, and systems (National Association of Clinical Nurse Specialists [NACNS], 2018). Having access to APNs such as CNSs is essential to the enculturation and sustainability of evidence-based initiatives. Depending on the organization and role delineation for APNs, such nurses can provide mentorship, guidance, facilitation, and dissemination for evidence-based nursing practice (Rycroft-Malone, 2008).

In the clinical story, the mentor for the CAUTI project is Mary, who is an MSN. Mary is the medical-surgical CNS who volunteers to work with Ann and the team on their project. She begins by helping them develop a PICO question and provides guidance on available resources for searching the literature. Mary also is available to answer questions and help develop an understanding of evidence-based practice. She helps the team to develop a protocol for catheterized patients and provides assistance with various committee approvals by attending meetings and supporting their project.

The clinical story demonstrates how an APN was accessible and supportive of the evidence-based initiative. Her ability to guide Ann through the processes helped move the project forward. If Ann did not have a mentor, guide, facilitator, and support system, she would have expended a large amount of time learning before doing, which could lead to frustration and discouragement, and to dropping the project. Of course, a project can be completed, and done well, without an APN; if the team is lacking knowledge of processes involved with evidence-based practice, an APN can provide needed mentorship. Research knowledge and mentoring support is an effective facilitator for evidence-based practice, especially when an APN is involved (Rycroft-Malone, 2008).

The i-PARIHS model suggests that you will more likely be able to implement evidence when the organizational culture, leadership, and evaluation processes are strong and facilitators such as CNSs have excellent skills, and clear roles and purposes (Harvey & Kitson, 2016). Until evidence-based practice processes are integrated and standardized into academic nursing curriculums, having a mentor who is knowledgeable and experienced in evidence-based practice is essential to the success of a project.

Involvement in Research Activities

Journal clubs have gained popularity in recent years. Such clubs are based on the premise that reading, reviewing, and discussing research, systematic reviews, and evidence-based practice protocols can generate an awareness of evidence-based practice. Although there is varied research on the success of journal clubs to increase the number of new research studies, understanding of how research affects nursing care by those attending is still a viable outcome. Members must attend regularly scheduled meetings and discuss the research using a standardized evaluation method in a nonthreatening and learning environment (Geerligs et al, 2018). A twist on the journal club is to hold open forums via a learning management system, e-mail subscriber list, online video meeting such as a Zoom meeting, or blog. Similar to e-learning, participants discuss the topic online as an interactive activity. This method allows participation at the nurse's convenience.

Information Seeking

Information seeking is an attribute of those nurses who question their clinical practice and actively seek out answers in the professional literature. Similar to the characteristic of the setting, the availability of databases can enhance information-seeking behaviors. The significance to the individual is the immediacy of information at the point of care, satisfying the internal need for appropriate clinical information, and encouragement for nurses to read available literature. For example, while caring for a patient you might question an intervention or practice. Possessing the characteristic of information seeking means you might consult reliable databases or repositories of information to actively seek out answers to your question. In addition, reviewing peer-reviewed journals from your professional organization can provide insights into how others addressed the same or similar issues specific to your area of nursing.

Individual barriers are just that; they arise from the value and worth placed on evidence-based practice by the individual. Such issues vary with the type of organization, educational level of nurses, and support structures available. The culture of an organization strongly affects the willingness of the nurse to participate in evidence-based initiatives. Whether addressing organizational, setting, or individual barriers to implementing evidence, adopting multifaceted and targeted methods for the variety of barriers is more effective than any single intervention (Farquhar, Stryer, & Slutsky, 2002; Geerlig et al, 2018; Glasgow, Lichtenstein, & Marcus, 2003; Pearson, 2004).

Sustaining Change

Once system barriers are minimized and facilitators are supported, the need to sustain change emerges. It is easy to fall back into the routine of what was always done. The challenge is to integrate changes into our everyday routine. This holds true for evidence-based practice initiatives as well. Once we make the change, how do we sustain it?

Having a dedicated person or team responsible for auditing the evidence-based practice protocol outcomes provides information on how well the initiative is working. Assigning this task ensures that data reflecting the outcomes are routinely gathered and analyzed. If the task is not clearly assigned, then who is actually monitoring the outcomes becomes muddled, with each person thinking the other is completing the task. It makes sense that the committee or nurse who initiated the evidence-based practice change also assumes the responsibility for gathering data. The team must also plan how they will feed the data back so that it is timely, does not punish, and is targeted and specific.

Piloting the evidence-based practice protocol with a small population is generally done to identify such issues prior to implementing on a larger scale (Geerligs et al, 2018). At this point, feedback from nurses is essential to identify potential problems and rework or retool the process you will use to make the practice change. The owner of the evidence-based practice project is typically the one to gather such information, make necessary changes, and reevaluate the process. This cyclical process is done prior to larger-scale implementation to identify and rectify potential problems. When you plan a practice change, you will want to find issues before they become problems. A small-scale pilot run allows you to fix issues that you might not have known existed before you start the large-scale implementation.

Another essential feature for sustaining change is the need to give feedback to those who are implementing the protocol or practice change as well as to the organizational committees. Feedback to nurses using the evidence-based practice protocol on data shows how the care influenced patient outcomes. Enabling nurses to see how their participation in the application of the evidence-based practice affected the outcomes of care received. Many times, nurses are asked to change their practice but are not told why or given information about how it affected their care outcomes. You can imagine the frustration you would feel if you were left out of the communication process. Consistently bringing data back to nurses reflecting care provided encourages engagement and commitment to the practice issue and EB protocol.

Evidence indicates that certain feedback techniques are more powerful than others to help start and sustain change and adherence to EB guidelines. When the audit team feeds the data back in a way that is individualized, nonpunitive, and timely, those who are trying to change their behavior are more likely to adhere to the EB guideline (Hysong, Best, & Pugh, 2006). In addition, the feedback may be most effective for those who were used to the EB practices before the change. In addition, the individualization and higher intensity of feedback work better (Jamvedt, Young, Kristoffersen, et al, 2009). Expert facilitators can help you craft the feedback message so that it does not place blame but is specific about where adherence is low and needs to improve and happens as close to the time of the data collection as possible.

Bringing audit data to the larger organizational committees demonstrates the impact of evidence-based practice on patient outcomes. Connecting the various layers to the direct care of patients helps bring the focus back to patient care outcomes. Different departments can begin to understand the importance of their role in nursing care. For example, in the clinical story, Ann brought the data back to a committee composed of department managers and directors. This action provided information on how the various non-nursing departments influenced the patient care outcomes. In addition, the process of disseminating data from initiatives links the strategic plan back to the direct care of patients.

The Impact of Magnet Recognition Program®

The American Nurses Credentialing Center (ANCC) developed and revised the **ANCC Magnet Recognition Program.**® This program is based on the Magnet model. Those organizations seeking Magnet recognition (or redesignation) find ways to overcome barriers to evidence implementation. The **Magnet model** requires organizations to demonstrate transformational leadership; structural empowerment; exemplary professional practice; and new knowledge, innovations, and improvements. Each piece is essential to achieving empirical quality outcomes, the central focus of the model. An **empirical quality outcome** is a measurement of a patient-centered and organizational health outcome and is the result of organizational commitment to excellence in nursing care. It is within the process of working toward Magnet recognition that an organization identifies areas of opportunity and develops structures to support nursing practice. Table 14■2 describes select forces and the impact on evidence-based practice implementation.

TABLE 14■2   **Forces of Magnetism and Impact on Evidence-Based Practice Integration**

Force of Magnetism	Types of Evidence	Impact on Evidence Integration
Transformational leadership	Strategic planning Advocating for resources Visibility, accessibility, and communication	Represent nursing's mission, vision, values at the organizational strategic plan level Meeting nurses' needs for evidence-based practice such as databases, time, mentors, etc. Maintains lines of communication with direct care nurses to identify and support practice changes
Structural empowerment	Professional engagement Professional development	Nurse involvement in decision-making entities through shared governance Educational activities that develop nursing knowledge of evidence-based practice processes

TABLE 14■2 **Forces of Magnetism and Impact on Evidence-Based Practice Integration** (continued)

Force of Magnetism	Types of Evidence	Impact on Evidence Integration
Exemplary professional practice	Interdisciplinary care	Nurse inclusion and leadership on interdisciplinary committees Interdisciplinary collaboration on quality improvement initiatives All levels of nurses involved in developing policies and standards of care
	Accountability, competence, and autonomy	Autonomous practice supported by access, routine use, current literature, and professional standards Nurse involvement in annual goal settings including participation in evidence-based practice initiatives Support for nursing involvement in practice decision making and autonomy Nurse accountability for clinical practice
	Culture of safety	Nurse-sensitive indicator data the mean of the national benchmarks used. Nurses participate in initiatives to reduce or eliminate barriers to safe patient care.
	Quality monitoring and improvement	Nurse responsibility for coordinating care among disciplines Trending care outcomes against national benchmarks to identify nursing practice issues Patient satisfaction is addressed using interdisciplinary methods with nurse involvement
New knowledge, innovations, and improvements	Research	Evaluating and using research findings in nursing practice Nurse participation on the Institutional Review Board for research studies Dissemination of knowledge from research studies
	Evidence-based practice	Structure and processes in place to allow the evaluation of current practice Clearly defined method for translating new knowledge into nursing practice Evaluation of how the translation of new knowledge affects patient outcomes

Adapted from American Nurses Credentialing Center. (2019). *2019 Magnet application manual.* Silver Spring, MD: Author.

■ Summary

In the clinical story, the group works for several months to implement the new protocol. They look at the number of CAUTIs during the next two quarters and are delighted to find that the number of CAUTIs fell to zero during a 6-month period. The CNO publicly thanked Ann and her group for taking the initiative to work on the problem. The unit director encourages the group to submit their protocol as a paper presentation to a nursing conference. Ann felt good about improving patient care outcomes and reflected on the experience, knowing that she received support and encouragement throughout the process.

The organizational culture depends on the type of leadership, available resources, enculturation of value for evidence-based practice, expectations of nurses, and the individual nurse. The culture, values, and norms of an organization all affect evidence implementation. As you develop an understanding of an organization, you will recognize both barriers and facilitators for evidence-based practice implementation at the organizational, setting, and individual levels. Such knowledge will prepare you to successfully navigate and direct an evidence implementation project.

CHAPTER QUESTIONS

1. Identify frequently encountered barriers found at the organizational, setting, and individual levels.

2. Describe facilitators that could counteract barriers found in the organizational, setting, and individual levels.

3. Explain how knowledge of setting barriers can facilitate evidence implementation.

4. Describe a plan for overcoming the following barriers:

   a. You identify a clinical practice issue. You ask another nurse what he thinks about investigating the problem further and receive the following response: "Only doctors can make changes to clinical practice."

   b. While caring for a patient on a ventilator, you wonder if your interventions are current and based on evidence. What resources could increase access to appropriate information?

   c. This is your fourth shift in a row with a different team of patients assigned to you.

   d. You want to join the research committee, but the meetings always occur during your scheduled time to work.

5. Think about one of your clinical experiences to answer the following questions:

   a. What formal structure was in place to facilitate the generation and movement of clinical issues?

C H A P T E R   Q U E S T I O N S (continued)

   b. How did the nurses use evidence to direct bedside care?

   c. What databases were available to the nurses for accessing systematic reviews?

   d. Do you know if the patient care policies were based on evidence? Why were they? or If they weren't why was that?

6. Reflect on your clinical experiences to answer the following questions:

   a. Based on the barriers discussed in the chapter and your own experiences in the clinical setting, do you think they are valid? Why?

   b. Would you have had time to incorporate evidence into your care of patients during your clinical experience?

   c. In your experience, what facilitation method would have helped you integrate evidence into your clinical practice?

7. If you are interviewing for a new position and you want to determine whether the organization has a culture of evidence-based practice, what questions would you ask during your interview?

References

American Nurses Credentialing Center. (2019). *2019 Magnet application manual.* Silver Spring, MD: Author.

Brown, C. E., Wickline, M. A., Ecoff, L., et al. (2009). Nursing practice, knowledge, attitudes and perceived barriers to evidence-based practice at an academic medical center. *Journal of Advanced Nursing, 65,* 371–381.

DiCenso, A. (2003). Evidence-based nursing practice: How to get there from here. *Nursing Leadership, 16* (4), 20-26.

Eccles, M. P., & Mittman, B. S. (2006). Welcome to implementation science. *Implementation Science, 1,* 1. doi:10.1186/1748-5908-1-1

Estabrooks, C. A., Floyd, J. A., Scott-Findlay, S., et al. (2003). Individual determinants of research utilization: A systematic review. *Journal of Advanced Nursing, 43,* 506–520.

Farquhar, C. M., Stryer, D., & Slutsky, J. (2002). Translating research into practice: The future ahead. *International Journal for Quality in Health Care, 14,* 233–249.

Forsetlund, L., Bjorndal, A., Rashidian, A., et al. (2009). Continuing education meetings and workshops: Effects on professional practice and health care outcomes. *Cochrane Database of Systematic Reviews, 2009*(2). doi: 10.1002/14651858.CD003030.pub2

Geerligs, L., Rankin, N. M., Shepherd, H. L., et al. (2018). Hospital-based interventions: A systematic review of staff-reported barriers and facilitators to implementation processes. *Implementation Science, 13*(36). doi:10.1186/s13012-018-0726-9

Glasgow, R. E., Lichtenstein, E., & Marcus, A. C. (2003, August). Why don't we see more translation of health promotion research to practice? Rethinking the efficacy to effectiveness transition. *American Journal of Public Health, 93,* 1261–1267.

Harvey, G., & Kitson, A. (2016). PARIHS revisited: From heuristic to integrated framework for the successful implementation of knowledge into practice. *Implementation Science, 11*(33). doi:10.1186/s13012-016-0398-2

HRSA. (2008). The registered nurse population: Findings from the National Sample Survey of Registered Nurses. Retrieved from http://bhpr.hrsa.gov/healthworkforce/reports/nursing/samplesurvey00/chapter2.htm

Hysong, S. J., Best, R. G., & Pugh, J. (2006). Audit and feedback and clinical practice guideline adherence: Making feedback actionable. *Implementation Science 1,* 9.

Institute of Medicine. (2003). *Health professions education: A bridge to quality.* Washington, DC: National Academies Press.

Jamvedt, G., Young, J. M., Kristoffersen, D. T., et al. (2006). Audit and feedback: effects on professional practice and healthcare outcomes. *Cochrane Database of Systematic Reviews, 2006*(2). doi:10.1002/14651858.CD000259.pub2

Kueny, A., Shever, L. L., Lehan Mackin, M., et al. (2015). Facilitating the implementation of evidence-based practice through contextual support and nursing leadership. *Journal of Healthcare Leadership, 7*, 29–39. doi:10.2147/JHL.S45077

Mannion, R., & Davies, H. (2018). Understanding organisational culture for healthcare quality improvement. *British Medical Journal, 363*, k4907. doi: https://doi.org/10.1136/bmj.k4907

National Association of Clinical Nurse Specialists. (2018). *2018 CNS census.* Retrieved from https://nacns.org/professional-resources/practice-and-cns-role/cns-census/

Pearson, A. (2004). Getting research into practice. *International Journal of Nursing Practice, 10*, 197–198.

Perry, C. K., Damschroder, L. J., Hemler, J. R., et al. (2019). Specifying and comparing implementation strategies across seven large implementation interventions: A practical application of theory. *Implementation Science, 14*, 32 doi:10.1186/s13012-019-0876-4

Powell, B. J., Waltz, T. J., Chinman, M. J., et al. (2015). A refined compilation of implementation strategies: results from the Expert Recommendations for Implementing Change (ERIC) project. *Implementation Science, 10*, 21. doi:10.1186/s13012-015-0209-1

Pravikoff, D. S., Tanner, A. B., & Pierce, S. T. (2005). Readiness of U.S. nurses for evidence-based practice. *American Journal of Nursing, 105*(9), 40–51.

Porter-O'Grady, T. (2019). Principles for sustaining shared/professional governance in nursing. *Nursing Management, 50*(1), 36–41.

Rycroft-Malone, J. (2008). Evidence-informed practice: From individual to context. *Journal of Nursing Management, 16*, 404–408.

Squires, J. E., Aloisio, L. D., Grimshaw, J. M., et al. (2019). Attributes of context relevant to healthcare professionals' use of research evidence in clinical practice: A multi-study analysis. *Implementation Science, 14*(1), 52. doi:10.1186/s13012-019-0900-8

Zwarenstein, M., Goldman, J., & Reeves, S. (2009). Interprofessional collaboration: Effects of practice-based interventions on professional practice and healthcare outcomes [Review]. *Cochrane Database of Systematic Reviews, 2009*(3). doi:10.1002/14651858.CD000072.pub2. http://ipls.dk/pdf-filer/ip_collaboration_cochrane.pdf

CHAPTER 15

Apply and Implement IV
National and International Systems of Evidence Implementation

Leslie Rittenmeyer

LEARNING OBJECTIVES

- Discuss the basic concepts of health-care policy.

- Explore health-care policy in the context of evidence-based practice.

- Describe how individual nurse decision making is influenced by larger systems.

- Discuss how evidence-based practice innovations can be driven by governmental policy.

KEY TERMS

Agency for Healthcare Research and Quality (AHRQ)
American Health Quality Association
Beveridge model
Bismark model
Care Quality Commission (CQC)
Centers for Disease Control and Prevention (CDC)
Centers for Medicare & Medicaid Services (CMS)
Children's Health Insurance Program (CHIP)

Core measures
Cost sharing
Deductible
Department of Health and Human Services (HHS)
Evidence-based health care
Health and Social Care (HSC)
Hospital-acquired conditions (HACs)
Indian Health Services (IHS)
Institute for Healthcare Improvement (IHI)
Lobbyists

(continues on page 224)

KEY TERMS (continued)

Medicaid
Medicare
Multipayer system
National health insurance
  model
National Health Service (NHS)
National Institute for Health and
  Clinical Excellence (NICE)
National Patient Safety Goals
  (NPSGs)
National Quality Forum (NQF)
National Service Framework
  (NSF)

Never events
Out-of-pocket model
Patient Protection and
  Affordable Care Act (PPACA)
Public policy
Single-payer system
Social policy
The Joint Commission (TJC)
TRICARE
Veterans Health Administration
  (VA)
World Health Organization
  (WHO)

Clinical Story

Winnifred is in her last semester of a BSN program. She is currently enrolled in a health-care policy course. Her final assignment is a project that will require her to integrate a multitude of concepts from the course. The grading rubric for this project indicates that Winnifred should address the following objectives:

- Describe the basic concepts of public policy and health-care policy.
- Describe the steps in how policy is made.
- Compare the different models of health-care delivery and provide some national and international examples.
- Compare the concept of regulatory responsibility in the United States to that in the United Kingdom.
- Describe how public policy influences quality, safety, and practice and explain why government would be interested in evidence-based health care.
- Choose a practice problem that is targeted by a governmental or accreditation policy that also has reimbursement or accreditation ramifications. Describe why an agency would target this problem.
- Explain how the policy has implications for practice change and the steps that might be taken to address the problem at the institutional level.

Think Before You Read

- When Winnifred examines a federal level health policy, do you think she will find that evidence played a major role in the development of that policy? Do you think she will find any difference in the role for evidence if she compares a federal policy with a local policy?
- What might be some common concepts when thinking about policies at the very local level (e.g., your clinical unit) up to the federal level? Do federal health policies impact the daily work of a clinical nurse?

- How do you think Winnifred might think about health policy if she lived in the United Kingdom where there is a nationalized health service versus how she might think about it living in the United States?

Introduction

Most health-care professionals would claim they want to provide their patients the best-quality health care possible. But what does *best quality* really mean in the context of health-care delivery? Who defines *best quality,* and how do you know if you are providing it? Is *best quality* framed differently from the practitioner's perspective than from a management perspective or governmental perspective? Does best quality always mean the care you are providing is evidence-based and flows directly from the best available evidence? Can you provide best-quality health care and make good clinical decisions without being aware of the best available evidence? Is best-quality care based on rigorous and scientific guidelines and standards generated with transparent methods? Does best-quality care mean safe health care?

Governmental and accrediting entities continue to develop health-care policy that affects how nurses practice. From a governmental perspective, the purpose of an evidence-based practice is to provide care that is less variable and more standardized, with emphasis on patient safety, better patient outcomes, continuing quality monitoring, and improvement. This chapter begins by explaining the dimensions of public policy, with a focus on health-care policy. A discussion of who influences the making of public policy follows. Health-care delivery models in both the United States and internationally are then compared and regulatory responsibilities discussed. This discussion leads to an exploration of the influence of public policy on health-care quality, safety, and practice. The chapter ends with an example of the implementation process for an evidence-based program that addresses a clinical problem that has safety and reimbursement ramifications.

What Are the Dimensions of Public Policy?

Winnifred starts her project by reviewing her notes and readings for the various definitions of public policy and health-care policy. She begins her paper with some basic definitions and explains the public policy process, including how different groups influence it.

Dye (1995) defines **public policy** as whatever governments choose to do or choose not to do. He points out that a lack of a policy is a policy statement in itself. Kilpatrick (2000) describes public policy as a system of laws, regulations, courses of action, and funding priorities in the context of a given issue promulgated by a governmental entity or its representative. Anderson (2006) defines policy as a planned course of action that is chosen for the purpose of addressing a problem.

The role of public policy in the health-care context is complex because it addresses issues such as health-care coverage, health-care cost, health-care philosophy, and health-care quality. These issues are emotionally charged, and the role of govern-ment in health-care policy is often debated along the lines of political ideology. Buse, Mays, and Watt state that health policy is "assumed to embrace courses of action (and inaction) that affect the set of institutions, organizations, services and funding arrangements of the health system" (2005, p. 6). Simply put, public policies are made to deal with public problems (Kraft & Furlong, 2010).

How Is Policy Made and Influenced?

Laws define public policy, and governmental entities enforce it. Elected politicians set the agenda and the regulatory framework. Health-care policy falls under the heading of **social policy** (policies that address things such as welfare, crime, education, and health care). Remember, governments also make economic and foreign policy. As you can see from the above definitions the development of any type of policy usually starts with the identification of a problem. Sometimes the government identifies the problem and sometimes other stakeholders identify it. Once the problem has been defined, the next step is debate between conflicting interest groups. These groups vary but can consist of stakeholders, politicians, consumers, and special interest groups. An example of a special interest group is the insurance industry itself. Special interest groups are represented by political activists and **lobbyists** (persons who attempt to influence legislation on behalf of special interests). Walt and Gilson (1994) claimed that health-care policy is about process, power, and influence, all of which are at play when policy is being made. Kilpatrick (2000) believes advocacy in the context of public policy is an attempt to influence policy through education, lobbying, or political pressure. Advocacy groups attempt to influence not only policy makers but the general public as well. An example of such a group is the American Nurses Association, which lobbies Congress and regulatory agencies on health-care issues. Another example is the **American Health Quality Association,** whose mission is to advance quality of care and patient safety nationwide. Box 15■1 contains a representative sample of health-care policy associations.

BOX 15■1 **Representative Sample of Health Policy Associations**

- Alliance for Health Reform
- Alliance to Improve Medicare
- American Association for Health Care Risk Management (ASHRM)
- American Association of Retired Persons (AARP)
- American Hospital Association (AHA)
- American Public Health Association (APHA)
- Citizen Advocacy Center (CAC)
- Henry J. Kaiser Family Foundation
- Institute for Health Policy Solutions
- National Rural Health Association

A study from the Center for Responsive Politics (CRP), Northwestern University, and the *Chicago Tribune* reported that lobbyists spent $862 million between 2008 and 2009 to influence senators and congressional representatives involved in the debate over health-care restructuring legislation (Martin, 2009). In addition, the drug industry spent $199 million on lobbying over a 9-month period, making the industry the second biggest spender next to the insurance companies. In 2019, Pharmaceutical Research and Manufacturers of America was the fourth top spender on federal lobby efforts, spending $22,762,00; the American Hospital Association followed next, spending $18,752,162; while the American Nurses Association spent just $349,045 (Center for Responsive Politics, 2019). You can see from this information how power, money, and competing interests can significantly slow the process of reaching consensus on health-care reform or health-care public policy.

If a policy is finally formulated at the end of the debate, legislators vote on it; if it passes the vote, the policy is enacted into law. Following the vote, the law is then signed or vetoed by the president, and it is then decided which governmental entity will enforce the policy.

The Role of Government in Health Care from a National and International Perspective: A Comparison

National Health-Care Policy (United States)

To understand the role of government in our national health-care system, it is necessary to understand how health care is structured in the United States. Simply put, at this time, the financing of health care in this country is shared by two entities, private insurance and the government. The United States is considered to have a **multipayer system.** In the private sector, employer-sponsored group insurance is the most common. Individuals who do not have employer-sponsored insurance are free to purchase private, nongroup insurance. This means these individuals pay out-of-pocket premiums. These premiums are usually very expensive and difficult for most people to afford, leaving many in this country uninsured or underinsured. More recently, because of the prohibitive cost of health care, it is not unusual for employers to ask employees to pay a portion of their health-care premium. This is called **cost sharing.** There is even some cost sharing in the federal programs (e.g., Medicare) in the form of **deductibles,** the amount of money an individual pays each year before his or her benefit payments begin.

Government-Funded Health Care in the United States: What Is It and Who Uses It?

The primary government funded health-care programs in the United States are **Medicare, Medicaid, Children's Health Insurance Program (CHIP), TRICARE,**

BOX 15■2 Functions of Federally and State-Funded Health-Care Programs

---

- **Indian Health Service (IHS)** is an operating division within the U.S. Department of Health and Human Services and provides medical and public health services to members of federally recognized Native American tribes and Alaskan tribes.
- **Medicaid** is a funded by both the federal government and the states. It is administered at the state level. It covers low-income children and their families.
- **Medicare** is a federally funded program that insures persons 65 years and older and some individuals with disabilities. Part A pays for hospital care, Part B for physician services, and Part D for prescription benefits.
- **Children's Health Insurance Program** (CHIP) is funded by both the federal government and the states to provide health care to children whose families earn too much income to qualify for Medicaid but do not have enough money to pay for private insurance. The program is administered by the states.
- **TRICARE** is a program that provides health coverage to all military retirees, their spouses, survivors, and other qualified dependents.
- **Veterans Health Administration** (VA) is a federally funded and administered program for veterans. Health care is delivered in government-run health-care facilities.

Veterans Health Administration (VA), and the **Indian Health Service (IHS).** Box 15■2 summarizes the function of each of these entities.

The Uninsured

The National Center for Health Statistics Report estimates health insurance coverage based on the National Health Interview Survey (Cohen, Terlizzi, Martinez & Cha, 2020). During the first half of 2019, 9.5% of Americans were uninsured, a larger proportion of adults (13.7%) than children aged 0 to 17 years (4.4%). More adult men (15.4%) than women (12.1%) were uninsured. Box 15■3 provides a summary of the distribution of insured by source and uninsured. Table 15■1 provides numbers and percentages of the uninsured in the United States. These data reflect significant decreases in uninsured since the 2010 Patient Protection and Affordable Care Act. Based on Census Bureau's America Community Survey, the Kaiser Family Foundation (2020) provides some further facts about the uninsured population based on 2018 data:

1. While 41% of the uninsured are non–Hispanic whites, people of color are at highest risk of being uninsured.
2. Hispanics and blacks have higher uninsured rates than whites.

BOX 15■3 **Distribution of Health Insurance Coverage in the United States for All Ages (2020)**

- Private insurance: 64.5%
- Public forms of insurance: 37.4%
- Uninsured: 9.5%

January 2020 – June 2020
Source: National Health Interview Survey Early Release Program (Cohen et al, 2020)

TABLE 15■1 **Numbers and Percentages of Uninsured in the United States**

Year	Number Uninsured (Millions)	Uninsured
2010	48.2	18.2%
2013 (Pre-ACA)	44.3	16.6%
2016	28.2	10.4%
2017	28.9	10.7%
2018	30.1	11.1%
2019	30.7	9.5%

Source: CDC National Center for Health Statistics. (2020) The National Health Interview Survey Early Release Program.

3. The uninsured are less likely than those with insurance to receive preventive care and treatment for major health conditions and chronic diseases.
4. Non-elderly adults without insurance coverage say they went without care in the past year because of cost.

Part of the reason for poor access among the uninsured is that many do not have a place to go when they are sick or in need for medical services.

Health-Care Reform

The **Patient Protection and Affordable Care Act (PPACA)** (2010) (Pub. L. No. 111-148) is a large bill with many provisions that offers rights and protections meant to make health care more fair, available, and affordable for citizens. Since the 2016 election, the current administration has challenged the bill after a campaign promise to repeal the bill. As of this writing, this goal has not been met although some provisions of the bill have been affected by attempts to weaken it. The PPACA created the health insurance marketplace where many people who do not have health insurance coverage through either private insurance or the government can purchase health insurance. The best place to search for a plan is on the marketplace

BOX 15■4 **Provisions of the Affordable Care Act**

- Requires insurance plans to cover people with pre-existing health conditions
- Provides free preventive care
- Gives young adults more coverage options
- Ends lifetime and yearly dollar limits
- Holds insurance companies more accountable
- Makes it illegal for health insurance companies to cancel health insurance
- Protects choice of doctors
- Protects from employer retaliation

at healthcare.gov. Refer to Box 15■4 for a list of some provisions of the bill that exist at this time.

Regulatory Responsibility

The U.S. **Department of Health and Human Services (HHS)** agency has the primary responsibility for protecting the health of Americans and providing essential human services, especially for the neediest populations. HHS represents close to a quarter of all federal outlay of funds and administers more grant dollars than all other federal agencies combined. The Medicare program, managed by HHS, is the nation's largest health insurer. Total expenditures for Medicare in 2018 were $750.2 billion (CMS, 2020). HHS works closely with state and local governments, and many HHS-funded programs are provided at the local level by state or county agencies or through private-sector grantees. The programs are administered through 11 operating divisions, which include 8 agencies in the U.S. Public Health Service and 3 human services agencies (see https://www.hhs.gov/about/agencies/index.html). Box 15■5 includes the agencies that make up the HHS.

Although describing all of the sub-agencies of the HHS is beyond the scope of this chapter, the following is a brief description of three of its sub-agencies that are a focus of this chapter:

- The **Agency for Healthcare Research and Quality (AHRQ)** supports research that helps people make more informed decisions and improves the quality of health-care services. AHRQ was formerly known as the Agency for Health Care Policy and Research (http://www.ahrq.gov).
- The **Centers for Medicare & Medicaid Services (CMS)** administers the Medicare program, providing health-care security and choice for aged and disabled people. Jointly with the state governments, CMS administers the Medicaid program and the **Children's Health Insurance Program (CHIP)**. CHIP provides health coverage to eligible children through both Medicaid and separate CHIP programs. States and the federal government jointly fund this program. CMS is the largest purchaser of health care in the United States. The

BOX 15■5 **Agencies of the U.S. Department of Health and Human Services**

- Administration for Children and Families (ACF)
- Administration for Community Living (ACL)
- Agency for Healthcare Research and Quality (AHRQ)
- Agency for Toxic Substances and Disease Registry (ATSDR)
- Center for Faith-Based and Neighborhood Partnerships (CFBNP)
- Centers for Disease Control and Prevention (CDC)
- Centers for Medicare & Medicaid Services (CMS)
- Food and Drug Administration (FDA)
- Health Resources and Services Administration (HRSA)
- Indian Health Service (IHS)
- National Institutes of Health (NIH)
- Substance Abuse and Mental Health Services Administration (SAMHSA)

Health and Human Services, HHS Agencies & Offices. (2016). Retrieved from https://www.hhs.gov/about/agencies/index.html

financial expenditures of CMS grew 4.6% to $3.6 trillion in 2018 and accounted for 17.7% of U.S. gross domestic product (GDP). Under current law, national health spending is projected to grow at an average annual rate of 5.4% for 2019 to 2028 and to reach $6.2 trillion by the year 2028 (CMS, 2020).

- The **Centers for Disease Control and Prevention (CDC)** collaborates to create the expertise, information, and tools that individuals and communities need to protect their health through health promotion; prevention of disease, injury, and disability; and preparedness for new health threats. The CDC seeks to accomplish its mission by working with partners throughout the nation and the world to monitor health, detect and investigate health problems, conduct research to enhance disease prevention, develop and advocate sound public health policies, implement prevention strategies, promote healthy behaviors, and foster safe and healthful environments (http://www.cdc.gov).

The health-care system in the United States is very complicated. Dialogue concerning health disparities, health access, efficiency, patient safety, value, and quality to some extent raises more questions than it provides answers to and certainly keeps the health-care reform debate alive. The next section provides a comparison of U.S. health-care policy with international health-care policy.

International Health-Care Policy

According to the Institute of Medicine of the National Academy of Sciences (2004), the United States is the only industrialized nation that does not offer universal medical insurance coverage for its citizens. Despite that fact, the United States spends more on health care than does any other country.

In his book on international health care, Reid (2010) states that health-care systems tend to follow patterns, creating four basic systems throughout the world. The first system he describes is called the **Beveridge model,** named for William Beveridge, the designer of the National Health Service (NHS) in the United Kingdom. It is also called a **single-payer system**—only a single entity pays the bill. In this system, health care is provided and financed by the government (the single payer) through a system of tax payments. In Britain, citizens never receive a bill for health-care services. Countries that adopt this model tend to have low costs per capita, because the government, as a sole payer, controls what doctors can do and charge for their services. The health insurance system in the UK is governed and guided by **National Health Services (NHS),** which aims to publicly fund the health-care entities in all of the different parts of the UK. According to the World Health Organization, government funding covers 85% of health-care expenditure in the UK. The remaining 15% is covered by private sector. Private insurance is usually accessed through employer groups or, more rarely, by wealthier individuals seeking additional benefits who access the carrier directly. The NHS includes **NHS** England, **NHS** Scotland, **NHS** Wales, and the affiliated **Health and Social Care (HSC)** in Northern Ireland, and there are some differences in their systems. Since 2013, operational responsibility is administered by **NHS** England. Examples of nations using the Beveridge model are the United Kingdom and almost all of the Scandinavian countries.

The second system is called the **Bismark model**. This model is more like segments of the U.S. system in that it uses an insurance system jointly financed by employers and employees. However, insurance companies in Bismark-type health insurance plans are mandated to cover all citizens, and they do not make a profit. Although this is a multipayer system, tight regulations give government as much cost-control clout as in the single-payer system. Germany, Japan, and Spain are three prominent nations that have adopted this model.

The third model is the **national health insurance model.** This model, Reid contends, has elements of both the Beveridge and Bismark models. It uses private-sector providers, but reimbursement comes from a government-run insurance company that is funded by all residents. Because there are no marketing costs, no financial motives to deny claims, and no profit to be made, these universal programs tend to be cheaper and simpler to manage. Canada is an example of this model.

The last system Reid describes is the **out-of-pocket model.** He suggests most nations are too impoverished to have any formalized health care. In these countries, rich citizens can pay out of pocket for health care, whereas the citizens with low incomes cannot afford care and usually stay sick or die. He provides examples of people in rural Africa, China, and India who have never seen a doctor in their entire lives.

Comparison of the U.S Health-Care System and International Systems

According to Reid (2010), America's health-care system is unique; the system is fragmented and has elements of all the models explained above. He compares our

VA system (which is a single-payer system) to the Beveridge model employed by the United Kingdom and Cuba. For those Americans over the age of 65, he compares the Medicare system to the national health insurance model employed in Canada and Taiwan. He compares employer-paid health insurance to the Bismarck model practiced in Germany, France, and Japan (even though those countries have strong government regulations controlling quality and cost). Finally, he compares the 9.5% of Americans who have no insurance and no ability to pay out of pocket to parts of Africa, China, and India. He believes the United States is unlike any other country because it maintains separate systems for separate classes of people. Other countries have settled on one model for everyone, which he believes is fairer and cheaper.

Despite differences in health-care delivery systems, Gray (2009) believes many of the problems and potential solutions to those problems are similar. His opinion is based on the belief that across the globe, despite the differences in the way health-care services are paid for and delivered, many of the major problems are the same. He cites some of the following as examples:

- Increasing cost
- Lack of capacity of any country to pay for the totality of health-care services
- Provision of inappropriate care
- Aging population
- Technological advances
- Rising professional and patient expectations

In addition to the macro problems listed above, Gray identifies the following eight problems that can be found in any health-care service:

1. Errors and mistakes
2. Poor-quality health care
3. Waste of resources
4. Variation in policy and practice
5. Patients' poor experience with health care
6. Overenthusiastic adoption of interventions of low value
7. Failure to find evidence and to put new interventions of high value into practice
8. Failure to manage ignorance and uncertainty (Gray, 2009, pp. 1–2)

Gray goes on to state, "In order to meet these powerful challenges, the principles of **evidence-based health care** can be applied to great effect, regardless of whether a health service is organized nationally (as in the United Kingdom [UK]), or by province (as in Canada) whether it is tax-based or insurance based (as in Japan), or whether the main source of funding is public or private (as in the USA)" (p. 3). Gray suggests the practice of evidence-based health care can have a great impact on some of the aforementioned challenges in any health-care delivery system.

The next section addresses how governmental policy influences health-care quality, safety, and practice, and the relationship to evidence-based health care.

The Influence of Governmental Policy on Health-Care Quality, Safety, and Practice: Why Evidence-Based Health Care?

Returning to this chapter's clinical story, Winnifred believes she understands the definition of *public policy* and its relationship to health care. She thinks she can give a good elemental description of the health-care delivery system in the United States and compare it to at least two international health-care systems. She also understands the structure of regulatory responsibility and now feels ready to tackle what she sees as the influence of government policy on quality, safety, and practice. She is beginning to see how larger systems and government policy can affect individual nurse practice.

There is great interest in evidence-based health care from both the private and public sectors because there is increasing concern about high cost, poor quality, and waste of resources. The imperative for evidence-based health care is more formalized and more embedded into public health-care policy in some countries than it is in others. For instance, the United Kingdom has taken a systematic approach to quality improvement in the NHS. Through formal public policy, the boards of NHS organizations have a duty to ensure the quality of health care is improved. To reach this goal, it has created new organizations such as the **National Institute for Health and Clinical Excellence (NICE), National Service Framework (NSF),** and the **Care Quality Commission** (CQC). Box 15▪6 summarizes the NHS quality assurance structure.

BOX 15▪6   **The Organizations That Make Up the United Kingdom's Quality Structure**

- **National Institute for Health and Clinical Excellence (NICE)** is an independent organization responsible for providing national guidance on promoting good health and preventing and treating ill health. NICE develops and defines the standards of health care that people can expect to receive. These standards will indicate when a clinical treatment (or set of clinical procedures) is considered highly effective, cost effective, and safe as well as being viewed as a positive experience by patients. (http://www.nice.org.uk)
- **National Service Framework (NSF)** program and strategies set clear quality requirements for care. These are based on the best available evidence of what treatments and services work most effectively for patients. (http://www.nhs.uk/nhsengland/nsf/)
- **Care Quality Commission (CQC)** independently regulates health and social care in England. Through their work they aim to protect the rights of vulnerable people and involve the public in health-care policies. They speak with an independent voice. (http://www.Cqc.org.UK)

In the United States, there are several agencies that recognize the value of evidence-based practice in improving health-care quality and safety. The **Agency for Healthcare Research and Quality (AHRQ)** is one of the subdivisions of the HHS, and its mission is to improve the quality, safety, efficiency, and effectiveness of health care for all Americans. AHRQ launched an initiative to promote evidence-based practice in everyday care through the establishment of 12 evidence-based practice centers (EPCs). The EPCs develop evidence reports and technology assessments on topics relevant to clinical, social science/behavioral, and economic areas, as well as other health-care organization and delivery issues—specifically issues that are common, expensive, and/or significant for the Medicare and Medicaid populations. With this program, AHRQ became a "science partner" of private and public organizations in an effort "to improve the quality, effectiveness, and appropriateness of health care" by synthesizing the evidence and facilitating the translation of evidence-based research findings (AHRQ, n.d., para. 1).

In an attempt to improve patient safety and control cost, the **Centers for Medicare & Medicaid Services (CMS)** implemented policies that attached reimbursement ramifications for facilities when patients experience certain secondary **hospital-acquired conditions (HACs)** (CMS, 2019). Medicare does not want to pay for medical complications that are the result of errors. Section 5001(c) of the Deficit Reduction Act of 2005 required the secretary of the Department of Health and Human Services to identify conditions that are (a) high-cost or high-volume or both, (b) result in the assignment of a case to a drug-related group that has a higher payment when present as a secondary diagnosis, and (c) could reasonably have been prevented through the application of evidence-based guidelines.

On July 31, 2008, in the Inpatient Prospective Payment System (IPPS) 2009, Final Rule, CMS included 10 categories of conditions that were selected for the HAC payment provision (Inpatient Prospective Payment System, 2009). See Box 15■7 for the current list of hospital-acquired conditions.

Never events or, as some have suggested calling them, serious reportable events are extremely serious, preventable patient safety incidents that should not occur if the relevant evidence-based practice measures are in place. The **National Quality Forum (NQF)** has identified 28 incidents that qualify as never events; the major categories are listed in Box 15■8 (NQF, n.d.). These incidents are very serious and costly from both a personal and fiscal perspective because people can and often do die from them. In 2007 (enacted October 2008), the CMS announced it would not reimburse the extra costs for complications caused by serious error. This is another example in which governmental policy influences clinical decision making and practice.

The Role of Accrediting Agencies

Accreditation of health-care organizations is technically voluntary. However, reimbursement by some entities, such as Medicare and Medicaid, requires organizations to be accredited. Therefore, if an organization wishes to be paid by Medicare and

BOX 15■7 **Current CMS List of Hospital-Acquired Conditions**

1. Foreign Object Retained After Surgery
2. Air Embolism
3. Blood Incompatibility
4. Stage III and IV Pressure Ulcers
5. Falls and Trauma
   - Fractures
   - Dislocations
   - Intracranial Injuries
   - Crushing Injuries
   - Burns
   - Electric Shock
6. Manifestations of Poor Glycemic Control
   - Diabetic Ketoacidosis
   - Nonketotic Hyperosmolar Coma
   - Hypoglycemic Coma
   - Secondary Diabetes with Ketoacidosis
   - Secondary Diabetes with Hyperosmolarity
7. Catheter-Associated Urinary Tract Infection (UTI)
8. Vascular Catheter-Associated Infection
9. Surgical Site Infection Following:
   - Coronary Artery Bypass Graft (CABG)—Mediastinitis
   - Bariatric Surgery
   - Laparoscopic Gastric Bypass
   - Gastroenterostomy
   - Laparoscopic Gastric Restrictive Surgery
   - Orthopedic Procedures
   - Spine
   - Neck
   - Shoulder
   - Elbow
10. Deep Vein Thrombosis (DVT)/Pulmonary Embolism (PE)
    - Total Knee Replacement
    - Hip Surgery

Source: Centers for Medicare and Medicaid Services, Hospital-acquired conditions (present on admission indicator). Retrieved from http://www.cms.gov/HospitalAcqCond/06_Hospital-Acquired_Conditions.asp#Top

Medicaid, it must seek accreditation. Accrediting agencies set certain standards and then evaluate the organization through a process of review to determine whether the organization meets those standards. Although not the only accreditation organization, **The Joint Commission (TJC)** is the agency of this chapter's focus. The Joint Commission is an independent, not-for-profit organization that accredits and certifies

---

BOX 15■8 **Current List of Major Categories of Serious Reportable (Never) Events**

---

1. Surgical or Invasive Procedure Events. Ex. Surgery performed on the wrong patient.
2. Product or Device Events. Ex. Patient death or serious injury associated with the use of contaminated drugs, devices, or biologics.
3. Patient Protection Events. Ex. Patient suicide, attempted suicide, or self-harm that results in serious injury.
4. Care Management Events. Ex. Patient death or serious injury associated with medication error.
5. Environmental Events. Ex. Patient or staff death or serious injury associated with electric shock.
6. Radiologic Events. Ex. Death or serious injury of a patient or staff associated with the introduction of a metallic object.
7. Potential Criminal Events. Ex. Abduction of a patient/resident of any age.

Note: For a complete list of events under each category, refer to (http://www.qualityforum.org/Topics/SREs/List_of_SREs.aspx)

---

more than 18,000 health-care organizations and programs in the United States. An accreditation or certification from TJC represents quality health care and recognition of the organization's commitment to meeting certain performance standards. Its mission, in collaboration with other stakeholders, is to continuously improve health care for the public by evaluating health-care organizations and inspiring them to excel in providing safe and effective care of the highest quality and value (http://www.jointcommission.org/). One example of how hospitals meet the TJC performance standards is to achieve Magnate® status. Magnate® recognition from the American Nurses Credentialing Center indicates excellent nursing practice, which leads to improved patient outcomes while providing a satisfactory professional work environment. Magnate® hospitals must demonstrate continual improved practice based on best available evidence. In this way quality care is intertwined with evidence-based practice.

Each year the TJC releases their **Joint Commission National Patient Safety Goals (NPSGs).** The 2020 NPSGs are readily found on the TJC Web site and include the following categories:

- Ambulatory health care
- Behavioral health care
- Critical access hospital
- Home care
- Hospital care
- Laboratory services
- Nursing care center (long term care)
- Office-based surgery

NPSGs are discussed later in the chapter.

The Joint Commission also developed a set of care processes called the **core measures.** The core measures were developed from a set of quality indicators defined by the CMS. The purpose of the core measures is to help institutions improve quality of patient care by focusing on outcomes. Although the core measures tend to be medically centered as opposed to nurse sensitive, the job of monitoring the measure often falls to nurses.

The role of government influence in health-care quality, safety, and practice is somewhat of a "carrot and stick" story. Public governmental policy can be influential in the use of an evidence-based practice model across a large spectrum of health-care agencies by using the "stick" of denied reimbursement and the "carrot" of incentives. The threat of delivering care that will not be reimbursed causes many organizations to pay attention, and the incentives keep that attention. Conversely, when there is not a "stick" and only a few "carrots" to go around, the influence of policy on practice diminishes. This means that some policies, even if based on solid evidence, are sometimes slow to trickle down or be embraced by the practice community.

In the clinical story, the last part of Winnifred's paper must provide an example of a potential clinical problem targeted by government policy that has safety and cost implications. She needs to explain the significance of the problem and also how she is going to use evidence-based knowledge to address it. She begins by looking at the CMS Web site to see the current list of HACs. She easily finds the list, and after some consideration, she chooses "surgical site infections, post orthopedic surgery," as her clinical problem (see Box 15■7 for a review of HACs). The rationale for her choice is both personal and academic; her grandmother suffered a surgical site infection after hip replacement surgery in which the cost in pain and suffering was high and she knows hospital-acquired infections should be preventable. Most important, she wants to know how she can ensure that her own nursing actions are based on the best available evidence and safe.

To learn more about the prevention of surgical site infection, Winifred decides to search the Web sites of the governmental and accrediting agencies that address this safety problem. She already knows that the CMS has identified surgical site infection after orthopedic procedures as an HAC. She also knows this condition has reimbursement ramifications because of that HAC designation. In looking at the Hospital NPSGs for 2020 from the Joint Commission, Winnifred notes that "prevent infection" is one of its safety goals as well (Box 15■9). However, TJC safety goals address hospital-acquired infections in general, whereas the CMS addresses surgical site infection specifically. She decides to stick with surgical site infection and theorizes how she would approach this problem in an actual clinical situation.

After reading the clinical guidelines for prevention of surgical site infection, she realizes she will not be able to address all of the recommendations found in the CDC guideline because they are extensive. For this particular project, she decides to narrow her scope to just one of the recommendations. She feels she can adequately illustrate how a government regulation can influence individual practice by following through with this one recommendation. She chooses Postoperative Incision Care.

BOX 15■9 **JC Hospital National Safety Goals**

■ Identify patients correctly
■ Improve staff communication
■ Use medicines safely
■ Use alarms safely
■ Prevent infections
■ Identify patient safety risks
■ Prevent mistakes in surgery

For more details on each goal, refer to https://www.jointcommission.org/-/media/tjc/documents/
standards/national-patient-safety-goals/2020/simplified_2020-hap-npsgs-eff-july-final.pdf
Source: https://www.jointcommission.org

This recommendation states, "Wash hands before and after changing dressings and any contact with the surgical site" (Mangram et al, 1999).

When you decide to address a clinical problem, you must first define the dimensions of the problems, as Winnifred's situation illustrates. For example, if you are concerned there is poor compliance to the hand hygiene policy or if there is a high rate of surgical site infections in your unit, you might decide to launch a hand hygiene and glove compliance intervention program. How would you do that? A good place to start would be the **Institute for Healthcare Improvement (IHI).** This organization offers a publication, "How-To Guide: Improving Hand Hygiene" (2006). This guide was developed in conjunction with the CDC, the Society of Healthcare Epidemiology of America, and the Association for Professionals in Infection Control and Epidemiology, and it provides a tool kit to implement such a program. Box 15■10 summarizes some of the recommendations. (The full program is part of the public domain and readily available at the IHI Web site.)

A part of any program (such as the one from the IHI) is data collection and analysis. Data are gathered to assess the extent of the problem and to measure improvement after implementation. Data are also gathered from the stakeholders as the program is being implemented to assess the process. Once you have analyzed the various types of data, you can search the literature to see if there are clinical guidelines based on the best available evidence that could inform you on the best way to frame a plan for implementing quality improvement measures and ultimately monitoring improvements. In the case of hand hygiene compliance, the CDC and **World Health Organization (WHO)** have well-established, evidence-based guidelines on hand hygiene. Box 15■11 provides the links to both the CDC and WHO hand hygiene recommendations, with explanations about the levels of evidence that informed the guidelines as well as the "How-to Guide" for hand hygiene from IHI.

The best available evidence should guide the implementation and evaluation of any program meant to improve hand hygiene compliance (Box 15■12). However, other considerations will enter into your decision making. Factors such as context, available resources, personal knowledge of the institution, facility limitations, and geographic location must all be considered in your planning.

BOX 15■10   **Approaches to Developing a Hand Hygiene and Glove Intervention Program**

- Give a diverse group of personnel a stake in the process, gather a multidisciplinary team, including physicians and administrators who can help remove barriers to implementation.
- Assess current practice and compliance.
- Perform a survey to determine hand hygiene and glove compliance rates. Determine how these rates compare to those in the literature.
- Set clear aims and time-specific improvement targets. Set the bar high.
- Allocate adequate resources and personnel to achieve target levels.
- Establish measures that will indicate whether changes are leading to improvement.
- Organize an educational program that teaches the core principles and hand hygiene and glove practice to clinical staff throughout the hospital.
- Assess satisfaction with current hand hygiene products.
- If alcohol-based hand products are not used by the hospital, have a select group of nurses and physicians test two or three products. Poorly functioning dispensers do not improve compliance.
- Introduce program to entire staff and have team members visit the units to answer questions.
- Provide a patient safety tip sheet for staff and families.
- Use measurement tools to monitor compliance.

Source: Institute for Healthcare Improvement (http://www.IHI.org).

BOX 15■11   **Links to the Centers for Disease Control and Prevention and World Health Organization Hand Hygiene Recommendations**

- WHO | The evidence for clean hands (http://www.who.int/gpsc/country_work/en/)
- CDC | Hand Hygiene in Healthcare Settings (http://www.cdc.gov/handhygiene/)
- Institute for Healthcare Improvement | How to Guide: Improving Hand Hygiene (http://www.ihi.org/resources/Pages/Tools/HowtoGuideImprovingHandHygiene.aspx)

BOX 15■12 **Interdisciplinary Rounds**

■ Pretend that you are responsible for putting a team together to plan and implement a hand hygiene program. How would you go about it? Who would you ask and why? What type of characteristics would you want the members of the team to have?
■ You are implementing a hand hygiene program and some of the physicians are not cooperating. What type of actions would you take to convince them of the value of the program?
■ What type of prompts would you design to remind everyone who enters the room to wash their hands?

BOX 15■13 **Tools for Learning and Practice**

■ Go the CDC Web site and locate the available tools to implement a hand hygiene program.
■ Using CINAHL and MEDLINE, search for evidence on hand hygiene. See if you can find a systematic review.
■ Go to the CDC Web site and sign up to be on their e-mail list.

■ Summary

By completing this project, Winnifred has learned the way public policy is made and how it influences health-care quality, safety, and practice. Of course, this influence varies somewhat according to the structure of the health-care delivery system. In the UK, for instance, the government (as single-payer system) has great influence on health-care practice. In the United States (a multipayer system), the government influence may vary from the private to the public sector. The government influence often comes in the form of reimbursement ramifications or incentives, which is the reason that public policy is able to influence change that trickles down to the individual practice level. For example, a nurse who practices poor hand hygiene has the potential to increase the rate of surgical site infections in the institution; the individual practice of the nurse has become part of the institution's noncompliance with the policy or standard. This, in turn, has both cost and accreditation ramifications for the institution. Hopefully, this example never happens, and the nurse, aware of the evidence-based guidelines for hand hygiene, adheres to those guidelines and, through her individual practice, increases the potential for a safe patient outcome.

Finally, Winnifred recognizes that despite the differences, all health-care systems experience some of the same problems centered on issues of affordability, cost, quality, safety, and continuous improvement and monitoring (Box 15■13). There is growing global interest in evidence-based health care as a way to address these concerns. This stems from the belief that use of the best available evidence will reduce errors, increase quality and safety, and result in better patient outcomes, while ultimately reducing both personal and fiscal costs.

CHAPTER QUESTIONS

1. Explain the process by which a policy is enacted into law.

2. Compare and contrast the U.S. health-care system with one other health-care system.

3. Analyze the difference between single-payer systems and multipayer systems. Make an argument in favor of one over the other.

4. Explain the role of the Department of Health and Human Services (HHS) in regulating health-care quality.

5. What is the mission of the Agency for Healthcare Research and Quality (AHRQ), and how is it connected to evidence-based practice?

6. In your opinion, what should the role of government be in controlling quality and safety in health care?

7. Write a one-page paper explaining briefly the relationship of evidence-based practice to health-care quality and safety.

References

Agency for Healthcare Quality and Research (AHRQ). (n.d.). About the effective health care program. Retrieved from https://effectivehealthcare.ahrq.gov/about/epc

Anderson, J. (2006). *Public policymaking: An introduction* (6th ed.). Boston, MA: Houghton Mifflin.

Buse, K., Mays, N., & Watt, G. (2005). *Making health policy*. Maidenhead, United Kingdom: Open University Press.

Centers for Disease Control National Center for Health Statistics. (2020). Health insurance coverage: Estimates from the national health interview survey. Retrieved from https://www.cdc.gov/nchs/nhis/healthinsurancecoverage.htm

Centers for Medicare & Medicaid Services (CMS). (2019). Hospital-acquired conditions (present on admission indicator). Retrieved from http://www.cms.gov/HospitalAcqCond/06_Hospital-Acquired_Conditions.asp#Top

Centers for Medicare & Medicaid Services (CMS). (2020). NHE Fact Sheet. Retrieved from https://www.cms.gov/Research-Statistics-Data-and-Systems/Statistics-Trends-and-Reports/NationalHealthExpendData/NHE-Fact-Sheet

Center for Responsive Politics. (2019). Top spenders. Retrieved from https://www.opensecrets.org/federal-lobbying/top-spenders

Cohen, R. A., Terlizzi, E. P., Martinez, M. E., & Cha, A. E. (2020). Health insurance coverage: Early release of estimates from the national health interview survey, January – June, 2019. Retrieved from https://www.cdc.gov/nchs/data/nhis/earlyrelease/insur202005-508.pdf

Dye, T. R. (1995). *Understanding public policy*. Englewood Cliffs, NJ: Prentice Hall.

Gray, M. (2009). *Evidence based health care and public health* (3rd ed.). London: Churchill Livingston Elsevier.

Health and Human Services (HHS). (2015). HHS agencies and offices. Retrieved from https://www.hhs.gov/about/agencies/hhs-agencies-and-offices/index.html

Inpatient Prospective Payment System (IPPS). (2009). Final rule. Retrieved from http://www.cms.gov/HospitalAcqCond/06_Hospital-Acquired_Conditions.asp#

Institute for Healthcare Improvement (IHI). (2006). How-to guide: Improving hand hygiene. Retrieved from http://www.ihi.org/resources/Pages/Tools/HowtoGuideImprovingHandHygiene.aspx

Institute of Medicine of the National Academy of Science. (2004). Insuring America's health: Principles and recommendations. Retrieved from www.iom.edu/.../Insuring-Americas-Health-Principles-and-Recommendations.aspx

Kirpatrick. D. (2000). Definitions of public policy and the law. Retrieved from www.musc.edu/vawprevention/policy/definition.shtml

Kaiser Family Foundation. (2020). Health insurance coverage of the total population. Retrieved from https://www.kff.org/other/state-indicator/total-population/?currentTimeframe=0&sortModel=%7B%22colId%22:%22Location%22,%22sort%22:%22asc%22%7D

Kilpatrick. D. (2000). Definitions of public policy and the law. Retrieved from www.musc.edu/vawprevention/policy/definition.shtml

Kraft, M., & Furlong S. (2010). *Public policy—politics, analysis, and alternatives* (3rd ed.). Washington DC: CQ Press.

Mangram, A.J., Horan, T. C., Pearson, J. L., Silver, L. C., & Jarvis, W. R. (1999). Hospital infection control practices advisory committee: Guideline for prevention of surgical site infection. *Infection Control and Hospital Epidemiology, 20*, 250–278.

Martin, P. (December 22, 2009). Health care profiteers: A billion-dollar lobby. Retrieved from https://www.wsws.org/en/articles/2009/12/lobb-d22.html

National Quality Forum. (n.d.). List of SREs. Retrieved from http://www.qualityforum.org/Topics/SREs/List_of_SREs.aspx

Reid, T. R. (2010). *The healing of America: A global quest for better, cheaper and fairer health care.* New York, NY: Penguin Press.

Walt, G. & Gilson, L. (1994). Reforming the health sector in developing countries: The central role of policy analysis. *Health Policy and Planning, 9,* 353–370.

CHAPTER 16

Assess and Evaluate

Outcome Measurement and Revision of Plan

Patti Ludwig-Beymer

LEARNING OBJECTIVES

■ Describe the components of an evaluation or measurement plan designed to assess the impact of evidence-based quality improvement initiatives.

■ Compare and contrast structure, process, and outcome measures.

■ Discuss data characteristics that should be considered as part of an evaluation plan.

■ Identify organizations that provide comparative data (benchmarks) for use in evaluating outcome measures.

KEY TERMS

Benchmarking	Prevalence
Common cause variation	Process measures
Data	Prospective data
Evaluation plan	Relative data
Incidence	Reliability
Magnet® recognition program	Retrospective data
Nursing-sensitive indicators	Special cause variation
Operational definition	Structure measures
Outcome measures	Validity

C l i n i c a l   S t o r y

Linda, the new manager of a medical surgical unit, reviews unit data related to infections. She is surprised to find that the unit has higher rates than the Centers for Medicare & Medicaid (CMS) Pay-for-Performance initiatives and the National Database of Nursing Quality Indicators (NDNQI) nursing-sensitive indicators for four clinical outcomes: catheter-associated urinary tract infections (CAUTIs), central line–associated bloodstream infections (CLABSIs), hospital-acquired *Clostridium difficile* (*C. diff*) infections, and hospital-acquired methicillin-resistant *Staphylococcus aureus* (MRSA). She notices that hand hygiene compliance on the unit, measured by secret observers, is low.

Think Before You Read

- What kind of data would you recommend that Linda gather to understand what might be contributing to higher infection rates on her unit? Considering the entire time from when patients are admitted until they are discharged, when might Linda gather data to understand the problem?
- What might be some of the challenges in collecting data related to hospital-acquired infections?
- What kinds of measurements related to safety need to be observed and what kinds of data may be already part of the electronic medical record that may help Linda figure out what is happening with infection rates?

Introduction

Evidence-based practice (EBP) can effectively improve patient outcomes, patient satisfaction, and organizational financial performance. Quality improvement (QI) is a framework used to systematically improve care delivery. Evidence should always be used to design and implement complex QI initiatives. QI involves continuous efforts to decrease process variation and improve the outcomes of the processes for patients, the health-care organization, and the health-care system (Agency for Health Care Quality and Research, 2013).

Nursing practice and health-care processes result in **data** that can be measured, analyzed, improved, and controlled. Data are used to determine whether care delivery goals are being met. Data are used to assess the quality of care and are reported to a variety of stakeholders, including consumers of care, purchasers of care, accreditation bodies, providers of care, and governing bodies. An evaluation plan, also known as a measurement plan, is an important component for both EBP implementation plans and QI initiatives. Ideally, the evaluation plan should include measures for structures, processes, and outcomes (Donabedian, 2003). Structures refer to the way in which care is delivered, such as supplies, equipment, and type and number of staff. Processes refer to actions taken in delivering care, such as policies and standards of care. Outcomes refer to the results of the care that was delivered. Outcomes may be clinical (e.g., catheter-associated urinary tract infection), functional (e.g., ability to perform activities of daily living), patient experience (e.g., patient or family satisfaction with care), safety (e.g., sentinel events), or financial (e.g., length of stay or hospital readmission rate). **Nursing-sensitive indicators** are outcome measures that reflect the structure, processes, and outcomes of nursing care. As part of the **Magnet® recognition** program, the American Nurses Credentialing Center (ANCC, 2017) requires that Magnet® facilities identify and provide data for nursing-sensitive indicators for practice in both acute and ambulatory care.

Evaluation or Measurement Plan

An **evaluation plan** should be developed before implementing a change. Otherwise, the effectiveness of the initiative cannot be measured. Baseline data should be collected before the process change and then re-collected post-implementation. To demonstrate sustainability, the AACN Magnet® program requires three data points after implementation (ANCC, 2017).

As seen in Table 16■1, an evaluation plan grid can be helpful for organizing data collection methods. When constructing a measurement plan, consider these questions:

- What structural changes occurred as part of the evidence implementation?
- What are the key process variables that are affected by the evidence implementation?
- What problem was the change intended to solve?

Structure Measures

Structure measures determine whether there have been changes in the environment of care. Several structural measures can be identified for the opening clinical story. For example, Linda may assess the number and placement of sinks and hand

TABLE 16■1   **Measurement or Evaluation Plan**

Measure	Operational Definition	Time of Collection	Person Responsible

hygiene dispensers on the unit. With the assistance of housekeeping, she might look at the amount of hand sanitizer used on the unit each month.

Process Measures

Process measures allow us to understand what is being done and determine whether we are doing the right thing. In the opening clinical story, secret observers document hand hygiene compliance for nurses, physicians, other clinicians, and visitors. These process measures allow Linda to determine where procedural improvements are needed.

Process measures could also be collected to examine care related to each of the infections described in the clinical story. For catheter-associated urinary tract infections (CAUTIs), Linda could examine process measures related to the insertion and maintenance of indwelling urinary catheters. For example, is the catheter inserted only for clinically appropriate reasons? Is it discontinued as soon as possible? Is the drainage bag kept consistently below the level of the bladder? While these process measures are an important part of quality improvement, they do not demonstrate actual improvement in a clinical outcome.

Outcome Measures

Outcome measure data are used to determine whether the right results occurred. In the clinical story, a reduction in CAUTIs, CLABSIs, hospital-acquired *C. diff* infections, and hospital-acquired MRSA rates will demonstrate improvements in clinical outcomes. Box 16■1 summarizes why outcome measurement is important and Box 16■2 lists common measurement foci.

Operational Definitions

Accurate measures require a clear description of what is being measured. **Operational definitions** describe in detail what is being measured, how it is being measured, who is measuring it, and when the measurement should occur. Operational definitions are clear and unambiguous and help to ensure that everyone is measuring the same

---

BOX 16■1 **Why Is Outcome Measurement Important?**

- Validation that existing policies and procedures are on target
- Increased quality
- Enhanced patient safety
- Increased patient satisfaction
- Cost containment
- Financial reimbursement from third-party payers
- Maintenance of managed care contracts
- Identification of staff education needs

BOX 16■2   Common Measurement Foci

Clinical Outcomes

- Catheter-associated urinary tract infections (CAUTIs)
- Central line–associated bloodstream infections (CLABSIs)
- Door-to-balloon time for acute MI
- Delay in treatment
- HbA1c level
- Hospital-acquired *C. diff*
- Hospital-acquired MRSA
- Hospital-acquired pneumonia
- Hospital-acquired pressure injury
- Mortality rates
- Patient experiences of care (patient satisfaction)
- Patient falls and patient falls with injury
- Postoperative pulmonary emboli (PE) or deep vein thrombosis (DVT)
- Sepsis
- Surgical site infections
- Surgical patient burns
- Venous thromboembolism (VTE)
- Ventilator-associated events (VAEs), including ventilator-associated pneumonia

Financial Indicators

- Cost per beneficiary
- Cost per case
- Readmission rate

Nursing Process Measures

- Adherence to care pathways/protocols
- Hand hygiene
- Medication errors
- Patient education
- Patient mobility
- Systematic skin inspections
- Wound care

---

thing. Creating an operational definition begins by searching the literature and examining definitions used by credible organizations.

Generating an operational definition is more difficult than it first appears. Consider the task of developing an operational definition for appropriate hand hygiene in the clinical story above. The World Health Organization (WHO, n.d.) created an evidence-based approach to hand hygiene that is applicable to all settings. The approach recommends health-care workers clean their hands five times: before touching a patient, before performing clean or aseptic procedures, after body fluid exposure or risk of exposure, after touching a patient, and after touching patient surroundings. Hand hygiene compliance by a validated observer through direct observation is considered the gold standard in hand hygiene compliance monitoring. It is the only method available to identify all hand hygiene opportunities, assess the appropriate timing of hand hygiene, and count the number of times when hand hygiene action is performed (WHO, 2009). The WHO further delineates when alcohol-based hand sanitizers can be used and when handwashing with soap and water is required. By establishing an operational definition for appropriate hand hygiene, accurate and detailed information can be collected.

Quality Data Considerations

As part of the evaluation plan, we must ensure that data are accurate, valid, reliable, secure, and timely and provide utility. To be accurate, data must be correct and complete. Data **validity** refers to ensuring that we are measuring what we really want to measure. For example, appropriate hand hygiene when caring for a patient with *C. diff* requires washing thoroughly with soap and water. Measuring the use of hand sanitizer for this patient population would not be an appropriate quality measure.

Reliability is also essential for data collection and data entry. For observations, it will be necessary to create specific measurement criteria and determine inter-rater reliability. For example, all secret observers must observe and document consistently so that we are confident that we'd get the same results in the same situation. In terms of security, data must be safely stored with patient confidentiality protected. Deadlines must be established and respected. Ultimately, the utility of data is based on providing the information needed to inform decisions. Accurate data allow us to make good decisions.

Types of Data

A variety of types of data may be collected. For example, the data may be retrospective or prospective. **Retrospective data** are easy to access because they use existing data. Retrospective data may be sufficient to meet the needs of the initiative. However, it cannot be manipulated, and the quality of the data cannot be controlled. We often use retrospective data from electronic health records. However, the documentation is not always complete. **Prospective data** are more labor intensive, as they require the creation of a data collection tool and people to collect the data. The data are only as good as the instrument that has been developed. However, prospective data collection can increase the completeness of documentation.

Data may also be absolute or relative. Absolute data, sometimes referred to as raw data, represent the true count or the actual numbers. Reporting actual numbers rather than rates could be misleading. For example, Linda may notice that the number of CAUTIs on her unit decreased during the month of July. She also knows, however, that half of the beds were closed on the unit that month for painting. As a result, the patient census was much lower than usual. For **relative data,** a denominator is provided, and a rate is calculated. A rate is a fraction, with the numerator being the number of cases and the denominator being the population at risk. For example, a CAUTI rate is generally reported as the number of CAUTIs per 1,000 catheter days during a month or a quarter.

Data may also be expressed as incidence or prevalence. **Incidence** is defined as the number of new cases occurring within a period of time reported as a fraction of the population at risk. Hospitals often report CAUTIs, CLABSIs, hospital-acquired *C. diff* and MRSA, and patient falls as incidences. **Prevalence** refers to the number of cases divided by the population during a period of time (period prevalence) or at a particular point in time (point prevalence). Hospital-acquired pressure ulcers are typically reported through a point prevalence study, because collecting the data on a daily basis for all patients would be difficult, and NDNQI requires they be reported in this way. One day is selected every quarter and each patient's skin is assessed for injury on that day. It is important to recognize whether data are incidence or prevalence.

Sources of Data

Data to measure the effectiveness of a QI or EBP initiative may be housed in a variety of areas. For example, data may be collected by staff in the quality, risk management, or infection prevention departments. Unit staff may also collect and store data. The finance department collects important information and can make the data available for QI and EBP initiatives. The medical staff office may have practitioner-specific data. Information systems can assist in retrieving data that have been documented in an electronic health record. This saves valuable time and avoids the need for a chart audit. At times, new data will need to be generated.

Comparative or Benchmark Data

When implementing evidence and making improvements, internal data are compared to results from reputable internal or external sources. This is referred to as **benchmarking**. The benchmarking tool has been used in the business world for many years. The Xerox Corporation used benchmarking in the 1970s to improve systemwide performance and implement the use of best practice in their industry (Tran, 2003). While financial benchmarking was historically conducted, benchmarking is also used in health care to evaluate quality care, safety, and patient experience. Benchmarking establishes a comparison that can then be used to judge care. The belief is that providing safe, high-quality care to patients will actually reduce the cost of care.

A benchmark can be established in many ways. In the clinical story, Linda might identify an internal unit with high rates of hand hygiene compliance and low rates of patient infections. She might compare her data and her processes of care to that unit to identify opportunities for improvement. Externally, Linda will start with a review of the literature (ROL). This review will encompass a strategic search for current knowledge on this topic. Published research is an example of previously generated knowledge and is useful for setting benchmarks. Quality organizations, like the Agency for Health Care Quality and Research (AHRQ), Centers for Disease Control and Prevention (CDC), and ANCC, also provide data that allow organizations to benchmark. An organization may set a goal to achieve outcomes that are better than the mean or median, upper quartile, or upper decile.

Benchmarking and the Nursing Process

Standards of nursing practice directly relate to nursing activities you carry out through the nursing process. This involves assessment, diagnosis, planning, implementation, and evaluation. As discussed in previous chapters, the nursing process is the basis for clinical decision making and drives all aspects of patient care. Standards of nursing practice are defined as "authoritative statements of the duties that all registered nurses, regardless of role, population, or specialty, are expected to perform competently" (ANA, 2015, p. 89). Standards are established by professional organizations, working groups, state boards of nursing, and other overseeing governing bodies.

Payors, such as CMS and insurance agencies, expect health-care delivery to be safe and of high quality. If this standard is not met, the payor may withhold reimbursement. In the United States, three CMS pay-for-performance programs add a financial incentive for hospitals to meet safety standards and quality benchmarks. Value-based purchasing rewards or penalizes hospitals for achievement and improvement scores for care processes, patient experience of care, outcomes, and efficiency. The readmission reduction program penalizes hospitals with excessive readmissions for common medical and surgical conditions. The hospital-acquired conditions reduction program penalizes hospitals that exceed benchmarks for several patient safety indicators, including CLABSIs, CAUTIs, and *C. diff* and MRSA infections. Linda's focus on reducing these infections on her unit is appropriate clinically, ethically, and financially.

Data Displays

Data can be displayed in a variety of ways, including line charts, pie charts, histograms, pareto charts, scatter plots, run charts, and control charts. While it is beyond the scope of this chapter to describe each tool in detail, the key is to present the data in a meaningful way. For EBP and QI projects, displaying data over time is often beneficial. Templates for creating many of these tools are available on The Joint Commission (TJC, 2019), Institute for Healthcare Improvement (IHI, 2019), and American Society for Quality (ASQ, 2019) Web sites.

As part of Magnet® documentation, each unit is required to submit a graph with eight quarters of nursing-sensitive data along with data from a nationally recognized database. This allows organizations to demonstrate how they perform against a respected comparison. Similarly, Magnet® requires a graph with four data points for QI and EBP initiatives: one data point before and three data points after implementation. This provides some indication of sustainability for the initiative. Magnet® requires two examples, with data, of an improved outcome associated with an evidence-based change made by clinical nurses in alignment with the organization's professional practice model and one example, with data, of an improved outcome associated with an interprofessional quality improvement activity led or co-led by a nurse (ANCC, 2017).

Interpreting Variations in Data

An important aspect of data measurement is the ability to understand variation. If we don't understand variation, we see trends where there are none, blame or give credit to people for things over which they have no control, try to explain natural variation as special events, and have limited ability to make improvements. W. Edwards Deming, a noted expert in quality improvement, stated, "If I had to reduce my message for management to just a few words, I'd say it all had to do with reducing variation" (quoted in Neave, 1990, p. 57).

There are two types of variation: common cause variation and special cause variation. **Common cause variation** is inherent in the design of the process and is due to regular, natural, or ordinary causes. Common cause variation is also known as random variation. **Special cause variation** is due to irregular causes that are not inherent in the process. This type of variation is also known as non-random variation. When implementing EBP and QI initiatives, we purposefully introduce changes that we hope will result in special cause variation. In research, the appropriate statistical test is used to determine whether the change is random (due to chance) or non-random (statistically significant). In QI and EBP initiatives, a run chart or control chart is used to determine the type of variation.

Returning to the opening clinical story will show why it is important to differentiate between common cause variation and special cause variation. Consider the following scenario: In one month, compliance with hand hygiene increased from 63% to 64%. Should Linda celebrate this improvement? No, this is normal variation. Similarly, Linda should not assume hand hygiene compliance is getting worse because it changed from 64% to 63%. Linda's goal is to decrease variation while increasing overall performance. In the case of hand hygiene, Linda wants each person to use appropriate hand hygiene with no variation. Using the WHO protocol will help to reduce practice variability.

Ask/Assess

Returning to the opening clinical story, Linda approaches her new position as a unit manager with an attitude of inquiry. She wonders what clinical outcomes are associated with nursing care delivered on the unit and how the care and outcomes can be improved. Her questions come from her practice as a nurse manager and are real and meaningful to her work and to improving care on her unit.

Linda recognizes that each patient who develops a CLABSI, CAUTI, hospital-acquired *C. diff* infection, or hospital-acquired MRSA infection has experienced a complication of care. Their length of stay may be longer, and they incur financial and personal hardships. They are at risk for long-term sequelae and even death. In addition, Linda knows that the hospital may be financially penalized for these poor outcomes. She also knows that poor compliance with hand hygiene protocols is a major contributing factor to all of these infections.

Linda needs to create an effective and practical plan to improve patient outcomes related to infections on her unit. She asks Paul, the clinical nurse specialist (CNS), to assist her in reviewing the literature and determining best strategies to increase hand hygiene compliance. Paul knows that the first step in conducting a literature review is to state a clear question that will lead to the right evidence. As a result, Linda and Paul construct the following PICO question: What are effective strategies for improving hand hygiene compliance on a medical-surgical unit?

Acquire/Diagnose

Linda and Paul do not have the time or resources to conduct a systematic review. Instead, they focus their search on existing systematic reviews and clinical practice guidelines. They find information on the AHRQ, CDC, WHO, and ASQ Web sites. They also find two JBI recommended practices on hand hygiene (Gyi, 2016, 2018) and one focused on education interventions (Fong, 2018) applicable to their patient population.

Appraise/Plan

Linda has identified four clinical problems and a process problem. She recognizes these problems by examining the unit data and comparing them to her hospital's data and national data from CMS and NDNQI. She knows that poor compliance with appropriate hand hygiene contributes to the suboptimal clinical outcomes. Linda and Paul have examined the literature and have used the appropriate tools to conduct a critical appraisal. They also realize that patient involvement is an important aspect of evidence-based practice and are happy to find a systematic review focused on patients partnering with health-care professionals for hand hygiene compliance (Butenko, Lockwood, & McArthur, 2017).

Linda prepares a project proposal and discusses it with her manager and with the director of the quality department. Everyone agrees that an interprofessional team should be chartered to address this issue. Linda and Paul serve as co-chairs and convene a team that includes nurses, physicians, nursing assistants, housekeepers, and an infection prevention practitioner.

Apply/Implement

Linda realizes that successful strategies require an interprofessional approach and is pleased that an interprofessional team has been convened. To fill one of the physician roles, a hospitalist volunteers to work on the initiative. Linda knows that the culture of the unit and the organization will affect the success of this initiative. To support the interprofessional team, she helps them examine barriers and facilitators from an organizational, unit, and individual level. The team receives strong organizational support. Preventing patient infections has high priority within the hospital. The chief nursing officer (CNO) supports evidence-based practice and expects nurses and other health-care providers to adhere to professional standards of care.

As part of the evidence-based change, Linda uses the Registered Nurses' Association of Ontario Toolkit (Registered Nurses' Association of Ontario, 2012) to analyze the unit's readiness for change. Because Linda recognizes that staff support and involvement are important to the overall success and implementation of the changes, Linda discusses the initiative at her monthly staff meetings. She shares the current data, conveys the importance of the initiative, and invites staff to provide suggestions to the chartered team. Linda's careful planning will help to ensure the success of the project.

Linda realizes that she will need to examine both process and outcome measures to evaluate the effectiveness of this initiative. Fortunately, the hospital is already collecting appropriate measurement data. Compliance with hand hygiene is a process measure; it is collected by secret observers and is tracked and trended by the infection prevention practitioner. The four hospital-acquired infections are also tracked by the infection prevention practitioner and are reported in graph form. The team prepares a data dashboard that displays the data for both process and outcome measures. Outcome measures are compared to national data from NDNQI.

The team convenes. Based on the evidence, they recognize that multimodal and interprofessional intervention strategies should be used to improve hand hygiene compliance. They agree to begin with education, followed by feedback and reminders. Simultaneously, they plan to assess the facility layout and the availability of hand hygiene products. They want to consider patient partnership and hand hygiene monitoring technology in the future.

Education is provided based on the World Health Organization's Five Moments for Hand Hygiene model (WHO, n.d.). Performance data for hand hygiene and the four hospital-acquired infections are posted on a graph in the unit break room. Historically, the data have been reported quarterly. During this initiative, however, the infection preventionist volunteers to update the data each month. After 100% of the staff and 90% of the physicians receive education, the graphs show a sharp increase in hand hygiene compliance and no change in CAUTI, CLABSI, MRSA, and *C. diff* rates.

The team notes that the number and placement of sinks is appropriate. However, some of the hand sanitizer dispensers are inconveniently located behind the patient's bed rather than close to the door. They ask for permission to purchase and install additional dispensers, which Linda approves. After the new hand sanitizers are installed, the team sees a small increase in hand hygiene compliance, a small improvement in CAUTI and CLABSI rates, and no change in hospital-acquired MRSA and *C. diff* rates.

Next, the team reviews how secret hand hygiene observers are trained. They work with infection prevention to implement additional training based on CDC guidelines for all observers. In addition, the observers are taught how to intervene to provide real-time feedback to staff, physicians, and visitors. Observers are deployed throughout the hospital. On Linda's unit, they make some interesting observations, particularly around patients in isolation for *C. diff* and MRSA. Staff, physicians, and visitors are not always compliant with isolation precautions and may even resist the feedback that is given to them.

When this information is brought to Linda and the team, they realize this will require additional interventions. Linda begins by discussing the situation with her peers. Linda learns that other unit managers have the same issue with isolation and have not identified an effective strategy to improve compliance. Linda and her manager discuss the situation with the CNO, who agrees to the request for a hospital-wide team to address this. Linda volunteers to be one of the pilot units for this initiative. Over time, as compliance with isolation protocols improves, hospital-acquired *C. diff* and MRSA rates decrease.

Linda's unit now has hospital-acquired infection rates that are close to CMS and NDNQI levels. Linda is not satisfied. The team continues to investigate options, including patient partnering. Based on a systematic review (Butenko et al, 2017), the team knows that partnership can enhance the performance of hand hygiene. They recognize that patients have differing levels of knowledge about hand hygiene and are fearful about influencing the caring relationship with their health-care providers. They also know that the culture, beliefs, and behaviors of health-care providers do not fully support this partnership. Linda knows that the hospital has a patient advisory committee, and she asks the CNO for some time on the agenda to discuss this issue with committee members. They provide valuable feedback and Linda and her team develop a plan for educating staff, physicians, and patients on partnership. Hand hygiene compliance reaches 98% to 100% and hospital-acquired infection rates drop below benchmark.

Linda recognizes that the use of secret observers is time consuming and expensive, and results in intermittent data. The team investigates the implementation of hand hygiene monitoring technology, including electronic and video monitoring systems. Through a JBI Evidence Summary (Pamaiahgari, 2018), they know that there is some evidence that the use of hand hygiene monitoring technology improves hand hygiene and/or reduces the incidence of hospital-acquired infections. However, the evidence is limited, and there is a risk of bias. To implement the technology at the hospital, it would need to be budgeted as a capital request, and there is strong competition for capital dollars. As a result, the team recommends the technology not be implemented at this time. Instead, they continue to focus on reminders, timely feedback, and patient partnerships. The graphs remain posted in the unit break room, and clinical staff are proud of their hard work and excellent clinical outcomes (Box 16■3).

■ Summary

The clinical story demonstrates many aspects of a successful improvement initiative. A passionate leader supported a strong interprofessional team. Evidence was used to develop tactics, and input was sought from staff and patients. The interprofessional

---

BOX 16■3 Interprofessional Rounds

- Plan a presentation in which you explain the concept of nursing-sensitive indicators to colleagues from other disciplines.
- Have a brainstorming session with several colleagues and discuss a benchmarking strategy to address an outcomes project.
- Compare and contrast the information on patient falls with injuries and hospital-acquired pressure injury on several health-care quality Web sites.

BOX 16■4 Tools for Learning and Practice

- Read the Hand Hygiene Toolkit located at https://www.ascaconnect.org/viewdocument/hand-hygiene-what-cms-surveyors-are-looking-for-asc-quality-collaboration-infection-prevention-toolkit and describe how the toolkit can be implemented by every member of the interprofessional team. Discuss strategies for implementing the toolkit. Identify how the effectiveness of the toolkit could be measured.
- Identify a nursing practice problem. Search the Internet and see if you can find a standard of care that addresses the problem.

---

team considered structures (the availability of sinks and hand sanitizer dispensers; the use of hand hygiene–monitoring technology), processes (performance of hand hygiene; education; consultation), and outcomes (rate of four hospital-acquired infections). Data were used to track performance and modify and augment improvement efforts. Improvement was viewed as ongoing and continuous.

Measuring outcomes to evaluate the effectiveness of EBP and QI initiatives is essential for maintaining and improving patient safety and quality. It is helpful to identify appropriate benchmarks to plan successful outcomes. Evaluating evidence-based quality improvement initiatives is complex. Evaluation plans must consider complexity, evolve as the initiative changes over time, and incorporate the local context (Parry, Coly, Goldman, et al, 2018). Outcome measures identify whether a process change has made a positive impact on care. On a regular basis, processes will need to be reevaluated. Health care is constantly evolving, influenced by new clinical knowledge, research results, and changes in patient needs. Measuring outcomes must be continual and ongoing (Box 16■4).

CHAPTER QUESTIONS

1. Why do we collect and use data in health care?
2. Why is it important to develop an evaluation or measurement plan for an evidence-based improvement initiative?

CHAPTER QUESTIONS (continued)

3. What are the differences between structure, process, and outcome measures? How do they relate to each other?

4. Why are operational definitions essential for data collection?

5. What is the difference between incidence and prevalence rates?

6. Where can benchmark data be found?

7. What is the purpose of standards of nursing practice?

8. What is the difference between common cause and special cause variation?

9. What are some examples of nursing-sensitive indicators?

References

Agency for Health Care Quality and Research. (2013). Module 4. Approaches to Quality Improvement. https://www.ahrq.gov/ncepcr/tools/pf-handbook/mod4.html

American Nurses Association. (2015). *Nursing: Scope and standards of practice* (3rd ed.). Silver Spring, MD: Author.

American Nurses Credentialing Center. (2017). *2019 Magnet application manual.* Silver Spring, MD: Author.

American Society for Quality. (2019). The global voice of quality. Retrieved from https://asq.org/

Butenko, S., Lockwood, C., & McArthur, A. (2017). Patient experiences if partnering with healthcare professionals for hand hygiene compliance: A systematic review. *JBI Database of Systematic Review and Implementation Reports*, 1645–1670. http://ovidsp.dc2.ovid.com/sp-4.04.0a/ovidweb.cgi?&S=NFOIFPFEPKEBNAHIIPCKMHEHGOEKAA00&Link+Set=S.sh.21%7c11%7csl_190

Donabedian, A. (2003). *An introduction to quality assurance in health care.* New York, NY: Oxford University Press.

Fong, E. (2018). Evidence summary. Prevention of health care associated infections: Educational interventions. The Joanna Brigs Institute EBP Database, JBI@Ovid. http://ovidsp.dc2.ovid.com/sp-4.04.0a/ovidweb.cgi?&S=NFOIFPFEPKEBNAHIIPCKMHEHGOEKAA00&Link+Set=S.sh.21%7c3%7csl_190

Gyi, A. A. (2018). Evidence summary. Hand hygiene: Strategies to improve compliance in healthcare settings. The Joanna Brigs Institute EBP Database, JBI@Ovid. http://ovidsp.dc2.ovid.com/sp-4.04.0a/ovidweb.cgi?&S=NFOIFPFEPKEBNAHIIPCKMHEHGOEKAA00&Link+Set=S.sh.21%7c7%7csl_190

Gyi, A. A. (2016). JBI recommended practice. Basic hand hygiene. The Joanna Brigs Institute EBP Database, JBI@Ovid. http://ovidsp.dc2.ovid.com/sp-4.04.0a/ovidweb.cgi?&S=NFOIFPFEPKEBNAHIIPCKMHEHGOEKAA00&Link+Set=S.sh.21%7c7%7csl_190JBI

Institute for Healthcare Improvement (IHI). (2019). Improving health and health care worldwide. Retrieved from http://www.ihi.org/

Neave, H. R. (1990). *The Deming dimension.* Knoxville, TN: SPC Press.

Pamaiahgari, P. (2018). Hand hygiene monitoring technology. The Joanna Briggs Institute EBP Database, JBI@Ovid. http://ovidsp.dc2.ovid.com/sp-4.04.0a/ovidweb.cgi?&S=NFOIFPFEPKEBNAHIIPCKMHEHGOEKAA00&Link+Set=S.sh.21%7c2%7csl_190

Parry, G., Coly, A., Goldman, D., et al. (2018). Practical recommendations for the evaluation of improvement initiatives. *International Journal for Quality in Health Care*, 30(S1), 29–36. https://academic.oup.com/intqhc/article/30/suppl_1/29/4852806

Registered Nurses' Association of Ontario. (2012). *Toolkit: Implementation of best practice guidelines* (2nd ed.). Retrieved from https://rnao.ca/bpg/resources/toolkit-implementation-best-practice-guidelines-second-edition

The Joint Commission (TJC). (2019). https://www.jointcommission.org/

Tran, M. N. (2003). Take benchmarking to the next level. *Nursing Management, 34*(1), 18–23. http://dx.doi.org.pnw.idm.oclc.org/10.1097/00006247-200301000-00009

World Health Organization (WHO). (n.d.) *My 5 moments for hand hygiene.* Retrieved from https://www.who.int/infection-prevention/campaigns/clean-hands/5moments/en/

World Health Organization (WHO). (2009). *WHO guidelines on hand hygiene in health care: First global patient safety challenge clean care is safer care.* Retrieved from https://www.ncbi.nlm.nih.gov/books/NBK144028/

Putting It All Together

This unit provides practical examples of evidence-based decision making in specialty nursing areas. Each chapter is structured in a parallel fashion to illustrate how an evidence-based approach can address nurse-sensitive outcomes. Nurse-sensitive outcomes are those that confirm nurses' contributions to patient care in areas such as quality of life, symptom management, safety, functional status, and utilization of nursing resources. The chapters in this unit integrate the evidence-based practice (EBP) process from problem identification to outcome evaluation and quality improvement. The specialty topics that are covered in this unit are medical-surgical nursing, maternal health nursing, nursing of children, mental health nursing, nursing care of the older adult, and community health nursing. Each chapter provides a unique lesson in evidence-based decision making.

CHAPTER 17

Medical-Surgical Nursing

Lisa Hopp

LEARNING OBJECTIVES

■ Given an ill-structured description of a common clinical case, apply all phases of the evidence-based practice process to guide decisions related to common medical-surgical nursing problems.

■ Analyze the challenges to making evidence-based decisions in complex health-care environments.

■ Generate next-step strategies to get better evidence into practice.

KEY TERMS

AGREE tools
Critical Appraisal Skills
  Program (CASP)
Hospital-acquired condition
  (HAC)
Incidence

Pay-for-performance
Pressure injury
Prevalence
Scale
Scope

Clinical Story

Sara has worked on an adult medical-surgical unit for 2 years. The patient population is a mixture of elderly, chronically ill patients with a variety of acute medical illnesses and general adult surgical patients. She is caring for LH, a 78-year-old female who is 5 days post-thoracotomy for lung cancer. LH was transferred from the intensive care unit to the Sara's unit 2 days ago. When helping LH to bathe, Sara noticed several areas of skin breakdown on her back and sacrum. The wounds on the skin covering her spine look as if a single layer of skin has been torn off, but the wound on her sacrum looks different. Sara observes that it is a shallow, full-thickness crater with a red to pink bed. Although LH walks about 15 feet twice per day and sits in a chair for 15 minutes after her walk, she spends the rest of the day in a standard hospital bed, requiring help to turn. She is still quite weak from her surgery and complicated early recovery and requires oral pain medication every 4 hours. She is consuming only clear liquids, tolerates them poorly, and has a distended abdomen. Sara wonders if there was something else that she and her fellow nurses could have done to prevent the breaks in LH's skin integrity.

Think Before You Read

- What are the steps of the EBP process?
- What PICO or PICo questions can you imagine that are relevant to the clinical story?
- What model can you use to structure how you approach implementing the evidence?
- What might be some key issues to consider as you search for and appraise the evidence?
- What might be some candidate implementation strategies?
- What do you need to consider to judge the success or failure of a project like the one in the clinical story?

Introduction

Skin care may seem like a very basic nursing task that does not merit a deep exploration of the evidence to support best practices. However, nurses should not reserve doing the right thing the right way only in complex interventions. Rather, nurses seek the best available evidence to support nursing care decisions and the best possible patient outcomes, regardless of how gripping the concern. In fact, often when you begin to think more about the reasons you do what you do, you find that there is more to understanding the simplest procedures than you had thought.

In this chapter, you will find a blueprint to apply the evidence-based practice process to one medical-surgical problem. To keep the focus sharp and the scenario as straightforward as possible, the chapter addresses only a small portion of the problem.

What Are the Key Issues?

According to international consensus and study, a **pressure injury** is "localized damage to the skin and underlying tissue usually over a bony prominence or related to a medical or other device. The injury can present as intact skin or an open injury and may be painful. The injury occurs as a result of intense and/or prolonged pressure or pressure in combination with shear. The tolerance of soft tissue for pressure and shear may also be affected by microclimate, nutrition, perfusion, comorbid conditions, and condition of the soft tissue" (Edsberg, Black, Goldberg, et al, 2016, p. 586). This definition provides hints about what a nurse needs to do to pay attention to and prevent pressure injuries, but it will be the evidence that indicates the correct thing to do.

The evidence-based practice process begins with a nurse being curious and skeptical. You can use the nursing paradigm to organize how you think about the care you provide. You need to pay close attention to the patient, his or her state of health, the environment, and the usual nursing care. By assessing and examining each element of the nursing meta-paradigm, you can uncover the key issues related to your decisions. For example, think about how patient and health-related factors of aging enter into your decisions about skin care. Consider the person's ability to move or even shift his or her weight, skin condition, continence, sensory function, nutritional status, or other issues.

Part of thinking about the person is to understand the patient's preferences. For example, some bed surfaces may reduce pressure, but the patient may find the surface uncomfortable. Patients have food preferences that can affect how to best meet their nutritional needs. It is important to find out and integrate patients' values, desires, and preferences in the decision-making process.

Next, question how the environment might influence your care. Is anything rubbing the skin to cause friction on the skin such as bed sheets, rails, or a device? What kind of surface is the patient sitting or lying on? Finally, consider how your nursing care can protect or pose a risk to the patient's skin integrity. For example, does the way you assist the patient to move in bed help or hurt? These are all key issues you must consider during the evidence-based practice process.

What Are the Scope and Scale?

When you have a curious attitude and are aware of how and why you make decisions, you can quickly become overwhelmed with the number of questions that underlie even basic nursing care. You can even run the risk of becoming paralyzed with inaction if you spend all of your time thinking rather than doing.

That is not the intent of evidence-based nursing practice. Rather, you need to be able to understand the **scope** (how big?) and **scale** (how much?) of the problem.

Scope

When you explore scope, you try to find the edges of the problem to determine its breadth. The "edges" may relate to age- or risk groups, disease, functional ability, setting, race, or even gender. In the case of skin integrity, the edges are very broad: all ages, all degrees of mobility, all settings, and all risk groups. However, in this chapter's clinical story Sara can narrow her concern to frail, poorly mobile, elderly patients in acute care facilities who are at high risk for impaired skin integrity because these factors all relate to LH's condition.

The scope of the question determines how you search and what type of evidence you find. For large questions, such as, What is the best way to care for any patient at risk for skin breakdown?, you are likely to find a clinical practice guideline that addresses many parts of the bigger problem. For smaller questions, such as, What is the best bed surface to reduce pressure in at risk older patients?, you are likely to find the answer in a systematic review of primary research or as part of a guideline.

Scale

To determine the scale of the problem, you need to determine whether your observation is an isolated occurrence or whether there is a trend that shows the nursing care simply isn't working. You may only focus on the care of particular patients for whom you are responsible, or you can expand your concern to a larger group of patients. To determine the scale of a problem in your unit, service line, or institution, you need to assess the **incidence** (the rate of new conditions) and/ or **prevalence** (the rate of a condition at any point in time) of the condition, as well as the contexts in which it is occurring. For example, you might assess the problem on a smaller scale and ask, Are elderly patients recovering from significant surgery experiencing too many pressure injuries on my unit? You may widen your view and ask, Are patients in certain areas such as the operating room or acute rehabilitation units acquiring too many pressure injuries? These two questions illustrate how the scope and scale of your curiosity will drive you to ask questions and assess and search to uncover the evidence.

Ask/Assess

Both the nursing process and evidence-based practice process begin when nurses assess the problem and then ask questions that lead to the best available evidence to inform their decisions. Sara's skin assessment demonstrated that, at least in one patient, several skin tears and a stage II pressure injury occurred. Her next steps will determine both what she can do as an individual and how she might work with others to find out if the problem is bigger than a single patient.

First, find out if an up-to-date, evidence-based resource already exists. Sara checks her policies and finds out that although there is a skin-care policy, the policy lacks references or any mentions of the evidence that informs it.

Second, find out if someone else is already gathering data that can help you determine the scale of the problem. Often quality improvement nurses, unit managers, risk managers, or clinical nurse specialists gather data on safety and quality-related outcomes such a pressure injury incidence and its prevalence. Use these local data as clues to help you understand the problem. If the incidence is less than benchmarks or at the level required by regulators, you would not receive much support to change practice. However, if the local data indicate there is a problem, then you need to find how best to intervene.

In 2008, the Centers for Medicare & Medicaid Services (CMS), the U.S. governmental agency administering several health programs, implemented a rule that the federal government will not pay additional costs associated with certain **hospital-acquired conditions (HACs),** meaning complications that could otherwise be prevented. Stages III and IV pressure injuries were among the first conditions that the CMS identified. This shift toward **pay-for-performance,** or reimbursement based on outcomes, makes pressure injury prevention a high priority for institutions and certainly for the patients themselves. In this case, *any* hospital-acquired pressure injury is unacceptable (Box 17▪1).

In the clinical story, the phrase "at-risk frail, elderly patients who are hospitalized in acute care areas" describes the scope of the problem. Using this scope, Sara talks with the quality officer, who provides her with the following data for the acute medical-surgical units in the facility and the latest national data:

- Monthly prevalence of all-stage hospital-acquired pressure injury rates on the medical-surgical units ranged from 5% to 12% over the past 6 months,

---

BOX 17▪1   Significance of Pressure Injuries

- Overall prevalence of pressure injuries = 11.9%
- Overall facility acquired pressures injuries = 5.0%
- Facility acquired rates were highest in critical care units:
  - 8.8% = general cardiac care units
  - 10.4% = surgical ICUs
  - 6% in medical and surgical step-down units
- In 2007, pressure injuries were estimated to cost $2.41 billion (HealthGrades, 2009).
- Pressure injuries cause pain and can lead to infection and sepsis.

From VanGilder, C., Amlung, S., Harrison, P., et al. (2009). Results of the 2008–2009 International Pressure Injury Prevalence™ survey and a 3-year, acute care, unit-specific analysis. *Ostomy Wound Management, 55,* 39–45. Retrieved from http://www.o-wm.com/content/results-2008-%E2%80%93-2009-international-pressure-injury-prevalence%E2%84%A2-survey-and-a-3-year-acute-care compared with 1.3% to 4% hospital-wide rates and a national benchmark of 5.0% for all types of U.S. hospitals in 2009 (VanGilder, Amlung, Harrison, et al, 2009).

- When stage I pressure injuries were excluded from the data, the units had hospital-acquired prevalence ranging from 3.2% to 7% compared with the national rate of 3.1% (VanGilder et al, 2009).

- Most pressure injuries in this hospital were on the sacrum or heels.

Given these data, Sara has good reason to pursue evidence to determine whether her nursing practice needs to change. To find the evidence, she needs to ask a well-formed question that points her to the target evidence. She decides that although all of the care related to preventing pressure injuries is important, she will begin with a limited focus.

The patient, LH, told Sara that she was on a different type of bed in the ICU. Sara suspects that transferring to a standard mattress in the medical-surgical unit may have contributed to the problem. Because the patient is weak and still experiencing pain, she does not move easily in bed; Sara often finds her crumpled at the bottom of the bed, needing a boost up toward the head of the bed. She assesses the patient's risk factors according to the hospital's policy, and she finds this patient is at high risk for pressure injuries due to limited activity, mobility, and nutrition and increased friction and shear (European Pressure Ulcer Advisory Panel [EPUAP], the National Pressure Injury Advisory Panel [NPIAP], and the Pan-Pacific Pressure Injury Alliance [PPPIA], 2019).

As Sara did, you will start with very broad questions that usually begin with, What is the best way to . . . ? As you define the focus, ask increasingly narrower questions until you can state the questions in a typical population, intervention, comparison, and outcome (PICO) format (Table 17■1).

Acquire/Diagnose

Sara suspects that her patient has impaired skin integrity related to inadequate pressure reduction and friction injury. Her diagnosis is based on her assessment of the patient's key risk factors: very limited mobility, increased friction caused by frequent repositioning, and very poor nutrition. Although Sara is not prepared to address the problems of the patient's nutrition, she recognizes the patient's poor intake contributes to her risk for skin breakdown. Sara's next step is to acquire the best available evidence based on her diagnosis and questions she suspects relate to caring for the patient's specific risk factors. She may search herself or call upon a librarian or more experienced searcher to help her.

Based on your PICO questions, generate a list of keywords and ideal sources of evidence. Take your PICO question apart, find the main words that will help you reach your target, and think about synonyms and alternate spellings for each (Table 17■2).

Now you are ready to search for your ideal source. Sara's questions relate to the effectiveness of interventions, so her ideal source would be an excellent clinical

TABLE 17■1 **Narrowing the Focus and Generating Questions**

Question Type	Example	
Broad	What are the best practices for preventing pressure injury?	
Narrow	What are the best bed surfaces for at-risk elderly patients?	
Narrow	What is the best way to help patients move up in bed to reduce friction?	
Searchable PICO	What is the effectiveness of pressure-reducing specialty beds versus standard hospital mattresses in elderly, at-risk patients on the incidence of pressure injuries?	P = elderly, at-risk patients I = pressure-reducing specialty beds C = standard hospital beds O = incidence of pressure injuries
Searchable PICO	What is the effectiveness of slip sheets versus helping elderly, at-risk patients move up in bed on the incidence of pressure injuries?	P = elderly, at-risk patients I = slip sheets C = helping patients move up in bed O = incidence of pressure injuries

practice guideline based on systematic reviews of randomized controlled trials that tested the interventions. If no guidelines exist that meet her requirements, she would need to search for systematic reviews or individual studies using bibliographic databases such as the Cumulative Index to Nursing and Allied Health Literature (CINAHL) or MEDLINE.

If you are consulting with a librarian, take your question and list of keywords and synonyms with you. If you are searching yourself, start by searching the "best-bet" sources. In the past, the librarian may have sent you to the online **National Guideline Clearinghouse** (NGC) to find full-text and abstracted versions of guidelines that societies, governmental groups, and agencies voluntarily submitted. Unfortunately, the Agency for Healthcare Research and Quality (AHRQ) no longer maintains the NGC because of federal funding cuts (AHRQ, 2018). Therefore, Sara will need to search multiple sources to find guidelines, and she may need to use simple to more complex search strategies.

Since no single comprehensive guideline index or catalog exists, Sara starts by reaching out to the wound and ostomy experts in her hospital to understand what societies and organizations produce guidelines relevant to a pressure injury prevention. In addition, she searches the CINAHL index using a basic strategy to find articles that may refer to guideline development or updates. She searches as follows: ("pressure injury" OR "pressure ulcer") AND (guideline). She discovers an editorial that mentions that in 2019 three international organizations (EPUAP/ NPIAP/PPPIP) revised their comprehensive guideline (Kottner, Carville, Haesler, et al, 2019). She goes to their Web site and easily finds both a quick reference guide

TABLE 17■2 **Keywords and Search Strategy for the Cochrane Library or a Bibliographic Database**

PICO	Synonyms	Search Strategy
What is the effectiveness of pressure-reducing specialty beds versus standard hospital mattresses in elderly, at-risk patients on the incidence of pressure injuries?		
I = pressure-reducing specialty beds	beds support surface specialty bed overlay sport bed gel bed low pressure static air pressure alleviat* pressure support pressure reliev* pressure reduc* waffle mattress alternat* pressure water suspension	Link with OR
C = standard hospital beds	bed foam standard	Link with OR
O = incidence of pressure injuries	pressure injury pressure ulcer decubitus pressure sore skin tear	Link with OR
I + C + O		Link with AND
I = slip sheets	reposition mobility aid slip sheet	Link with OR
O = incidence of pressure injuries	pressure injury pressure ulcer decubitus pressure sore skin tear	Link with OR
I + O		Link with AND

and a complete guideline (https://npiap.com/) and decides to review this guideline to see if it should be appraised. In addition, she searches the Registered Nurses' Association of Ontario (RNAO) Best Practice Guideline library and the National Institute for Health and Care Excellence (NICE) for their most up-to-date guidelines. She selected these organizations because her clinical nurse specialist and quality improvement nurse told her that they publish high-quality and thorough guidelines. When Sara scans the guidelines, she decides to prioritize the most recent guideline first (EPUAP/NPIAP/PPPIA), but she will also consider the 2014 NICE guideline (NICE, 2014). The RNAO guideline on prevention has not been updated since 2002.

Finally, Sara searches the Cochrane Library to see if any more recent systematic reviews have been published. If Sara uses the basic search using just "pressure ulcer" as the search term (the Medical Subject Heading remains pressure ulcer), she gets over 700 results. She needs to narrow the search using the advanced search tools. If she uses the advanced search and some logic, she can narrow the results quickly. She uses the following Boolean strategy to first capture common terms for the outcome and intervention and then to link them together in the same review: ("pressure injury" OR "decubitus" OR "pressure ulcer") AND ("bed" OR "support surface" OR "mattress" OR "lift" OR "reposition") AND ("prevent*"). She also selects "abstract" to filter results to those where the support surface, lift or reposition would be most relevant. She is able to view by type of source because the results are organized by systematic review, protocol, trials, and other types of nonsystematic review publications. She nets 12 reviews, but only two are clearly relevant and one was not included in the guidelines she has selected (McInnes, Jammali-Blasi, Bell-Syer, et al, 2015).

Busy clinicians usually do not have time to conduct exhaustive searches using all of the potential synonyms and spellings. Your librarians can help you search the bibliographic databases if you can articulate what evidence you are looking for. It is helpful to talk with them to help them discover the words that might be used in various evidence sources. To obtain the right results, the search experts will link synonyms and alternate spellings for each key element together with the Boolean operator "OR" to expand the search, and they will glue the PICO elements together with "AND" to narrow the search toward your target (see Table 17■2).

Appraise/Plan

Sara has selected two clinical practice guidelines and two systematic reviews to evaluate to determine whether the recommendations represent the best available evidence. The comprehensiveness of the search determines the *available evidence*. Now Sara will need to appraise the evidence to find out if it is the *best evidence*. Because she has searched at the top of the effectiveness hierarchy (guidelines as meta-sources and systematic reviews), she has already obtained a more powerful type of evidence. But she still needs to appraise the evidence before she can use it to inform her nursing practice.

To appraise evidence, you will use a standardized tool that matches the type of evidence you have selected. Generally, these are the overall questions you will address when appraising evidence:

- How clear is the focus?
- How transparent and rigorous were the methods?
- Can I apply the recommendations to these patients?

When Sara appraises the two practice guidelines and the systematic review, she uses two tools that others have developed and validated: the **AGREE II tool,** a standardized appraisal tool for practice guidelines, rigorously developed by an international group of experts, and the tools from the **Critical Appraisal Skills Programme (CASP),** part of the Oxford Centre for Triple Value Healthcare portfolio in the United Kingdom. These tools were created to develop appraisal skills, to standardize criteria, and to make appraisals easier because they have hints about what to look for while reading guidelines and reviews (AGREE Next Steps Consortium, 2013; Critical Appraisal Skills Programme, 2018). When Sara appraises both practice guidelines using the AGREE II tool, she finds that both were strong in all of the following criteria:

- Scope and questions are clear and focused.
- Diverse stakeholders were an integral part of the process.
- Both used rigorous and transparent methods including systematic methods to search and appraise the evidence.
- A panel of experts reviewed the appraised and extracted evidence and considered the benefits and risks to reach a consensus on recommendations.
- Both identified the levels of evidence or recommendations and used external reviewers.
- Both have an update plan.
- Both are clear and have synopses that are freely available online, but the full EPUAP/NPIAP/PPPIA guideline requires purchase, whereas the entire NICE guideline is free online.

Next, Sara uses the CASP tool for systematic reviews (Critical Appraisal Skills Programme, 2018) to appraise the meta-analysis of support surfaces, published after the most recent practice guideline. She finds the following strengths of the review by McInnes et al (2015), in which the authors evaluated the effectiveness of various support surfaces for preventing pressure injuries:

- Objectives were clear, and the authors selected appropriate study designs to include in the review (randomized controlled trials).
- A comprehensive search of four databases and hand searching were used.
- Study appraisal and data extraction were fairly strong, although a second author was used to check decisions rather than a blinded, dual reviewer method; the authors transparently identified and used rigorous criteria to decide what to include in the study.

- The authors used appropriate statistical methods to determine the effectiveness of different surfaces with good precision (using confidence intervals).
- Because of study designs, the authors were unable to find significant benefit among the various mattresses and overlays, but they did find that some kind of pressure support device is superior to standard foam mattresses.
- The studies did not consistently address patient comfort or caregiver preferences; therefore, the authors could not address these outcomes.

Once you have appraised your sources, you need to look for consistencies, summarize the bottom-line recommendations, and identify the strengths of each recommendation. For her question, Sara combines recommendations from the two practice guidelines and the systematic review to answer the questions about support surfaces and how to decrease friction during repositioning. Her bottom-line determination for patients at risk for pressure injuries is the following:

- Do not use a standard foam hospital mattress (level A) (EPUAP/NPIAP/PPPIA, 2019; McInnes et al, 2015; NICE, 2014).
- Use a mattress or overlay that reduces interface pressures, such as high-density foam. In patients at higher risk, consider an active support surface (e.g., alternating pressure, air-fluidized or low-air-loss beds). There is no good evidence to recommend one of these higher-technology surfaces over the others (level A) (EPUAP/NPIAP/PPPIA, 2019; McInnes et al., 2015)
- Use lifting devices or slip sheets; avoid dragging the skin over another surface to reduce friction and shear (level C) (EPUAP/NPIAP/PPPIA, 2019).

You will note that each recommendation has a rating of the level of recommendation. As you learned in Chapter 11, many systems exist to represent levels of evidence and strength of recommendations. Levels of evidence usually indicate the degree of confidence you can have in the underlying approach to answer the question. Degrees may vary from strong—a systematic review—to weak—an expert opinion. Grades of recommendations should relate to the level of evidence and usually make a qualified statement about how urgently you should adopt the practice or avoid the practice altogether. International efforts exist to standardize the rating of evidence and recommendations and, increasingly, guideline groups are using or adapting the system (Gyatt, Oxman, Kunz, et al, 2008).

Sara's institution uses an A through D hierarchy in which recommendations are based on the body of the evidence:

- Grade A = strong support that merits application; evidence from a systematic review or precise randomized controlled trial
- Grade B = moderate support that merits consideration; evidence from single, well-designed studies
- Grade C = Moderate support that merits consideration: evidence from case series or expert consensus
- Grade D = Evidence cannot support the adoption of the practice

Apply/Implement

Armed with evidence about support surfaces and how to move patients in bed, Sara can now make decisions when she intervenes with at-risk patients. Sara recognizes that these are just two of a larger set of interventions to prevent pressure injuries, but she can still individualize her care by assessing each person's risk and preferences. Because the best available evidence does not indicate that one surface is superior to another, she can offer alternatives based on the availability of different products at her facility. When patients are at risk, she offers one of the support surfaces available and includes their preferences in her selection decision. When patients need to move in the bed, she makes sure she uses a slip sheet to avoid any friction or shear, enlists help, or uses a lift device to avoid dragging the patient over the bed surface.

Implementation within a system is complex. If Sara is the only nurse making decisions based on the evidence, her impact will be limited. She will need to work with a team to change the practices of others (Box 17■2). You will need to seek out a clinical nurse specialist or skin care advanced practice nurse to aid the practice change throughout the hospital. If advanced practice nurses use the Integrated Promoting Action on Research Implementation in Health Services (i-PARIHS) framework, they will assess the strength of the context and the characteristics of the innovation (including the strength of the evidence) and the recipients (including stakeholders) to determine how to facilitate the practice change (Harvey & Kitson, 2015). Nurses who deliver bedside care are key stakeholders and need to be involved in the process of changing practices system-wide.

In Sara's situation, the evidence has already been appraised as strong. The advanced practice nurses may use tools that are just being developed to assess the

---

BOX 17■2 **Interdisciplinary Rounds**

Pressure injury prevention is a team effort. Involve the following members in your plans:

- Registered nurses providing professional nursing care at the bedside
- Nursing assistants who contribute to patient hygiene and mobility
- Physiotherapists who intervene to progress mobility
- Wound and ostomy specialists with expert knowledge
- Clinical nurse specialists with expert knowledge and change and project management skills
- Hospitalists or other physicians with vested interest
- Safety and quality officers
- Clinical educators
- Risk managers

Ensure that the key stakeholders have a voice and engage their clinical expertise appropriately.

context based on characteristics that will either help or hinder implementation of the evidence. These characteristics relate to a system's leadership, evaluation systems, and organizational culture. If the context is strong, advanced practice nurses can best facilitate practice change by enabling and empowering others to use the evidence. If the context is weaker, they may need to facilitate practice change by providing more directions and technical, practical, and task-driven help (Harvey & Kitson, 2015; Kitson, Rycroft-Malone, Harvey, et al, 2008).

Advanced practice nurses could also develop evidence-based strategies to help the organization adopt the guidelines in nursing practice. For Sara's question about pressure injury prevention or any other guideline implementation, the following are some examples of research-based strategies to move evidence into practice. You may use them alone, but they may be more effective in combination:

- Interactive education sessions about when and how to use support surfaces and lift devices (Forsetlund, Bjørndal, Rashidian, et al, 2009; O'Brien, Rogers, Jamtvedt, et al., 2007)
- Educational outreach via one-to-one education and support at the bedside from the clinical nurse specialist or skin-care specialist (Forsetlund et al, 2009; O'Brien et al, 2007)
- Prompts or reminders as simple as a magnet on the door signifying the patient within is at high risk for pressure injuries or as high-tech as a pop-up electronic reminder when a patient reaches high risk as well as some type of visual prompt in the care plan (O'Brien et al, 2007)
- Audit and high-intensity feedback about how frequently the unit uses the proper surface and lift devices in at-risk patients (Jamtvedt, Young, Kristoffersen, et al, 2006)
- The Apply phase of the evidence-based practice process includes both application of the evidence supporting the nursing intervention and the evidence supporting strategies to change practice

Assess/Evaluate

Both the nursing and evidence-based practice processes require assessment to evaluate the effectiveness of interventions used with patients. Sara assesses all of LH's skin but carefully focuses on the pressure points of her sacrum, heels, scapula, hips, elbows, ears, and occipital region. She also follows the stage II pressure injuries to make sure that they begin to heal. If the depth, color, or size of the injuries worsens, she will need to intensify her efforts and consult further with wound specialists.

Patient outcomes are the highest priority, but the process of care is important to assess as well. The manager or advanced practice nurse will help audit the key interventions to determine whether the right patients receive the right care at the right time.

■ Summary

Every day, nurses make both basic and complex clinical decisions. In this chapter's clinical story, Sara systematically assessed the patient and determined whether the problem was an isolated event or part of a trend. She asked the questions to find the best available evidence. She searched and acquired the evidence to fit her diagnosis. She appraised the relevant evidence and was able to select synthesized sources to help her plan. Finding similar answers among those sources that met her criteria of excellence, she implemented the evidence and considered patient preferences when making decisions with other at-risk patients. Beyond her individual application of the evidence, she consulted with advanced practice nurses and wound and skin specialists for their clinical expertise and their influence over change on a larger scale within the institution. Finally, Sara evaluated the effectiveness of implementing the evidence in her individual patients by following the important clinical outcomes, and she helped monitor how other nurses used the evidence-based guidelines (Box 17■3). Thus, the evidence-based nursing practice and the nursing process aligned to produce optimal patient outcomes.

BOX 17■3 Tools for Learning and Practice

- Generate additional PICO questions related to pressure injury prevention.
- Search for additional evidence based on the keywords in your PICO question using the strategy supplied in this chapter as a template.
- Go to international guideline repositories such as the National Institute for Health and Care Excellence (http://www.nice.org.uk/) and compare the guideline recommendations with those from the National Pressure Injury Advisory Panel (https://npiap.com/). Use the AGREE collaboration tool to appraise the guidelines (https://www.agreetrust.org/resource-centre/).
- Compare and contrast levels of evidence and levels of recommendations from organizations such as the RNAO, the JBI, and the Centers for Disease Control and Prevention.
- Help gather data by participating in the national pressure injury prevalence study.
- Develop a simple audit tool that allows you to observe for adherence to key evidence-based strategies or use criteria that may already have been developed.
- Conduct an audit, summarize the data, and present feedback to colleagues.
- When mentoring other nurses, discuss the evidence related to pressure injury prevention with mentees; role-model best practices such as selecting appropriate pressure-reducing surfaces and using friction-reducing techniques to reduce sheer.

CHAPTER QUESTIONS

1. In this chapter's clinical story of pressure injury prevention, what were the steps of nursing process that Sara took? What were the steps of the evidence-based process?

2. What were the strengths of the evidence that Sara found?

3. What were the differences in how Sara approached the problem of pressure injury prevention as an individual nurse and when she consulted with advanced practice nurses to solve the problem on a broader scale?

4. Understanding that there is more to pressure injury prevention than support surfaces and how to move a patient in bed, what are other PICO questions that you could ask?

5. Using these PICO questions, search for a practice guideline and a systematic review. Using the criteria for critical appraisal, make a decision to use or discard the evidence you found. Support your reasoning and identify the strength of the evidence using a hierarchy.

6. If you found more than one guideline or systematic review, compare them and identify if they found similar recommendations or differed.

7. Given the implementation strategies that were listed, what are some creative ways that you could use to put these strategies into practice?

8. Consider a scenario in which the evidence indicates that a certain bed surface is effective in preventing pressure injuries but the patient refuses to use it because it is uncomfortable. What would you do next?

9. Given the evidence that Sara found, construct a simple audit tool to observe adherence to these interventions. Make sure that your criteria can be observed or identified in documentation and that they can be answered with a simple yes or no. Determine what the next steps would be to improve performance on those items where adherence was low. For high-performing criteria, plan a creative celebration to acknowledge good work among your peers.

References

Agency for Healthcare Research and Quality. (2018). About NGC and NQMC. Retrieved from https://www.ahrq.gov/gam/about/index.html

AGREE Next Steps Consortium. (2013). *The AGREE II Instrument* [Electronic version]. Retrieved from http://www.agreetrust.org

Centers for Medicare & Medicaid Services. (2008). Hospital-acquired conditions: Statute regulations program instructions. Retrieved from http://www.cms.hhs.gov/HospitalAcqCond/02_Statute_Regulations_Program_Instructions.asp

Critical Appraisal Skills Programme. (2018). CASP systematic review checklist. Retrieved from https://casp-uk.net/wp-content/uploads/2018/03/CASP-Systematic-Review-Checklist-2018_fillable-form.pdf

Edsberg, L. E., Black, J. M., Goldberg, M., et al. (2016). Revised National Pressure Injury Advisory Panel pressure injury staging system. *Journal of Wound Ostomy Continence Nursing, 43*, 585–597. doi:10.1097/WON.0000000000000281

European Pressure Ulcer Advisory Panel, National Pressure Injury Advisory Panel, and Pan-Pacific Pressure Injury Alliance (EPUAP/NPIAP/PPPIA). (2019). Prevention and treatment of pressure ulcers/injury: Clinical practice guideline. Retrieved from https://npiap.com/page/2019Guideline

Forsetlund, L., Bjørndal, A., Rashidian, A., et al. (2009). Continuing education meetings and workshops: Effects on professional practice and health care outcomes. *Cochrane Database of Systematic Reviews, 2009*(2). doi:10.1002/14651858.CD003030.pub2

Guyatt, G. H., Oxman, A. D., Kunz, R., et al. (2008). Going from evidence to recommendations. *British Medical Journal, 336*, 1049. doi:https://doi.org/10.1136/bmj.39493.646875.AE

Harvey, G., & Kitson, A. (Eds.). (2015). *Implementing evidence-based practice in healthcare: A facilitation guide.* New York, NY: Routledge.

HealthGrades. (2009). The sixth annual HealthGrades patient safety in American hospitals study. Retrieved from http://www.healthgrades.com/media/dms/pdf/PatientSafetyInAmericanHospitalsStudy

Jamtvedt, G., Young, J. M., Kristoffersen, D. T., et al. (2006). Audit and feedback: Effects on professional practice and health care outcomes. *Cochrane Database of Systematic Reviews 2006*(2). doi:10.1002/14651858.CD000259.pub2

Kitson, A., Rycroft-Malone, J., Harvey, G., et al. (2008). Evaluating the successful implementation of evidence into practice using the PARIHS framework: Theoretical and practical challenges. *Implementation Science, 3*. doi:10.1186/1748-5908-3-1

Kottner, J., Carville, K., Haesler, E., et al. (2019). Second update of the International Clinical Practice Guideline for the prevention and treatment of pressure ulcers/injuries 2019. *Wounds International, 10*(1), 6–7.

McInnes, E., Jammali-Blasi, A., Bell-Syer, S. E. M., et al. (2015). Support surfaces for pressure injury prevention. *Cochrane Database of Systematic Reviews, 2015*(9). doi:10.1002/14651858.CD001735.pub5

National Institute for Health and Care Excellence (NICE). (2014). Pressure ulcers: Prevention and management. Retrieved from https://www.nice.org.uk/guidance/cg179

O'Brien, M. A., Rogers, S., Jamtvedt, G., et al. (2007). Educational outreach visits: Effects on professional practice and health care outcomes. *Cochrane Database of Systematic Reviews, 2007*(4). doi:10.1002/14651858.CD000409.pub2

VanGilder, C., Amlung, S., Harrison, P., et al. (2009). Results of the 2008–2009 International Pressure Injury Prevalence™ survey and a 3-year, acute care, unit-specific analysis. *Ostomy Wound Management, 55*, 39–45. Retrieved from https://www.o-wm.com/content/results-2008-%E2%80%93-2009-international-pressure-ulcer-prevalence%E2%84%A2-survey-and-a-3-year-acute-care-

CHAPTER 18

Evidence Implementation to Provide Safe Nursing Care to Laboring Women

Cheryl Moredich, Amanda Kratovil

■ Examine the role of evidence-based practice in the promotion of patient safety in the context of caring for a laboring mother.

■ Analyze the effect of ethical principles on evidence-based decision making.

■ Establish a prototype for change toward evidence-based practice.

■ Facilitate shared decision making as a means toward implementing evidence in the workplace.

Advocate
Autonomy
Beneficence
High-alert medications

Nonmaleficence
Professional standards
Shared decision making
Safety huddle

$Clinical\ Story$

Freda is caring for a 26-year-old nulliparous woman who is at 38 weeks and 2 days' gestation. The patient has not experienced complications during this pregnancy and appears nervous about her labor being induced today. Both her mother and husband are accompanying her. Freda overhears the patient and her husband questioning why she is being induced today when her due date is not for two more weeks. Freda has worked in labor and delivery for over 3 years, witnessing both positive and negative responses to induction of labor. According to the patient's gestational age, Freda also questions the order for induction in this apparently healthy pregnant woman. She decides to discuss her concerns with the attending obstetrician. As she approaches the obstetrician, she overhears her discuss her travel plans for the next two weeks. When questioned about the reason for the induction of her patient, the obstetrician states, "The patient stated she wants me to deliver her baby and I will not be available for the next two weeks." Remembering that she also overheard her patient's confusion about her induction, Freda wonders if there was a miscommunication between the health-care provider and the patient.

Think Before You Read

- What are the steps of the EBP process?
- What PICO or PICo questions can you imagine that are relevant to the clinical story?
- What model can you use to structure how you approach implementing the evidence?
- What might be some key issues to consider as you search for and appraise the evidence?
- What might be some candidate implementation strategies?
- What do you need to consider to judge the success or failure of a project like the one in the clinical story?

Introduction

The goal of any elective induction of labor is to facilitate a vaginal birth without causing harm to the mother or fetus. Medical indications for inducing labor exist; however, when induction of labor is implemented solely for provider or patient convenience, it is termed *elective*. Although a variety of methods are available for induction of labor, we focus here on the use of oxytocin. Oxytocin is used to induce or augment labor in approximately 50% of U.S. pregnant women (Declercq, Sakala, Corry, et al, 2014; Heuser Knight, Esplin, et al, 2013). This drug works by increasing the contractility of the uterus and has been shown to decrease the length of labor (Bugg, Siddiqui, & Thornton, 2013). However, oxytocin can cause dangerous side effects such as uterine hyperactivity that may lead to uterine rupture, fetal hypoxia, and postpartum hemorrhage (Heuser et al, 2013; Simpson & James, 2008). Therefore, it remains on the high-alert medication list (Institute for Safe Medication Practices, 2018). **High-alert medications** are those medications that can cause significant harm if administered incorrectly. Because oxytocin is a high-alert medication, practitioners need to be astute in identifying the indications for its use during labor, including risk versus benefit, contraindications, best practices, and patient preferences.

Professional organizations have developed recommendations to promote the safe use of oxytocin during induction and augmentation of labor (Agency for Healthcare Research and Quality [AHRQ], 2017a, 2017b; American College of Obstetricians and Gynecologists [ACOG], 2019a; Association of Women's Health, Obstetric, and Neonatal Nurses [AWHONN], 2019). However, administration decisions for oxytocin have traditionally been at the discretion of the individual obstetrician. Breaking away from tradition and moving toward evidence-based practice will facilitate safety in elective induction and augmentation of labor.

This chapter's clinical story demonstrates the immediate and subsequent actions that the nurse can take to ensure the care delivered to the laboring patient is safe and includes the patient's preferences. Immediate actions (i.e., steps taken immediately to correct a safety concern), occur as the clinical story unfolds. Subsequent actions are those taken after the identification of a clinical problem but will take time to develop and implement. This chapter provides a depiction of how the identification and selection of resources lay the foundation for providing the best patient care. Freda uses the processes of ask, acquire, appraise, apply, and assess as she builds a plan for safe patient care.

Ask/Assess

Freda is trying to reconcile what she believes to be safe patient care with the current clinical situation. Freda questions whether the patient truly understands the risks of elective induction of labor, especially before 39 gestational weeks, compared to the benefit of having her desired obstetrician available for her delivery. Freda questions if she is adequately prepared to **advocate** for the patient's wishes. To advocate is to champion or support the patient to meet her needs and wishes. Is this choice the best for the baby? Could she advocate on behalf of the unborn child? What are the unit policies regarding induction and are those policies current? All of these thoughts race through Freda's mind as she assesses the situation.

Freda wants to provide safe, evidence-based, quality patient care. She knows the desired outcome, yet has many questions concerning the care of this patient. The significance of the problem is discussed in Box 18■1.

The first question is the rationale for this patient's ordered induction of labor. Freda recalled reading a recent peer-reviewed article suggesting against the elective induction of labor before 39 completed gestational weeks. ACOG (2019a) defines full-term pregnancy as 39 weeks and 0 days through 40 weeks and 6 days. Freda is also aware that because oxytocin is a high-alert medication, she needs to be particularly cautious and informed about how to use the drug safely. She wonders if the unit's oxytocin protocol matches the current national guidelines. Staffing

---

BOX 18■1 **Significance of the Problem**

- Fifty percent of pregnant women in the United States receive oxytocin to induce or augment labor; it is the most common method to induce labor worldwide.
- Oxytocin, being considered a high-alert medication, can cause dangerous maternal–neonatal side effects such as uterine hyperactivity that may lead to uterine rupture, fetal hypoxia, and postpartum hemorrhage.
- Steps to reduce obstetrical adverse events with oxytocin must be in place and include appropriate patient selection, considering risk, benefit, and contraindications; up-to-date oxytocin protocol bundles; clear communication between members of the care team; and appropriate nurse:patient staffing.

patterns also concern Freda. If this patient becomes her second labor patient, Freda worries that she will not be able to be adequately vigilant, which could jeopardize the patient's safety. She wants to be proactive in creating an environment that promotes the safe use of oxytocin in laboring patients, but how does this journey begin? Freda recognizes the presence of a moral dilemma. She can use an ethical guide to help her sort out the best solution (Table 18■1).

To begin, Freda takes immediate action by informing either her charge nurse, nurse manager, or nurse supervisor about her concerns regarding safe patient care. Following her chain of command, Freda knows that the first line of help comes from those in a direct supervisory position closest to the point of care. When critical incidents escalate, a formalized channel of communication helps stakeholders interact cooperatively. Frequently, immediate actions are taken to minimize patient risk and maximize safe patient care. An example of an immediate action is for the charge nurse to change Freda's assignment to reflect the acuity of care required by the patient. Additionally, Freda may ask the obstetrician to further discuss the elective induction with the patient and her family to clarify the risks and benefits. If attempts to encourage further discussions between the patient and obstetrician are met with resistance, Freda could consult with the ethics committee. Some organizations have specific committees designed to come together when a critical incident arises. Such committees allow a real-time decision on a patient care issue. The benefits include working through a critical issue as it occurs rather than afterward.

Freda also questions whether the oxytocin protocol on her unit mirrors the national guidelines. Because the scope and scale of her concerns are broad, Freda's question is quite comprehensive. Her question is, What is the best available evidence for elective induction of labor in healthy pregnancies at 38 weeks and 2 days' gestation? Potential roadblocks to safe administration of oxytocin include outdated protocols that do not reflect the evidence, less than adequate staffing, and inappropriate patient selection. On review, Freda realizes that her unit protocol is missing gestational age limits and staffing guidelines, and has not been updated in 5 years. Freda hears

TABLE 18■1 **Guide for Moral Decision Making**

Step	Guideline	Relevance to Clinical Situation
Recognize the moral issue	Understand that there is a moral/ethical issue.	Current practice is not based on the best evidence and could cause harm.
Identify the participants/stakeholders	Identify those who have a stake in the issue. Consider those with obligations or special considerations to the issue.	Mother, baby, father, patient's mother, physician (OB-GYN and Peds), nurse, unit director, charge nurse, nursing assistants, pastoral care, patient advocate (if present), ethics committee representative
Distinguish the values involved	Think through the values associated with the issue (autonomy, justice, advocacy, beneficence, nonmaleficence, confidentiality).	Autonomy, advocacy, beneficence, nonmaleficence
Weigh the benefits and burdens	Benefits include outcomes from choices that are positive. Burdens involve results from actions that cause physical, emotional, or other pain/suffering.	Positives: Patient satisfaction, convenience for mother/father and physician Negatives: Increased risk to the baby both immediate and later developmentally
Look for analogous situations	Identify similar cases; examine the decisions made and outcomes. Was it a good decision? Look at the similarities and differences between the cases.	Freda can consult with the ethics committee, unit director, and charge nurse as well as her professional organization to identify similar situations.
Discuss with appropriate people	Time permitting, discuss the case with as many participants as possible to understand their opinions of the case. Rules of confidentiality must be adhered to.	Freda needs to discuss with the physician, ethics committee, charge nurse, unit director, and unit practice council.
Ascertain organizational rules and legal codes	Consider the legality of the case and options, ethics of the professional organization, and institutional policies.	Freda should consult the policies, her professional organization (AWHONN), and, if possible, the legal and ethical departments.

TABLE 18▪1   **Guide for Moral Decision Making** (continued)

Step	Guideline	Relevance to Clinical Situation
Examine own comfort with the decision	Questions to be asked in this regard might include the following: 1. If I carry out this decision, would I be comfortable telling my family about it? My pastor? My mentors? 2. Would I want children to take my behavior as an example? 3. Is this decision one that a wise, informed, virtuous person would make? 4. Can I live with this decision?	While making a decision about the ethical issue, Freda should consider her responses to the questions.

Adapted from http://www.ethicsweb.ca/guide/

other nurses voice a concern that this oxytocin protocol is sometimes forfeited in favor of physician preference.

Based on the evidence she has gathered, Freda has good reason to question the clinical practice on her unit. She decides to ask her supervisor if she can form a team of nurses to investigate the evidence. This would be considered a subsequent action.

Acquire/Diagnose

As described in Chapter 17, Freda's next step is to acquire the best available evidence relating to her questions. She can conduct a search of the evidence herself or consult with a more experienced person such as a librarian. Freda is fortunate that she has access to professional practice recommendations that address her clinical problem. She finds an AWHONN recommendation stating that elective induction of labor should be reserved for patients who are at 39 completed weeks of gestation unless medically indicated (AWHONN, 2019). Appropriate staffing patterns for laboring patients are also addressed by AWHONN (2010). Other professional organization recommendations address the frequency of nursing assessments for laboring women (American Academy of Pediatrics & American College of Obstetricians and Gynecologists, 2017; AWHONN, 2018). Freda continues her search of the literature. She finds an *Elective Induction of Labor* bundle that matches AWHONN's recommendation from the Institute for Healthcare Improvement (IHI) Web site (IHI, 2009), but wonders if this recommendation is still valid since it is from 2010. As she continues to search, she finds a Safety Program for Perinatal Care from the Agency for Healthcare Research and Quality that includes a toolkit for safe oxytocin administration (AHRQ, 2017a, 2017b). She also finds a systematic review and meta-analysis in the

Cochrane Library that explored the neonatal and pregnancy outcomes of full-term (i.e., 39 weeks and 0 days to 40 weeks and 6 days) and uncomplicated pregnancies after an induction of labor (Saccone, Della, Maruotti, et al, 2019).

In every patient situation, nurses are obliged to follow the principles of the American Nurses Association (ANA) Code of Ethics (Fowler, 2015). The ethical concepts of **beneficence** and **nonmaleficence** must govern when nurses participate in elective induction of labor. Simply put, beneficence is a moral obligation to help another, and nonmaleficence is a moral obligation not to harm (Butts & Rich, 2020). If induction of labor may cause undue risk to the mother or baby, then, ethically, the nurse must act. Informed consent requires that we fully disclose to the patient, who is competent to make a consent decision. In the case of a pregnant woman, the patient is making a decision for both herself and her unborn baby. Therefore, we must be sure that a health professional provided her full disclosure about the risks and benefits of elective induction.

Autonomy in health care is respected and honored as a basic ethical right of the patient. The importance of patient autonomy is reflected in the current practice recommendations of both major perinatal professional organizations, AWHONN and ACOG. Both professional organizations promote patient autonomy through shared decision making in the perinatal setting (ACOG, 2019a, 2019b; AWHONN, 2019). **Shared decision making** occurs when the patient and health-care providers review patient health challenges, discuss the benefits and risks of treatment, and determine together the best treatment plan based on the evidence and patient preference. Decision aids, in the form of videos, pamphlets, or health-care Web pages, assist decisions when there are multiple treatment choices that have similar effect yet may be valued differently (Stacey, Légaré, Lewis, et al, 2017). The role of the nurse is to facilitate shared decision making (AWHONN, 2019). In the clinical story, shared decision making can be achieved immediately through informed and effective communication between the patient and her obstetrician. Shared decision making can also be incorporated into the practice and culture of the unit.

Freda is not sure how to facilitate a culture of shared decision making on her unit. Again, she uses the resources she has available to her. She finds a tool developed by AHRQ designed to help implement shared decision making (AHRQ, 2018). The SHARE Approach consists of a five-step process for shared decision making. A carefully planned discussion of the benefits, risks, and harms of each available option is a major component of the SHARE Approach (AHRQ, 2018). Freda feels that the discussion between her patient and the obstetrician related to the risks and harms of an induction before 39 weeks of gestation is a good first step to facilitating shared decision making. She also realizes that to implement a change in practice and culture on her unit, she will have to develop a long-term plan.

Appraise/Plan

In addition to her role as a facilitator of shared decision making for her own patients, Freda thinks about her role as a professional nurse and the strength of the **professional standards** in nursing that promote quality and safety in the provision of care. Professional organizations develop appropriate standards of care based on the *Nursing Scope and Standards of Practice* (ANA, 2015). This document provides a framework for each state's professional practice act, which defines the legal obligation for nursing. Each state prescribes an appropriate scope of practice for a registered nurse. When confronted with a complex nursing situation, these documents help determine the best course of action. Freda considers the professional standards of nursing as well as the ANA Code of Ethics as she considers updating the policies on her unit.

According to the ANA Code of Ethics (Fowler, 2015), nurses have a duty to participate in the advancement of the profession through contributions to practice and collaboration with other health professionals (provisions 7 and 8). Just as Freda began by examining current practice and comparing it to national recommendations, an interdisciplinary committee on policies and procedures for the obstetric unit should do the same. On Freda's unit, members could include Freda, the nursing assistant, charge nurse, nurse manager, respiratory therapist, obstetrician, neonatologist, pharmacist, social worker, pastoral care provider, and other stakeholders.

Collaborating with other disciplines brings a multidimensional aspect to the provision of care. Each perspective provides valuable insights on facets of the clinical concern. Although an interdisciplinary team approach in health care may improve the safety and well-being of patients, it is difficult to implement evidence-based practices in the clinical setting (Flodgren, O'Brien, Parmelli, et al, 2019). Freda considers the information she found as she strategizes how she can integrate the best available evidence into policies and practices on her unit. She decides to ask the nurse managers to help her identify the stakeholders with whom she should collaborate to update the unit's policies and practices.

Armed with the clinical recommendations and the best available evidence, the committee can appraise the literature. Freda appraises the practice recommendations using the AGREE II tool (see Chapter 17); she determines that the recommendations were strong in all of the following criteria:

- The scope and questions are clear and focused with a definitive population.
- Appropriate multidisciplinary stakeholders were part of the process.
- A variety of professional organization recommendations were incorporated.
- A risk/benefit analysis for recommendations was completed.
- The levels of evidence and recommendations used external reviewers.
- The guideline provides advice and/or tools on how the recommendations can be put into practice, describing facilitators and barriers to its application.

After appraising the recommendations using the AGREE II tool, the team can construct a new protocol on elective induction of labor, one that reflects the best available evidence.

Apply/Implement

Once they write a new protocol, the team can begin the process of implementing it. Dissemination of the new protocol will need to be well thought out and involve the entire perinatal team. All members need to be educated about the new oxytocin guideline. As Freda learned, implementing new evidence into practice is difficult. Including opinion leaders (i.e., members of each discipline who are influential and trusted members of the associated community) in interdisciplinary teams and in the education of clinicians has been shown to be an effective way to improve compliance among health-care professionals when new clinical practices are being introduced (Chen, Opiyo, Tavender, et al, 2018; Flodgren et al, 2019). Posting a clinical checklist that reflects the new protocol can also serve as a reminder to staff and improve compliance (Clark, Meyers, Frye, et al, 2015) (Fig. 18■1).

As the new oxytocin protocol is implemented, challenges in communication may develop for nurses and physicians. The foundation of communication is a clear and common goal that is understood by all parties (nurses, physicians, midwives, parents, etc.). For example, in the clinical story, Freda and the other stakeholders clearly understand the common goal of safely delivering the mother without harming either the mother or baby. AHRQ identified process problems with communication and suggested ways to address such issues. According to AHRQ (2019), communication should be timely, complete, and accurate and result in closure. Multiple structured channels are fundamental to effective communication. A primary tool for nurse–physician communication is situation-background-assessment-recommendation (SBAR). The use of this tool structures communication to enhance its effectiveness. Box 18■2 provides an example of Freda's use of the SBAR tool to communicate information from the clinical story to her supervisor.

Another tool that enhances clear communication between disciplines is the multidisciplinary safety huddle. Supported by the National Academy of Medicine (NAM), previously the Institute of Medicine (IOM), safety huddles are intended to facilitate interdisciplinary communication, reduce medical errors, and promote patient safety. **Safety huddles** are short (up to 15 minutes), planned, and purposeful stand-up meetings, typically held at the beginning of a shift, that help teams actively manage quality and safety of care through communication (The Joint Commission, 2017; Scoville, Little, Rakover, et al, 2016). The implementation of safety huddles in perinatal units has proven helpful for improving the quality and safety of care for women and children (Driscoll & Metwally, 2014; Thompson, Krening, & Parrett, 2018). Table 18■2 provides an example of a safety huddle in a perinatal care setting.

Assess/Evaluate

The effect of the new practice guideline implementation requires assessment to evaluate outcomes in elective induction processes. In this chapter's clinical story, a key element is the auditing of interventions to determine that the right patient receives the right care at the right time. The clinical nurse specialist, manager, or even staff nurses may audit key interventions that include safe oxytocin administration to the appropriate patient and staffing ratios that reflect the care required when patients receive oxytocin. Chart audit reviews provide evidence of safe oxytocin administration to the appropriate patient. Cross-referencing daily staffing and team

Elective Induction of Labor Safety Checklist

Patient selection appropriate

☐ Gestational age 39 weeks as evidenced by ＿＿＿＿＿＿

☐ Absence of contraindications to labor

Consent guidelines followed

☐ Elective induction of labor video watched by patient

☐ Risks and benefits of elective induction of labor discussed by primary care provider (PCP)

☐ Consent signed after shared decision-making with PCP

AWHONN staffing guidelines for registered nurses followed

☐ 1:1 nurse-patient ratio for women receiving oxytocin for labor induction

☐ Physician capable of performing a cesarean delivery available

Standardized oxytocin protocol followed

☐ Uniform mixed preparation of oxytocin established for all patients

☐ Standard dosing established that includes initial dose, incremental dose increase, frequency of increase and maintenance dose

☐ Oxytocin delivered via a calibrated pump as secondary line inserted into the proximal port of the mainline IV

Approach to Assessment of Changes to FHR Changes

☐ Baseline fetal heart rate assessment done established before induction

☐ Frequency of continued maternal and fetal status established

☐ Physician notification of changes in maternal-fetal status

☐ Standing orders for Category II or III FHR changes

　　☐ Provider notification criteria

　　☐ Criteria for stopping induction

　　☐ Standard for maternal oxygenation

　　☐ Position changes

Patient Care Team Communication

☐ Provider will be available at: ＿＿＿＿＿＿＿＿＿

☐ Neonatal care unit/surgical team notified of adverse patient status

☐ Chain of command will be followed in the event of disagreements

FIGURE 18■1 Example of an elective induction of labor safety checklist

---

BOX 18■2   **SBAR Use in the Clinical Story**

"Hi Ann (nursing supervisor), I am calling about a situation that is occurring on the OB unit. I need some guidance on how to proceed."

Situation

"I received a patient for an elective induction, and I just don't feel right about it. The problem is she is at 38 weeks and 2 days' gestation, and Dr. Z is planning on inducing her labor with oxytocin today. I am concerned that the patient is not an appropriate candidate for elective induction, and I do not feel she has been properly informed of her options. She appears nervous about her labor being induced and the patient and her husband are questioning why she is being induced today when her due date is not for two more weeks. In addition, she will be my second labor patient."

Background

The patient is here with her husband and mother and is voicing concern about being induced birth before her due date.

Assessment

Her physical assessment is normal, and the baby is presenting appropriately; however, the patient has not signed the consent for induction of labor.

Recommendations

"I feel that the obstetrician should further discuss the induction with the patient and her family to clarify the risks and benefits of an elective induction prior to the consent being signed."

SBAR tool. (Courtesy of Kaiser Permanente.)

---

assignment with oxytocin patients provides evidence of safe staffing levels that adhere to the guidelines. Finally, safe delivery of a healthy baby and the maintenance of a healthy mother are the most important clinical outcomes.

■ Summary

In the clinical story, Freda identified a clinical problem that may have put her patient and the patient's unborn infant at risk of an adverse outcome. To remedy the immediate clinical problem and prevent future occurrences, Freda employed the systematic process of ask, acquire, appraise, apply, and assess to change practice. Throughout the process, Freda maintained a focus on her ethical obligations to provide optimal care, ensured that the patient understood the risks and benefits of the elective induction, and sought to base her actions on current evidence (see Box 18■3). She also took action that promoted collaboration with interdisciplinary teams, including opinion leaders, to establish and implement guidelines based on the best available evidence.

TABLE 18■2   **Safety Huddle**

Steps	Description	Rationale	Examples
1. The nurse leader starts at a designated time with an agenda.	■ The time is consistent for the safety huddle ■ Involves a multidisciplinary team ■ Members stand	■ Consistent time encourages prompt attendance, planning of workday, and adherence to routine huddles	At 0700, the nurses from labor and delivery, postpartum, neonatal intensive care, and antenatal units meet with the designated leader from the obstetrician group, anaesthesia, and respiratory care in a private area in an agreed upon location.
2. One person from each discipline discusses patients for the day, identifying any safety issues.	■ Identifies unit safety concerns	■ Focuses on complex clinical cases to ensure collaboration and the safe provision of care	The nurse leader calls on the designated person from each discipline to present the unit census, any expected admissions, discharges, and safety concerns (e.g., staffing, high-risk patients, social concerns, complex clinical cases).
3. The nurse leader closes the huddle.	■ Thank the team ■ Say, "Huddle is now over" ■ Provide summary and/or announcements that affect the team	■ Demonstrates courtesy ■ Provides information applicable to the patient care teams	The nurse leader states: "I want to make sure everyone is aware that OR 2 will be closed until tomorrow at 0500. All deliveries will be performed in OR 1 and 3 until then. Thank you for your time. Huddle is now over."

Adapted from AHRQ. (2017). *Daily Huddle Component Kit*. Rockville, MD: Author. Retrieved from https://www.ahrq.gov/hai/tools/ambulatory-surgery/sections/sustainability/management/huddles-comp-kit.html

BOX 18■3 **Tools for Learning and Practice**

■ Find comprehensive evidence related to a problem such as maternal labor, search AWHONN guidelines; compare them with guidelines from American College of Obstetricians and Gynecology, and other organizations.
■ Appraise the guidelines using the AGREE tool.
■ Use checklists, reminders, and alerts to help health-care providers implement evidence-based guidelines.
■ Use communication tools such as SBAR and the Safety Huddle to provide structure and develop routines.
■ Use guides such as those in Table 18■1 to help structure ethical thinking and decision making.
■ Audit criteria based on the evidence and feedback directly to those engaged in the care to improve implementation.
■ Know your unit's performance related to patient outcomes such as safe delivery rates, complications, and vaginal delivery rates.

CHAPTER QUESTIONS

1. Apply the ethical principles from the ANA *Code of Ethics* to Freda's clinical situation.

2. Discuss how the nurse might use a safety huddle or chain of command when working through the following clinical situation:
   a. Dr. X prescribes oxytocin that contradicts the newly established protocol without medical indication.

3. You know that a policy guiding the care of the postpartum patient is outdated. Develop a plan to address the issue.

4. Select one of your patients from a recent clinical experience. Using the SBAR format, create a report to a physician.

5. A safety huddle is a way to improve communication and patient safety. How could you contribute to the information shared in the safety huddle? Create a plan for communicating your perspective to the interdisciplinary group.

References

Agency for Healthcare Research and Quality. (2017a, May). *AHRQ safety program for perinatal care: Experiences from the frontline* (AHRQ Publication No. 17-0003-23-EF). Retrieved from https://www.ahrq.gov/sites/default/files/wysiwyg/professionals/quality-patient-safety/hais/tools/perinatal-care/perinatal_care_toolkit_fullcolor.pdf

Agency for Healthcare Research and Quality. (2017b, May). *AHRQ safety program for perinatal care: Safe medication administration oxytocin* (AHRQ Publication No. 17-0003-19-EF). Retrieved from https://www.ahrq.gov/sites/default/files/wysiwyg/professionals/quality-patient-safety/hais/tools/perinatal-care/modules/strategies/medication/tool_safe–oxytocin.docx

Agency for Healthcare Research and Quality (2018, July). *The SHARE approach—Putting shared decision making into practice: A user's guide for clinical teams.* Retrieved from https://www.ahrq. gov/health-literacy/curriculum-tools/shareddecisionmaking/tools/tool-8/index.html

Agency for Healthcare Research and Quality (2019, September). *Communication between Clinicians.* Retrieved from https://psnet.ahrq.gov/primer/communication-between-clinicians

American Academy of Pediatrics & American College of Obstetricians and Gynecologists. (2017). *Guidelines for perinatal care* (8th ed.). Itasca, IL: Author.

American College of Obstetricians and Gynecologists. (2019a). Definition of term pregnancy. Committee Opinion No. 579. *American College of Obstetricians and Gynecologists. Obstetrics & Gynecology, 122,* 1139–1140. https://www.acog.org/-/media/Committee-Opinions/Committee-on-Obstetric-practice/co579.pdf?dmc=1&ts=20191222T0537262785

American College of Obstetricians and Gynecologists. (2019b). *Practice Advisory: Clinical guidance for integration of the findings of The ARRIVE Trial: Labor induction versus expectant management in low-risk nulliparous women.* Retrieved from https://www.acog.org/Clinical-Guidance-and-Publications/Practice-Advisories/Practice-Advisory-Clinical-guidance-for-integration-of-the-findings -of-The-ARRIVE-Trial?IsMobileSet=false

American Nurses Association. (2015). *Nursing: Scope and standards of practice* (3rd ed.). Nursesbooks.org.

Association of Women's Health, Obstetric, and Neonatal Nurses. (2010). *Guidelines for professional registered nurse staffing for perinatal units.* Retrieved from https://c.ymcdn.com/sites/www. awhonn.org/resource/download/20150923_084518_19352/SG-910.pdf

Association of Women's Health, Obstetric and Neonatal Nurses. (2018). AWHONN position statement: Fetal heart monitoring. *Journal of Obstetric, Gynecologic, & Neonatal Nursing, 47*(6), 874–877. https://www.jognn.org/article/S0884-2175(18)30322-8/pdf

Association of Women's Health, Obstetric and Neonatal Nurses. (2019). Elective induction of labor: Position statement. *Journal of Obstetric, Gynecologic, & Neonatal Nursing, 48*(2), 227–229. https:// doi.org/10.1016/j.jogn.2019.01.004

Bugg G. J., Siddiqui, F., & Thornton, J. G. (2013). Oxytocin versus no treatment or delayed treatment for slow progress in the first stage of spontaneous labour. *Cochrane Database of Systematic Reviews, 2013*(7). https://www.ncbi.nlm.nih.gov/pubmed/21735408

Butts J. B., & Rich, K. L. (2020). *Nursing ethics across the curriculum and into practice* (5th ed.). Burlington, MA: Jones & Bartlett Learning.

Chen, I., Opiyo, N., Tavender, E., et al. (2018). Non-clinical interventions for reducing unnecessary caesarean section. *Cochrane Database of Systematic Reviews, 2018*(3). https://www.ncbi.nlm.nih. gov/pubmed/?term=10.1002%2F14651858.CD005528.pub3

Clark, S. L., Meyers, J. A., Frye, D. K., et al. (2015). Recognition and response to electronic fetal heart rate patterns: Impact on newborn outcomes and primary cesarean delivery rate in women undergoing induction of labor. *American Journal of Obstetrics and Gynecology, 212*(4), 494.e1-6. https://www.ncbi.nlm.nih.gov/pubmed/?term=10.1016%2Fj.ajog.2014.11.019

Declercq, E. R., Sakala, C., Corry, M. P., et al. (2014). Major survey findings of listening to mothers (SM) III: pregnancy and birth: report of the third national U.S. survey of women's childbearing experiences. *Journal of Perinatal Education, 23*(1), 9–16. https://www.ncbi.nlm.nih.gov/pubmed/ ?term=10.1891%2F1058-1243.23.1.17

Driscoll, C. H., & Metwally, D. E. (2014). A daily huddle facilitates patient transports from a neonatal intensive care unit. *BMJ Quality Improvement Reports, 3*(1), u204253.w1876. https://www.ncbi.nlm. nih.gov/pubmed/?term=10.1136%2Fbmjquality.u204253.w1876

Flodgren, G., O'Brien, M. A., Parmelli, E., et al. (2019). Local opinion leaders: Effects on professional practice and health care outcomes. *Cochrane Database of Systematic Reviews, 2019*(5). https:// www.ncbi.nlm.nih.gov/pubmed/?term=10.1002%2F14651858.CD000125.pub5

Fowler, M. D. M. (2015). *Guide to the code of ethics for nurses with interpretive statements* (2nd ed.). Silver Spring, MD: American Nurses Association.

Heuser, C. C., Knight, S., Esplin, S. M., et al. (2013). Tachysystole in term labor: incidence, risk factors, outcomes, and effect on fetal heart tracings. *American Journal of Obstetrics & Gynecology, 209*(1), 32.e1–32.e6. https://www.ajog.org/article/S0002-9378(13)00353-0/fulltext

Institute for Healthcare Improvement. (2009). *Elective induction and augmentation bundles.* Retrieved from http://www.ihi.org/IHI/Topics/PerinatalCare/PerinatalCareGeneral/EmergingContent/ ElectiveInductionandAugmentationBundles.htm

Institute for Safe Medication Practices. (2018, August 28). *High-alert medications in acute care settings.* https://www.ismp.org/recommendations/high-alert-medications-acute-list

The Joint Commission. (2017, June). *Daily safety briefings—A hallmark of high reliability.* Retrieved from https://www.jointcommission.org/-/media/tjc/documents/newsletters/quick_safety_issue_34_2017_safety_briefings_finalpdf.pdf?db=web&hash=9464C65B495614616CC30CDD8D7D42F8

Saccone, G., Della, C. L., Maruotti, G. M., et al. (2019). Induction of labor at full-term in pregnant women with uncomplicated singleton pregnancy: A systematic review and meta-analysis of randomized trials. *Acta Obstetricia et Gynecologica Scandinavica, 98*(8), 958–966. https://obgyn.onlinelibrary.wiley.com/doi/full/10.1111/aogs.13561

Scoville, R., Little, K., Rakover, J., et al. (2016). *Sustaining improvement* (IHI White Paper). Institute for Healthcare Improvement. Retrieved from http://www.ihi.org/resources/Pages/IHIWhitePapers/Sustaining-Improvement.aspx

Simpson, K., & James, D. C. (2008). Effects of oxytocin-induced uterine hyperstimulation during labor on fetal oxygen status and fetal heart rate patterns. *American Journal of Obstetrics and Gynecology, 199*(1), 34e1–34e5. https://www.ncbi.nlm.nih.gov/pubmed/?term=10.1016%2Fj.ajog.2007.12.015

Stacey, D., Légaré, O. F., Lewis, K., et al. (2017). Decision aids for people facing health treatment or screening decisions. *Cochrane Database of Systematic Reviews, 2017*(4). https://www.ncbi.nlm.nih.gov/pubmed/28402085

Thompson, L., Krening, C., & Parrett, D. (2018). Interdisciplinary team huddles for fetal heart rate tracing review. *Nursing for Women's Health, 22*(3), 240–249. https://10.1016/j.nwh.2018.03.002

CHAPTER 19

Nursing Care of Children

Ellen Moore

- Examine the role of evidence-based practice (EBP) in the promotion of patient safety in the context of caring for infants in acute care and community settings.

- Apply all phases of the EBP process to guide decisions for the promotion of safety through safe sleep practices for caregivers and parents of infants to decrease infant mortality rates.

- Considering the complexity of scoping and scaling an attitude of inquiry question, develop a plan to facilitate the implementation of using the best available evidence to inform decision making.

- Generate next step strategies to get the best available evidence into practice.

Attitude of inquiry
Accidental suffocation or strangulation in bed (ASSB)
Baby box
Barriers
Clinical expertise
Context
Facilitators
Implementation science
Infant mortality rate (IMR)

Local data
Promoting Action on Research Implementation in Health Services (PARIHS)
Safe sleep practices
Sudden infant death syndrome (SIDS)
Sudden unexpected infant death (SUID)

Clinical Story

Nursing students Sanida, John, and Michael are in the final semester of their nursing program and are a little bit anxious about the capstone course, one of the final courses before their long-anticipated graduation. They have heard this is an evidence-based practice (EBP) course that involves integrating previous nursing knowledge to complete a team-driven EBP project. From conversations with previous graduates, they learned that the course involves being able to work effectively within a team to accomplish each phase of the evidence-based practice process.

Sanida, John, and Michael have previously worked together on class projects and have decided to work together to complete this task successfully. They are eager to begin their EBP assignment. The student team has chosen a project with an objective to focus on **safe sleep practices** (ways of putting infants to sleep to prevent sleep-related deaths) to reduce infant mortality among teen mothers. As part of their team, they will be collaborating with their course instructor, a project director, and an advanced practice nurse from a regional community hospital. In fact, it was the project director who had the curiosity to consider questioning safe sleep practices among teen mothers in the community. They realize that their instructor and the project director would be very important members of the team to provide direction, feedback, and ultimately, to help them gain the confidence to become EBP champions in the workplace.

The team examined international, national, state and local data related to infant mortality rates (IMR). The county where Sanida, John, and Michael reside is ranked in the top 10 counties for having the highest infant mortality rate (IMR of 8.5 per 1,000 infants) in their state. From prior classes they recall that EBP focuses on identifying best practices to improve patient outcomes. This includes using the best available evidence, clinical expertise, preferences of patients/families, and the resources available to answer their question.

They are ready to begin by developing a PICO question. They start by setting up a schedule for team meetings, signing a team contract that defines ground rules, and developing a project management plan that includes status reports deadlines and meetings with their instructor and project director.

Sanida, John, and Michael wonder what the best practices for infant safe sleep are and how can they implement a program to educate caregivers, parents, and teen mothers to lower the infant mortality rates in their community. Based on their past knowledge of the evidence-based practice process, they recognize the importance of scoping and scaling their PICO question to develop a realistic timetable for implementation.

Think Before You Read

- What are the steps of the EBP process?
- What PICO or PICo questions can you imagine that are relevant to the clinical story?

- What model can you use to structure how you approach implementing the evidence?
- What might be some key issues to consider as you search for and appraise the evidence?
- What might be some candidate implementation strategies?
- What do you need to consider to judge the success or failure of a project like the one in the clinical story?

Introduction

During 2017, more than 22,000 infants died in the United States. **Infant mortality rate** (IMR) is defined as the number of infant deaths (less than 1 year of age) per 1,000 infants. In 2017, the IMR in the United States was 5.8 deaths/1,000 births (Centers for Disease Control and Prevention [CDC], 2019). This is much higher compared to countries like Japan and Finland, both with IMRs of 2.0 deaths/1,000 (United Health Foundation, 2020). On examining state data for this clinical story, the IMR for the state in which the students live ranks 40 out of 50, indicating only 10 states have a worse IMR (CDC, 2020b).

Infant deaths can result from birth defects, preterm birth, maternal complications, **sudden infant death syndrome (SIDS),** and injuries such as suffocation (CDC, 2020a). SIDS is defined as sudden death of an infant less than 1 year of age that cannot be explained after an examination of the death scene, a review of the case history, and a complete autopsy. SIDS is considered a diagnosis of exclusion, meaning all other causes need to be evaluated and ruled out first. **Sudden unexpected infant death** (SUID) occurs in a previously healthy infant with no obvious cause of death prior to investigation. It is an umbrella term that includes three types: SIDS, unknown cause, or **accidental suffocation or strangulation in bed (ASSB)** (CDC, 2020c). Given the rate of infant mortality in their state, the students need to seek the best available evidence that may lower mortality rates for infants and find ways to educate caregivers and parents about SUID. SUID is a major problem related to maternal and infant health at the national, state, and local levels. Given how devasting the loss of an infant would be for parents and the problems in their state, the students did some preliminary reading and discovered that sleep practices were important. They wondered if cases could be prevented using safe sleep practices.

There are many factors in the population that have been associated with high infant mortality rates, including race or ethnicity, age, gender, education, income, and geographical location (CDC, 2020c). Notably, mothers between 15 and 19 years of age experience significantly higher infant death rates when compared to mothers 25 to 29 years of age (Xu, Murphy, Kochanek, et al, 2016).

In this chapter, you will find a blueprint to apply the EBP process to a children's health problem—promoting safe sleep practices to reduce infant mortality. This chapter is a "snapshot" of a very comprehensive 5 As process to implement a sustainable infant safe sleep program from asking through assessing.

What Are the Key Issues?

Infant mortality is defined as the death of a baby before his or her first birthday. The **infant mortality rate (IMR)** gives us key information about maternal and infant health and is an important indicator of the overall health and wellness of a given population.

Sanida, John, and Michael examine 2017 local data from the county they live in and find that it has one of the highest infant mortality rates in their state with an IMR of 10.5. This compares with the state's IMR of 7.3 deaths/1,000 births, which exceeds the average for the United States of 5.3 deaths/1,000 births (ISDH, 2017).

To add to this problem, the state has one of the highest teen birth rates, ranking 12th of the 50 states for the number of teen births among females aged 15–19 in the year 2013 (CDC, 2020d) contributing to higher risk of infant mortality (Xu et al, 2016). Therefore, infant mortality and teen pregnancies are growing concerns for the county.

Infant mortality due to SUIDS may be influenced by education and health promotion activities that promote safe sleep practices. The Safe to Sleep® campaign (formerly known as the Back to Sleep campaign) brings public attention to SIDS/SUIDS and educates caregivers on ways to reduce SIDS risk through the *ABC's of Safe Sleep*. The acronym *ABC* stands for "Alone on my Back in a Crib." The mnemonic device has expanded to aid caregivers in remembering specific safe sleep practices. *ABCDEF* stands for "**A**ll by myself, on my **B**ack, in a **C**rib, **D**ressed for sleep, in an **E**mpty crib, **F**lat on my back" (https://www.nichd.nih.gov/sts) (Box 19■1).

The EBP process begins by being curious and having an **attitude of inquiry.** The team begins to ask questions:

- What are the best practices for promoting safe sleep for infants?
- Who are the infant caregivers?
- Is mom a teen?
- What information do caregivers and parents need to have to promote safe sleep?
- What are the sleep practice preferences of the parents/caregivers?

    Next, they question how the environment might influence safe sleep:

- What is the safest sleeping environment?
- What factors may be related to limited knowledge as new parents/caregivers?
- What are the living arrangements?
- What cribs, mattresses, and supplies are safe?
- Where does the baby sleep?
- Does bed sharing occur?
- What additional socio-economic factors need to be considered?

What Are the Scope and Scale?

As Sanida, John, and Michael begin to review the key issues that may influence caregiver decision making and infant sleep safety, they quickly become overwhelmed. There are many questions and pieces of the puzzle that need to be put together

BOX 19■1 **Significance of Problem**

■ Infant mortality is defined as the death of an infant before the age of 1 year. The infant mortality rate in the United States is 5.8 deaths/1,000 live births (CDC, 2016).
■ Sudden unexpected infant death (SUID) occurs when an infant less than 1 year old unexpectedly dies (CDC, 2016).
■ 3,500 babies die unexpectedly in the United States (CDC, 2016).
■ Safe sleeping conditions are part of the preventive solution.

after their quick review of the key issues. How can they develop an effective evidence-based practice safe sleep program for infants to lower infant mortality rates? They try to remain calm as they remember the importance of scope (How big is this problem?) and scale (How much of this problem can be addressed and accomplished in a brief time? [in this case, the class semester is 15 weeks long]).

To begin to discuss the scope, they schedule a weekly meeting with their instructor and project director for guidance through each step of the EBP process. They have realized that promoting safe sleep is a complex problem that may extend through several phases for a realistic and sustainable implementation plan for the community. They come prepared with a list of questions based on their initial search for evidence related to safe sleep practices. With help from their instructor, an agenda for an initial meeting is made to keep everyone focused on safe sleep practices.

The next step is a meeting with the clinical project director, an advanced practice nurse at the community agency. The project director is a primary stakeholder who is extremely passionate about safety and safe sleep initiatives for infants to lower infant mortality rates. They realize that the project director has **clinical expertise,** is very knowledgeable of the **context** of the organization, and is aware of some of the barriers and **facilitators** for a successful implementation. This information will be invaluable as they develop a project management plan to scale the EBP project to into reasonable phases.

The student team reflects on the importance of scoping a question to design a search strategy to locate and appraise the best available evidence. Larger questions, such as best practices for infant safe sleep, may be found in clinical practice guidelines or expert opinion recommendations from national organizations, such as the American Academy of Pediatrics (AAP), that address many parts of the bigger problem. For smaller questions, such as, What is the effect of a specific type of crib, bed surface, bed padding, or sleeping positions on infant mortality?, a systematic review of primary research may be a better source. Alternatively, a specific aspect of a comprehensive guideline may be an option.

Ask/Assess

The team remembers that the EBP process begins with asking questions of inquiry after a problem has been identified that requires evidence-based decision making.

Questions will lead to a structured search for the best available evidence. At this point, initial data have been collected about infant mortality rates, teen pregnancy rates, and causes of infant mortality locally and nationally. Sanida, John, and Michael have their weekly meeting with their instructor to discuss crafting their PICO question.

They start by identifying what evidence-based resources are already available for caregivers and parents. Systematic reviews, clinical practice guidelines, AAP recommendations, and Safe to Sleep® resources through the National Institutes of Health may be potential sources to inform their thinking. They remember that finding pre-appraised evidence would be very helpful since this has been appraised by experts in the field.

Next, the team will examine **local data** that may be available from quality improvement nurses, pediatric nurse practitioners, clinical nurse specialists, nurse managers, risk managers, and other health-care professionals. The CDC may be one evidence-based resource for health indicator data. The National Vital Statistics System (NVSS) is an intergovernmental data-sharing system by which the National Center for Health Statistics (NCHS) collects and disseminates the Nation's official vital statistics and is available at https://www.cdc.gov/nchs/nvss/index.htm.

The team began to generate their PICO question. They started with a very broad question: What are the best practices for creating a safe sleep environment to reduce infant mortality due to sudden unexplained infant death? During the initial meeting with their instructor and project director, the team learned that a team of students from the previous semester already found extensive background information. They had searched comprehensively to identify the best available evidence related to teen pregnancy, infant mortality, and infant safe sleep environments. That team found that significant independent risk factors for SIDS include a soft sleep surface, maternal smoking in pregnancy, prone sleeping position, pillow use, not using a pacifier, and bed sharing. After adjusting for several confounding variables like marital status, maternal education, age of parents, and prenatal care, these risk factors tell the story of an unsafe sleeping environment that could be modified (Hauck, Herman, Donovan, et al, 2003).

The AAP SIDS campaigns have been very effective for avoiding infant prone sleep positioning (AAP, 2020). It is very important that parents are educated and are receptive to understanding and implementing safe sleep practices (Gelfer, Cameron, Masters, et al, 2013). Populations with high IMR rates include women with a maternal age under 20 years, less than 12 years of education, lack of prenatal care, multiparous pregnancy, and smoking while pregnant (Carlberg, 2013).

The previous team of students evaluated a study conducted in a 100-bed neonatal intensive care unit (NICU) after a program was developed by staff to implement safe sleep practices that the AAP recommends. The researchers designed an educational program to teach NICU health-care workers and parents about SIDS and techniques to decrease infant mortality rates. They used multiple methods including mandatory education requirements for nurses and new hires, "Back to Sleep" crib cards for hospital staff and cards developed for parents to use at home, SIDS educational videos for parents, a discharge instruction sheet including safe sleeping practices, and a questionnaire completed by a telephone call to parents post discharge. They found that after 3 months, parents increased the frequency of placing their infants in supine position to sleep from 39% to 83%. Firm sleeping surfaces improved from 5% to 96%. The crib cleared of any objects increased from 45% to 75%. Overall, parents increased their use of safe sleep practices from 23% to 82% (Gelfer et al, 2013).

Through a rigorous search of research evidence in the United States and internationally, the phase one team identified that the use of a "baby box" provided a safe sleep environment and met the product safety requirements. The **baby box** is a reusable and sustainable and a safe resource for teen mothers and their infants to use as a protective sleeping environment. The baby box was one measure taken in Finland for reducing infant mortality. Evidence supported the use of the Baby Box (Baby Box, 2019) to meet standards for preventing SIDS, suffocation, and strangulation deaths when used appropriately.

This first meeting was very helpful for understanding the scope of the problem and progress that had been made to date. The PICO question was adjusted to find the best available evidence about the effectiveness of an evidence-based intervention to promote safe sleep and lower infant mortality rates. The PICO resulted in a question with a narrower focus: For caregivers, parents, and pregnant teens, what is the effectiveness of implementing a safe sleep education program to reduce infant mortality rates?

Acquire/Diagnose

The team now sets out to acquire the best available evidence based on their narrowed PICO question. They consider two potential focus areas: (1) a rigorous search for evidence to develop an evidence-based implementation plan based on **implementation science**, and (2), to use that evidence to implement a safe sleep education program for caregivers, parents, and pregnant teens.

Initially, the team searched for clinical guidelines and recommendations from the Agency for Healthcare Research and Quality (AHRQ) and did a Google Scholar search on the AAP safe sleep recommendations. They discovered the Safe to Sleep® Campaign resources (2014) available through the National Institute of Child Health and Human Development (NICHD) (http://safetosleep.nichd.nih.gov). Sanida, John, and Michael decided to consult with the research librarian for guidance with developing a more systematic search strategy to acquire the research evidence. They generated a list of keywords and synonyms based on their PICO question. Together with the librarian, they constructed the following search strategy:

1. "Sudden Infant Death Syndrome" OR SIDS OR "Sudden Unexpected Infant Death" OR SUID
2. Parent* OR nurs*
3. "safe sleep" OR sleep
4. "Implementation strateg*" OR "knowledge transfer" OR "knowledge translation" OR educat*

5. "infant mortality" OR "infant death"
6. 1 AND 2 AND 3 AND 4 AND 5

They searched the following databases: MEDLINE (EBSCO), CINAHL (EBSCO), JBI EBP Database, Cochrane Library, and PubMed. The results from these database searches yielded articles to support the PICO question.

Appraise/Plan

The team selected a set of relevant articles to critically appraise using the appropriate JBI appraisal checklist or **CASP** tool that corresponded with the type of study or article. They then ranked each article using the JBI Levels of Evidence (2014).

With the help of their instructor, the team begins to practice the skill set necessary for critical appraisal. As students with limited experience in critical appraisal, the team remembers that the purpose of critical appraisal was threefold: to assess the validity of the study and determine whether the evidence is of high enough quality to consider for a practice change; to determine whether the results would fit into their local context; and to determine whether the results would help caregivers, parents, and teen moms implement infant safe sleep practices.

The capstone team appraised the evidence to design an evidence-based implementation plan. Many studies were obtained that supported the PICO question.

Barriers to implementing infant safe sleep practices are well documented in primary research studies. Inadequate knowledge of newborn care among health providers, a lack of leadership support for evidence-based, low-cost interventions, and a critical lack of trained staff all contribute to ineffective implementation (Aliganyira, Kerber, Davy, et al, 2014).

A 4-year infant safe sleep environment study found that engaging all levels of management early in the process would have made the implementation process go more smoothly. Staff turnover and cultural variances were barriers to implementation.

Investigators identified the importance of education for safe sleep in a study of 255 sleep-related deaths. Chu, Hackett, and Kaur (2015) found that having a crib in the home does not decrease the risk for a sleep-related injury. However, these themes for sleep-related deaths emerged: situational (the infant needed care and was found outside the crib because the caregiver fell asleep); preference (the infant cried when placed in the crib or the caregiver wanted to watch the infant more closely); and lack of knowledge (the caregivers were knowledgeable of the importance of safety but didn't realize that what they were doing was potentially harmful).

Grazel, Phalen, and Polomano (2010) found that parents mimic behaviors of nurses at home after hospital discharge and that education for nurses is equally important as it is for parents. The study found that most nurses can identify SIDS risk-reduction strategies while some nurses still have a knowledge deficit. "Misconceptions and unfounded fears may contribute to nurses' reluctance to integrate evidence-based SIDS reduction strategies into the clinical setting" (Grazel et al, 2010, pp. 338–339).

As an educational intervention, Shaefer et al (2010) designed a pretest/posttest study to assess knowledge of SIDs and infant safe sleep practices among nurses. Findings showed no significant difference of nurses' knowledge of SIDs reduction after the educational intervention, but they did find a significant increase in posttest scores about infant safe sleep practices.

Andreotta, Hill, Eley, et al (2015) identified that the most influential intervention in changing the sleep practice was role-modeling and interactive education with parents. Socioeconomic status, age, and ethnicity were shown to influence parental perception of safe sleep. "The most consistent variables among SIDs victims were sharing a sleep environment, use of surfaces that were not intended for infants and extraneous soft objects in the sleep environment" (Andreotta et al, 2015, p. 197).

Several studies were appraised that targeted vulnerable populations for high infant mortality. The investigators gathered data on self-efficacy (to assess the confidence level), educational status, race, and social support (living arrangements and who is the source of income). Findings showed that when young mothers valued the importance of education, they may also understand that knowledge of infant safety and infant safe sleep is important (Turney, Conway, Plummer, et al, 2011). Chablani and Spinney (2011) examined engaging high-risk mothers using Prochaska and DiClemente's cycle of change model. They identified that most young mothers are in the earlier stages of change as compared to older mothers who are in later stages. This may be one reason they do not participate in the same prenatal classes that appeal to older mothers.

Finally, the team appraised evidence from the NICHD materials titled *Sudden Infant Death Syndrome (SIDS) and Other Related Causes of Infant Death: Question and Answers for Health Care Providers* (2014) using JBI's appraisal tool for narrative, expert opinion, and text.

Sanida, John, and Michael were pleased with their progress in expanding their skill set for critical appraisal. Appraising "SIDS and Other Sleep-Related Infant Deaths: Updated 2016 Recommendations for a Safe Infant Sleeping Environment," the AAP Task Force on Sudden Infant Death Syndrome (2016) recommendations, was their last task. They used the AGREE II tool to evaluate three basic questions: How clear is the focus? How transparent and rigorous were the methods? Can I apply the recommendations to caregivers, parents, and teen mothers?

Once the capstone team acquired and appraised the extensive amount of best available evidence, they remembered the importance of evidence hierarchies as a system to rank the evidence and to determine the confidence in the recommendation or source of evidence. They applied the JBI Levels of Evidence (2014) to rank the evidence from level 1 to level 5.

Apply/Implement

The students are now ready to meet with their instructor and project director for guidance with the next step of the evidence-based practice process—Apply and Implement. Before their meeting, they completed a status report and created an agenda with a list of questions for discussion. From their extensive review of the evidence, they identified two potential innovations for implementation to address their PICO question: For caregivers, parents, and pregnant teens, what is the effectiveness of implementing a safe sleep education program to reduce infant mortality rates?

Originally, the student group wondered if they should pursue the implementation of equipment such as the box for babies or if they should focus on educating caregivers, parents, and teens about evidence-based practices for a safe sleep environment for infants. After reviewing the "O" (outcome) portion of the PICO question—"to reduce infant mortality rates"—and the evidence they sought through their search, the team determined a need for an infant safe sleep environment educational program. As a first step, they decided to target the nursing staff in the NICU. They would then move forward to implementation in the community with area obstetrical and pediatric clinics.

They were familiar with a variety of evidence implementation models and selected the **Promoting Action on Research Implementation in Health Services (PARIHS)** because it was a practical framework that they determined would help guide them through the implementation process (Kitson, Harvey, & McCormick, 1998). In 2015, the authors modified the original model to i-PARIHS. The modified model integrates change theory typically reflected in many implementation models. The new model recognizes that the strength of the evidence is key but so are the characteristics of the innovation based on the evidence. In addition, the authors expanded on the role of facilitation. That is, successful implementation is a function of the active ingredient of facilitation and the characteristics of the innovation (including the strength of the evidence), the stakeholders, and the context. The authors depicted the framework with this schema: $SI = Fac^n(I + R + C)$ where successful implementation (SI) is a function of the active ingredient of facilitation (Fac^n) and the nature of the innovation (I), including the evidence, the recipients' engagement (R), and the quality of the context (C) (Harvey & Kitson, 2015). Successful implementation is more likely to occur when (1) the scientific evidence and the innovation that emerges from it are of high quality, are compatible with professional and patient beliefs, are perceived as beneficial, can be observed and trialed, and are less complex. (2) The health-care context is receptive to implementation, including supportive leadership, culture, and evaluation systems. (3) Those who facilitate provide the "active ingredient" by selecting strategies that allow them to assess, align, and integrate the other elements (Harvey & Kitson, 2015; Rycroft-Malone, 2004).

The team identified the stakeholders of the safe sleep education program to be newborn intensive care nurses and staff, advanced practice nurses, clinical educators, unit managers, quality improvement directors, nursing students, and county residents including caregivers, parents, teen moms, infants, and family members of teen moms. Because the issue of preventable infant death is very emotionally laden, the team felt that all the stakeholders would be aligned with their values and their belief that prevention strategies would be seen as beneficial and as long as the educational strategies were straightforward, they would be seen as less complex and they could be trialed.

The students ranked the recommendations of the AAP's "SIDS and Other Sleep-Related Infant Deaths: Updated 2016 Recommendations for a Safe Infant Sleeping Environment" as strong evidence after applying the AGREE II appraisal tool. The students found that the NICHD Safe to Sleep® campaign provided a variety of educational materials for developing an educational intervention, and it aligned with the evidence from the guideline. Armed with the evidence, the structure of the implementation model, and guidance from the project director and their instructor, the students developed an educational intervention (NICHD, 2016).

The project director was a nurse leader in the hospital system; she was able to provide guidance on the context for developing a successful implementation plan. This included an assessment of the characteristics that relate to a system's leadership, evaluation systems, and organizational culture.

The team determined that they were the active ingredient of the model as they would take on the role of facilitation, focusing on making the implementation of evidence into practice a little easier while considering the characteristics of the innovation, context, and the stakeholders. After collaborating with their instructor and project director, they decided to develop an interactive educational program and to use prompts and reminders as a first step toward implementation.

From their search of the evidence, they remembered that nurses are often the first contacts parents see about safe positioning and safe sleep environments for their infants. Many times, what is an example of practice provided by the nurse is not the best practice according to the evidence (Price, Gardner, Hillman, et al, 2007).

The students developed an implementation plan incorporating the AAP recommendations for safe sleep and the Safe to Sleep® campaign educational materials (AAP Task for on Sudden Infant Death Syndrome, 2016; NICHD, 2016). They designed an educational program to aid nurses, caregivers, and parents in remembering safe sleep practices by using the *ABCDEF* mnemonic.

They created a literacy-sensitive education program for the NICU professional staff. Understanding that the i-PARIHS model predicts that "trialability" fosters implementation, the team decided to pilot the program with senior nursing students currently enrolled in maternal/child health and students in the capstone course. Along with the interactive educational session, they planned to measure knowledge before and after the program. The pretest would provide a baseline to determine the staff's current knowledge and the posttest would demonstrate whether or not the interactive education worked. This would help determine not just the effectiveness of the teaching but also lend observability to the innovation as recommended by i-PARIHS. In addition to the *ABCDEF* memory device, they provided the nurses with a supplemental pamphlet and a safe sleep badge to serve as prompts or reminders.

The students reflected on the Apply/Implement step in the evidence-based practice process. They acknowledged that the evidence about what should be done (the safe sleep evidence of the guidelines), the structure of the i-PARIHS model and the evidence about how to implement the intervention (the interactive education, prompts and reminders and memory device) were all important to support the practice change (Box 19■2).

BOX 19■2 **Interdisciplinary Rounds**

AAP Recommendations (2016) for creating a safe sleep environment impact all disciplines. They include the following:

■ Place the baby on his or her back on a firm sleep surface such as a crib or bassinet with a tight-fitting sheet.
■ Avoid use of soft bedding, including crib bumpers, blankets, pillows, and soft toys. The crib should be bare.
■ Share a bedroom with parents, but not the same sleeping surface, preferably until the baby turns 1 but at least for the first 6 months. Room sharing decreases the risk of SIDS by as much as 50%.
■ Avoid baby's exposure to smoke, alcohol and illicit drugs.

Other recommendations include the following:

■ Offer a pacifier at naptime and bedtime.
■ Do not use home monitors or commercial devices, including wedges or positioners, marketed to reduce the risk of SIDS.
■ Infants should receive all recommended vaccinations.
■ Supervised, awake tummy time is recommended daily to facilitate development.

Assess/Evaluate

Sanida, John, and Michael recognized that the last task to complete the EBP process requires assessment to evaluate the effectiveness of the infant safe sleep practice interventions used with NICU nurses and students. To evaluate the effectiveness of their safe sleep education, they compared the baseline test of knowledge with a test conducted after their interactive education program. In addition, they ensured understanding through a question-and-answer session.

Of course, the ultimate goal of their project was to impact IMRs among teen mothers' rates related to SUID. The unit manager, quality improvement staff, and the advanced practice nurse committed to auditing the outcomes and sustained safe sleep practices among their parents after discharge.

■ Summary

There is a multitude of factors that can contribute to infant mortality. One of the key practices to reduce infant mortality is to promote safe sleep interventions for health-care providers, caregivers, parents, and teen mothers. This team discovered that safe sleep practices are one important intervention to decrease infant mortality rates.

During the final week of classes, Sanida, John, and Michael presented their evidence-based project to stakeholders, faculty, staff, classmates, and community representatives. The team was confident that they learned so much from their project that they will become EBP champions in the workplace after graduation.

Health care in the 21st century is increasingly being delivered within a rapidly changing environment. Nursing graduates are expected to become change agents, transformational leaders, and active members of the nursing profession. Understanding and implementing evidence-based practice is essential for making sustainable practice changes. Working through all the phases of the EBP process through active learning, team engagement, an attitude of inquiry, the spirit of facilitation, and knowledge of what works to manage change will improve patient outcomes and encourage the use of the best available evidence in every practice setting (Box 19■3).

BOX 19■3 **Tools for Learning and Practice**

- Generate additional questions related to infant safety and measures to reduce infant mortality rates among teen mothers.
- Since this is a team project, develop a plan to work effectively as a team to design and implement an evidence-based project.
- Develop a simple audit tool that allows you to observe infant safe sleep environments in the NICU using evidence-based strategies recommended by the American Academy of Pediatrics.
- Using the i-PARIHS framework to develop an implementation plan, make a list of three facilitation strategies to empower others to use the evidence in the practice setting.
- Considering your role as an evidence-based champion, develop three ways to improve the uptake of evidence into practice.

CHAPTER QUESTIONS

1. In this chapter, what were the steps that Sanida, John, and Michael took to complete the evidence-based practice process?

2. Recognizing the importance of scoping and scaling a PICO question related to infant safe sleep practices, develop a realistic timetable for implementing safe sleep practices for infants in community maternal/child health clinics.

3. Ensuring safe sleep habits in the NICU is a team effort. Interdisciplinary rounds are a way to include the staff in the implementation process. Who should be included? How can they assess for compliance of the "ABDEF" of safe sleep?

4. Since this is a team-driven evidence-based project that focuses on Ask, Acquire, Appraise, Apply, and Assess, how can the workload be divided among team members to complete the project?

5. Develop a plan to bring the educational intervention to clinics in the community and to engage teen mothers in attending prenatal classes that focus on patient safety.

References

Aliganyira, P., Kerber, K., Davy, K., et al. (2014). Helping small babies survive: An evaluation of facility-based kangaroo mother care implementation progress in Uganda. *The Pan African Medical Journal, 19,* 1–7. doi:10.11604/pamj.2014.19.37.3928

American Academy of Pediatrics (AAP) Task Force on Sudden Infant Death Syndrome. (2016). SIDS and other sleep-related infant deaths: Updated 2016 recommendations for a safe infant sleeping environment. *Pediatrics, 138*(5), e20162938. https://doi.org/10.1542/peds.2016-2938

American Academy of Pediatrics. (2020). Safe sleep. Retrieved from https://www.aap.org/en-us/about-the-aap/aap-press-room/campaigns/Safe-Sleep/Pages/default.aspx

Andreotta, J., Hill, C., Eley, S., et al. (2015). Safe sleep practices and discharge planning. *Journal of Neonatal Nursing, 21,* 195–199. http://dx.doi.org/10.1016/j.jnn.2015.04.003

Baby Box Company (2019). Retrieved from https://www.babyboxco.com

Centers for Disease Control and Prevention. (2020a). About SUID and SIDS. Retrieved from https://www.cdc.gov/sids/data.htm

Centers for Disease Control and Prevention. (2020b). Infant mortality rates by state. Retrieved from https://www.cdc.gov/nchs/pressroom/sosmap/infant_mortality_rates/infant_mortality.htm

Centers for Disease Control and Prevention. (2020c). Sudden unexpected infant death and sudden infant death syndrome: Data and statistics. Retrieved from https://www.cdc.gov/sids/data.htm

Centers for Disease Control and Prevention. (2020d). Teen birth rate by state. Retrieved from https://www.cdc.gov/nchs/pressroom/sosmap/teen-births/teenbirths.htm

Chablani, A., & Spinney, E. R. (2011). Engaging high-risk young mothers into effective programming: The importance of relationships and relentlessness. *Journal of Family Social Work, 14*(4), 369–383. doi:10.1080/10522158.2011.588544

Chu, T., Hackett, M., & Kaur, N. (2015). Exploring caregiver behavior and knowledge about unsafe sleep surfaces in infant injury death cases. *Journal of Health Education & Behavior, 42*(3), 293–301. doi:10.1177/1090198114547817

Eunice Kennedy Shriver National Institutes of Child Health and Development (NICHD). (2014). Sudden Infant Death Syndrome (SIDS) and other sleep-related causes of infant death: Questions and answers for health care providers. Retrieved from https://www.nichd.nih.gov/sites/default/files/publications/pubs/Documents/SIDS_QA_HealthCareProviders.pdf

Eunice Kennedy Shriver National Institutes of Child Health and Development (NICHD). (2016). Safe to Sleep® Public Education Campaign. Retrieved from https://safetosleep.nichd.nih.gov/resources/shareable-content

Gelfer, P., Cameron, R., Masters, K., et al. (2013). Integrating "back to sleep" recommendations into neonatal ICU practice. *Pediatrics 131*(4), e1264–1270. doi:10.1542/peds.2012-1857

Grazel, R., Phalen, A. G., & Polomano, R. C. (2010). Implementation of the American Academy of Pediatrics recommendations to reduce sudden infant death syndrome risk in neonatal intensive care units: An evaluation of nursing knowledge and practice. *Advances in Neonatal Care, 10*(6), 332–342. doi:10.1097/ANC.0b013e3181f36ea0

Harvey, G., & Kitson, A. (Eds.). (2015). *Implementing evidence-based practice in healthcare: A facilitation guide.* New York, NY: Routledge.

Hauck, F. R., Herman, S. M., Donovan, M., et al. (2003). Sleep environment and the risk of sudden infant death syndrome in an urban population: The Chicago infant mortality study. *Pediatrics, 111*(5), 1207–1214.

Indiana State Department of Health (ISDA). (2017). Infant mortality. Retrieved from https://www.in.gov/isdh/27470.htm

Joanna Briggs Institute. (2014). JBI levels of evidence. Retrieved from https://joannabriggs.org/sites/default/files/2019-05/JBI-Levels-of-evidence_2014_0.pdf

Kitson, A., Harvey, G., & McCormick, B. (1998). Enabling the implementation of evidence-based practice: A conceptual framework: *Quality and Safety in Healthcare, 7,* 149–158.

Price, S. K., Hillman, L., Gardner, P., et al. (2007). Changing hospital newborn nursery practice: results from a statewide "Back to Sleep" nurses training program. *Maternal and Child Health Journal, 12*(3), 363–371.

Rycroft-Malone, J. (2004). The PARIHS framework—A framework for guiding the implementation of evidence-based practice. *Journal of Nursing Quality, 19*(4), 297–304.

Shaefer, S. J. M., Herman, S. E., Frank, S. J., et al. (2010). Translating infant safe sleep evidence into nursing practice. *Journal of Obstetric, Gynecologic & Neonatal Nursing, 39,* 618–626. doi:10.1111/j.1552-6909.2010.01194.x

Turney, H. M., Conway, P., Plummer, P., et al. (2011). Exploring behavioral intentions among young mothers. *Journal of Family Social Work, 14,* 298–310. doi:10.1080/10522158.2011.588552

United Health Foundation. (2020). America's health rankings: 2018 rankings. Retrieved from https://www.americashealthrankings.org/learn/reports/2018-annual-report/findings-international-comparison

Xu, J., Murphy, S. L., Kochanek, K. D., et al. (2016). Deaths: Final data for 2013. *National Vital Statistics Report, 64*(2). Retrieved from https://www.cdc.gov/nchs/data/nvsr/nvsr64/nvsr64_02.pdf

CHAPTER 20

Psychiatric–Mental Health Nursing

Leslie Rittenmeyer

LEARNING OBJECTIVES

- Given an ill-structured description of a serious clinical problem, apply all phases of the evidence-based practice process to guide decisions related to the psychiatric–mental health domain.

- Analyze the challenge of making evidence-based decisions in complex health-care environments.

- Generate next-step strategies to get better evidence into practice.

KEY TERMS

Acute care setting
Local data
Occupational hazard
Occupational Safety and Health
  Act of 1970

PARIHS framework
i-PARIHS framework
Workplace violence

Clinical Story

Adam is a psychiatric liaison nurse at a large, acute care hospital. He provides services to the medical-surgical acute care units, including nursing staff consultation and education. During a weekly meeting with the nurse managers, Adam expresses concern about three different incidents of aggressive behavior in the past 6 weeks for which security staff presence was required. Two incidents were patient related, and one was family related. In the first case, the patient was transferred to the psychiatric unit; in the second case, the patient was given anti-anxiolytic medication; and in the third case, the offending family member was banned from visiting. In one incident, a staff nurse sustained an injury when she was shoved against a wall. The nurse managers share Adam's concern, but they fear the staff is ill equipped to provide intervention that prevents or manages aggressive behaviors. They feel this is an increasing problem and admit they lack a cohesive plan for addressing the issue. They ask Adam to assist them in addressing this vexing problem.

Think Before You Read

- What are the steps of the EBP process?
- What PICO or PICo questions can you imagine that are relevant to the clinical story?
- What model can you use to structure how you approach implementing the evidence?
- What might be some key issues to consider as you search for and appraise the evidence?
- What might be some candidate implementation strategies?
- What do you need to consider to judge the success or failure of a project like the one in the clinical story?

Introduction

Internationally, workplace violence is an increasing problem in the health-care environment (Beech & Leather, 2006). According to McPaul and Lipscomb (2004), it is a complex one as well, presenting an **occupational hazard** (danger of sustaining harm because of one's occupation) for nurses and other health-care workers. McPaul and Lipscomb believe that the complexity is due, in part, to a health-care culture that resists the idea that health-care workers are truly at risk and treats workplace violence as "just part of the job." Lack of formal training in violence prevention and intervention adds to the problem and leaves the nursing staff with few resources to combat this growing issue. According to the Occupational Safety and Health Administration (OSHA), approximately 75% of nearly 25,000 workplace assaults reported annually happened in health-care and social services settings (U.S. Department of Labor and Occupational Safety and Health Administration [OSHA], 2016). To complicate this further, episodes of violence in all categories are underreported because the ways in which health-care injuries are reported lack consistency (Arnetz, Hamblin, Ager, et al, 2015).

As Adam starts developing a plan to address the increasing violence in the medical-surgical units at his facility, he realizes he needs to search for the best available evidence before he can make any recommendations about the right thing to do and the right way to do it. He also realizes that this is a complex problem because it affects both the well-being and safety of patients as well as of staff. Adam wants to ensure he uses the best available evidence when crafting his recommendations because he understands that any recommendations he makes will likely lead to changes in facility policy and new program development.

In this chapter, you will find guidelines for applying the evidence-based practice process to a growing mental health problem: workplace violence. To manage the complexity of this problem, the focus here is on the effectiveness of prevention and management interventions for aggressive behaviors in patients in the **acute care setting.** An acute care setting, such as a medical or surgical unit, provides services to patients with acute needs as opposed to chronic, rehabilitative, or palliative needs.

What Are the Key Issues?

Searching for information that will help solve clinical problems begins by asking basic questions. When considering the problem of workplace violence in the health-care setting, a list of initial questions might include the following:

1. What is workplace violence?
2. What are the scale and scope of the problem in the health-care setting?
3. Are there prevention guidelines already in place?
4. If there are guidelines in place, what type of evidence informed those guidelines?
5. Are there systematic reviews available to inform this topic?
6. What does the primary research literature say about this topic?
7. What do the experts say about this topic?

To start gathering information to answer these questions, you might first search the Internet for societies and groups that consider workplace violence in the health-care setting a problem. In doing so, you would find entities such as the World Health Organization (WHO), the U.S. Department of Labor Occupational Safety and Health Administration (OSHA), the Canadian Centre for Occupational Health and Safety (CCOHS), National Institute for Occupational Safety and Health (NIOSH), the American Nurses Association (ANA), the American Association of Occupational Health Nurses (AAOHN), and the U.S. Department of Justice (DOJ). All of these organizations consider workplace violence a serious problem in the health-care setting and recognize the need for prevention and education.

Although the wording might vary slightly, the definition of **workplace violence** is consistent across the organizations. The term is defined as any act in which a person is abused, threatened, intimidated, and/or assaulted as a result of their employment. The acts that constitute workplace violence include being threatened, either verbally or in writing; harassment; verbal abuse; or physical attack. Workplace violence is not just limited to the traditional workplace and can occur off site—for example, employees receiving threatening phone calls at home. Workplace violence can result in injury, psychological distress, and, in some cases, even death.

The next step is to identify the scale and scope of the problem. *Scope* is identifying the breadth of the problem, and *scale* is determining whether the problem is an isolated experience. In the case of workplace violence, the DOJ and the Bureau of Labor Statistics (BLS) gather relevant national statistical data related to the problem. Available data from the DOJ and BLS reveal that health-care workers are at increased risk to become victims of workplace violence and have the highest rate of non-fatal injury of any industry. These data suggest that workplace violence in the health-care setting is not unique to Adam's institution in this chapter's clinical story. Adam begins to see that the problem is large in both scope and scale. Having gathered some baseline data and having a better idea of the scale and scope of the problem, Adam begins to develop a question that will guide him in his search for the best available evidence.

Ask/Assess

Both the nursing process and the evidence-based practice process begin with assessment, which should result in questions that lead to the best available evidence. To begin his assessment, Adam attempts to find out how many aggressive incidents occurred at his facility over the past 2 years. In most facilities, the risk management department should have a reliable system in place for recording and storing these types of data. These data would constitute **local data** and can provide a better understanding of the problem at Adam's particular institution. Unfortunately (and to his disappointment), Adam finds the record-keeping in his facility has been somewhat lax. The most he can ascertain is that security was called to the medical-surgical units 26 times in the past 2 years for reasons ranging from theft to threats of aggression. Adam makes a mental note to recommend more accurate and verifiable reporting mechanisms for aggressive incidents at his workplace. After some research he finds that lack of reporting standards is a problem nationally. He knows that collecting reliable local data will lead to better planning and policies.

Adam recognizes the next step he needs to take is to find out if there is an existing policy on workplace violence prevention at his institution. Once existing policies are located, they can be evaluated to determine what type of evidence, if any, informed the policy. In some cases, policies are produced without being informed by any evidence, usually leading to ineffective programs or infrastructure. On searching the procedure manuals of his facility, Adam finds policies that generally address issues of patient and employee safety, as well as policies that outline procedures for dealing with aggressive incidents after they occur. However, none of the policies specifically addresses workplace violence prevention and intervention before or as it occurs.

While searching for more information, Adam finds that OSHA published updated guidelines entitled *Guidelines for Preventing Workplace Violence for Healthcare and Social Service* Workers (OSHA, 2016). These guidelines were updated from 2004. As in the 2004 guideline, OSHA does not have a mandatory compliance standard for the prevention of workplace violence because the guidelines are only advisory in nature. The compliance standard is the **Occupational Safety and Health Act of 1970.** This act mandates that, in addition to compliance with hazard-specific standards, all employers have a general duty to provide their employees with a hazard-free workplace. Adam also discovers that, although there is no federal standard that specifically requires workplace violence protections, The Joint Commission has attached hospital accreditation to the meeting of Standard 3.01.01 that requires leaders to create and maintain a culture of safety and quality. This standard requires that (1) leaders develop a code of conduct that defines acceptable behavior and behaviors that undermine a culture of safety and (2) leaders create and implement a process for managing behaviors that undermine a culture of safety. This illustrates how policy development is often cross-walked to accreditation standards (The Joint Commission, 2012).

After reviewing this information, Adam believes he has ample reason to pursue the development of a policy and program aimed at the prevention of workplace violence. He is ready to ask a well-formed question that will help him find the best available evidence to accomplish his task. After some thought, he forms the following two PICO questions:

1. What is the effectiveness of interventions in the prevention of aggressive behaviors in patients admitted to an acute care hospital setting?
2. What is the effectiveness of interventions in the management of aggressive behaviors in patients admitted to an acute care hospital setting?

To understand how he developed these questions, please refer to Table 20■1.

Acquire/Diagnose

Once you have used the assessment data to identify a problem and you have clarified your question, you begin to pursue the next step of the process: how to acquire the best available evidence. Based on your PICO questions, you should generate a list of keywords to start a search. If your questions are based on the effectiveness of interventions, the ideal source of evidence is a clinical practice guideline based on systematic reviews of randomized controlled trials (RCTs) that tested the interventions. If no such guidelines exist, search for systematic reviews or individual studies using bibliographic databases such as CINAHL and MEDLINE. It is usually wise to ask the hospital librarian to assist you in searching. This is what Adam did, and Table 20■2 provides an outline of Adam's proposed search strategy and keywords.

TABLE 20■1 **Narrowing the Focus and Generating Questions**

Broad	What are the best practices for preventing workplace violence?	
Narrow	What are the best practices to prevent and manage workforce violence in the health-care sector?	
Narrow	What is the best way to prevent and manage aggressive behaviors in the acute care setting?	
Searchable PICO	What is the effectiveness of interventions in the prevention of aggressive behaviors in patients admitted to an acute care hospital setting?	P = admitted patients I = interventions to reduce aggressive behavior C = no comparison O = reduction of aggressive behavior
Searchable PICO	What is the effectiveness of interventions in the management of aggressive behaviors in patients admitted to an acute care hospital setting?	P = admitted patients I = interventions to manage aggressive behaviors C = no comparison O = management of aggressive behavior

Adam has previously identified that OSHA has published revised guidelines on violence prevention and intervention but wishes to determine how these guidelines were developed (OSHA, 2016). A good guideline will demonstrate validity, reliability, reproducibility, and transparency. In examining the OSHA 2016 guidelines, Adam observes that they do not seem to have been developed from synthesized sources of evidence like systematic reviews but were informed more by individual research studies and the opinion of experts.

Adam decides to broaden his search to look for available synthesized evidence to help with his task. Synthesized evidence is the effect of pooling the results of research findings to make a judgment about what interventions, activities, or phenomena the evidence supports. The hospital librarian assists him in broadening his search and the results reveal what he previously observed: there is more evidence that addresses violence prevention in the mental health setting than in the acute care setting. Finally, after conducting an extensive search, Adam finds one systematic review on the prevention and management of workplace violence in the acute care setting. (Kynoch, Wu, & Chang, 2009). The objective of the review was to establish best practice in the prevention and management of aggressive behaviors in patients admitted to acute care settings, and Adam is hopeful that this systematic review will report reliable synthesized evidence.

As a last step, Adam asks the librarian to search the Cochrane Library and JBI Database of Systematic Reviews for any other systematic reviews that could assist him. In the end, he focuses on the OSHA guideline because it is the only practice guideline he found related to his question and the systematic review because it

TABLE 20■2 **An Example of Keywords and Search Strategy for Searching the CINAHL Bibliographic Database for a PICO Question**

What is the effectiveness of interventions in the prevention and management of aggressive behaviors in patients admitted to an acute care hospital setting?

1.	(MH "Nurses") or (MH "Nurse Patient Relations")
2.	Nurs*
3.	S1 or S2
4.	(MH "Violence") or (MH "Workplace Violence")
5.	Aggress* or abus* or violen* or danger* or assault*
6.	S4 or S5
7.	(MH "Patients")
8.	Patient*
9.	S7 or S8
10.	(MH "Hospitals") or (MH "Hospital Units")
11.	(acute, or medical surgical) (ward* or hospital or setting*)
12.	S10 or S11
13.	(MH "Psychotherapy") or (MH "Chemical restraint") (MH "Psychopharmacological treatment") ("Physical restraint") (MH "Music therapy") (MH "Staff education")
14.	Intervention or prevention or restrain*
15.	S13 or S14
16.	S3 and S6 and S9 and S12 and S15
17.	S3 and S6 and S9 and S12 and S15

provided the most complete form of synthesized evidence. Adam is confident that his comprehensive search has led him to best available evidence, but now he needs to appraise the evidence to judge its quality.

Appraise/Plan

There are numerous tools available for the critical appraisal of clinical guidelines. Standardized appraisal tools assist with evaluating practice guidelines and systematic reviews to answer the following basic questions (Public Health Research Unit [PHRU], 2007):

- How clear is the focus?
- How transparent and rigorous were the methods?
- Can the recommendations be applied to this situation?

Adam appraises the OSHA (2016) guideline first. Although there are numerous tools available for the critical appraisal of clinical guidelines, he chooses the Appraisal of Guidelines for Research and Evaluation Tool (AGREE II) (AGREE Collaboration, 2013). This tool and its revisions are developed by an international collaboration of researchers and policy makers whose goal is to improve the quality and effectiveness of clinical practice guidelines (Box 20■1).

Adam appraises the OSHA guideline against the AGREE II criteria and found the following:

- The scope and questions seemed clear and focused.
- Diverse stakeholders such as doctors, nurses, academics, researchers, psychologists, and consumers were an integral part of the process.
- The use of rigorous and transparent methods, including systematic methods to search and appraise the evidence, was not readily evident. Single-study papers were used to develop the guideline, but it was not synthesized research.
- Although stakeholders and experts were involved in the development of the guideline, there did not appear to be a formal process in which a panel of experts appraised and extracted the evidence, considered the benefits and risks, and reached consensus on the recommendations.
- The level of evidence was not identified in the guideline.
- The U.S. Inspector General's office performed an evaluation of OSHA's handling of workplace violence issues and made recommendations. There seems to be no formal update plan.
- The guideline is understandable and readily available online.

Adam chooses the Critical Appraisal Skills Program (CASP) tool for systematic reviews (CASP, 2018) to appraise the systematic review (Box 20■2).

He identifies the following strengths of the review:

- The review asked two clearly focused PICO questions and selected appropriate study designs to include in the review (RCTs, controlled prospective, prospective cohort).
- There was a comprehensive search of eight databases and the gray literature as well as hand searching.
- The study appraisal and data extraction were strong. The authors used a blinded duel review method and transparently used rigorous criteria to include in the study.
- The researchers used appropriate data analysis techniques. Because of the type of studies conducted, a meta-analysis was not undertaken, but as there was

BOX 20■1 **AGREE II Appraisal Instrument**

Scope and Practice

The overall objective(s) of the guideline is (are) specifically described.

The health questions(s) of the guidelines is (are) specifically described.

The population to whom the guideline is meant to apply is specifically described.

Stakeholder Development

The guideline development group includes individuals from all the relevant professional groups.

The views and preferences of the target population have been sought.

The target users of the guideline are clearly defined.

Rigor of Development

Systematic methods were used to search for the evidence.

The criteria for selecting the evidence are clearly defined.

The strengths and limitations of the body of evidence are clearly defined.

The methods for formulating the recommendations are clearly described.

The health benefits, side effects and risks have been formulated in the recommendations.

There is an explicit link between the recommendations and the supportive evidence.

The guideline has been externally reviewed by others.

A procedure for updating the guideline is provided.

Clarity of Presentation

The recommendations are specific and unambiguous.

The different options for management of the condition or health issue are clearly presented.

Key recommendations are easily identifiable.

Applicability

The guideline is supported with tools for application.

The guideline describes facilitators and barriers to its application.

The potential resource implications of applying the recommendations have been considered.

The guideline presents monitoring and/or auditing criteria.

Editorial Independence

The views of the funding body have not influenced.

Competing interests of guideline development group members have been recorded and addressed.

BOX 20■2 **Critical Appraisal Skills Program (CASP) (2018)**

Critical Appraisal of Systematic Review Criteria
- Did the review ask clearly focused questions?
- Were all of the relevant studies included?
- Did the reviewers try to identify all relevant studies?
- Did the reviewers assess the quality of the included studies?
- If the results of the studies have been combined, was it reasonable to do so?
- What are the overall results of the review?
- How precise are the results?
- How can the results be applied to the local population?
- Were all important outcomes considered?
- Are benefits worth harms and costs?

considerable variation in the measured outcomes in the trials identified, data were therefore presented in a narrative summary.
- The results of the study were reported according to the study intervention participants (e.g., staff training program, music, chemical restraint).
- There is limited evidence to support the use of staff training, chemical and/or physical restraint, and music therapy.
- The results of this study could be applied to a local population.

After reviewing the evidence he has gathered, Adam is disappointed that there is not more synthesized evidence but is confident that this is the best evidence available to him at this time. He agrees with the conclusions in the systematic review that state "further quality research is needed to assist staff with identifying appropriate interventions to prevent and manage aggressive behavior in acute hospitalized patients" (Kynoch et al, 2009, p. 196).

Because the systematic review represents stronger evidence than the 2016 OSHA guideline, Adam compares the two to look for consistencies in recommendations. From both the OSHA guideline and the systematic review, Adam identified the following bottom-line recommendations:

- A training program for staff about managing patient aggression improves self-efficacy and assists staff in managing aggressive and/or violent patients (Kynoch et al, 2009 p. 195).
- Effective violence preventions programs have the following components (OSHA, 2016):
  1. Management commitment and worker participation
  2. Worksite analysis
  3. Hazard prevention and control
  4. Safety and health training
  5. Record-keeping and program evaluation

- Administration of medication reduces the incidents of aggressive and/or violent behavior in patients in the acute care setting (Kynoch et al, 2009, p. 195).
- Physical restraints are effective in reducing harm to patients and staff and have minimal complications when used for short periods of time (Kynoch et al, 2009 p. 195).
- Individual interventions such as music therapy have been shown to decrease aggressive/and or agitated behaviors (Kynoch et al, 2009, p. 195).

Apply/Implement

The next step in the process is planning to implement changes in policy or programs. Remember that the whole point of evidence-based practice is to move evidence to the point of care. Because the evidence illustrates the benefits of staff training programs, Adam thinks he will focus his efforts on staff training. He begins thinking about how he can best facilitate this process, He decides to be guided by the **i-PARIHS framework.** The i-PARIHS framework, a revision of the original PARIHS framework, provides a way to implement research into practice. The original **PARIHS** framework posits that the successful implementation of evidence into practice has as much to do with context or setting where the new evidence is being introduced and how the evidence is introduced (facilitated into practice) as it has to do with the quality of evidence (Kitson, Harvey, & McCormack 1998). In the revised i-PARIHS model, facilitation is the ingredient that integrates action around the innovation so that it can be successfully implemented in the appropriate context. Adam understands that the success of any program he wishes to implement will likely be compromised if he is the sole planner (Box 20■3). He realizes his role will be that of a facilitator who is sensitive to the context and can also guide others to be good facilitators. He knows, as the OSHA (2016) guideline suggests, that he needs to elicit management commitment and employee involvement. Adam proceeds to create a steering

---

BOX 20■3 **Interdisciplinary Rounds**

In the acute care setting, it is essential to involve a diverse group of stakeholders. Participation by the following is vital. Can you think of any others?

- Vice-president of nursing service
- Nurse managers of the acute care units
- Registered nurses providing professional nursing care at the bedside
- Licensed practical nurses providing technical nursing care at the bedside
- Nursing assistants
- Risk managers

committee with broad representation of upper management, risk control staff, unit managers, professional nurses, and other appropriate staff. He knows that initially, as Harvey and Kitson (2015) suggest, he will need to facilitate change by providing direction along with technical, practical, and task-driven help. Eventually, he hopes his role will be to support and empower others to facilitate and evaluate the workforce prevention-training program.

With the emphasis on the development of a training program, Adam wants to discuss with others what he is envisioning. He knows he must provide strong leadership to create a culture sympathetic to the creation and implementation of the program.

As the systematic review did not make specific recommendations about the content of a training program, Adam focuses on the recommendations in the OSHA (2016) guideline. Although he would prefer to have a guideline developed with stronger synthesized evidence, he knows that this guideline is the best evidence that is available to him at this time. Adam also understands that time is of the essence with this problem, and he cannot afford to wait for better evidence to emerge. He reviews the OSHA (2016) recommendations related to essential training program content, as listed below:

- Presence of a workplace violence prevention policy
- Risk factors that cause or contribute to assaults
- Early recognition of escalating behavior or recognition of warning signs or situations that may lead to assault
- Ways to prevent or diffuse volatile situations or aggressive behavior, manage anger, and appropriately use medications as chemical restraints
- A standard response action plan for violent situations, including the availability of assistance, response to alarm systems, and communication procedures
- Ways to deal with hostile people other than patients and clients, such as relatives and visitors
- Progressive behavior control methods and safe methods to apply restraints
- The location and operation of safety; devises such as alarm systems, along with required maintenance schedules and procedures
- Ways to protect oneself and coworkers, including the use of a buddy system
- Policies and procedures for reporting and recording
- Information on multicultural diversity to increase staff sensitivity to racial and ethnic issues and differences
- Policies and procedures for obtaining medical care, counseling, workers' compensation, or legal assistance after a violent episode or injury

Adam uses his own clinical knowledge and expertise to judge the OSHA recommendations, and he finds them theoretically consistent with what he believes should be part of an effective training program. In addition, although he does not want to recommend more than the steering committee can handle at one time, Adam feels that designing a better record-keeping system to gather better local data is also a priority. He also knows that they must design a good program evaluation system so that they can measure the effectiveness of their program. He is confident

---

BOX 20■4   **Tools for Learning and Practice**

■ Generate PICO questions that narrow the focus of prevention/management of workplace violence in acute care settings.
■ Generate your own list of keywords and search for evidence in CINAHL and MEDLINE pertaining to prevention/management of workplace violence in acute care settings.
■ Search the Internet for the AGREE II Collaboration tool.
■ Search the Internet for the CASP tool.
■ Find OSHA's (2016) *Guidelines for Preventing Workplace Violence for Healthcare and Social Service Workers* (No. OSHA 3148-06R) and appraise them using the AGREE Collaboration tool.
■ Conduct a search for workplace violence prevention and management programs and assess what evidence the program is based on.
■ Search the Centers for Disease Control and Prevention (CDC) Web site and see if it has any data about workplace violence in the heath-care setting.

---

that he can successfully navigate the complexities of implementing evidence into practice and improve staff and patient safety at his facility (Box 20■4).

■ Summary

As Adam searched for the best available evidence, he discovered there is often a need for more primary research that can be pooled on a particular subject. Research generation is part of the evidence-based practice model and is certainly vital to Adam's quest for evidence about the prevention and management of aggressive patients in acute care settings. One of the benefits of an evidence-based practice model is that it identifies when there is a need for more evidence generation. Another common problem Adam encountered was learning there are instances when guidelines are based more on expert opinion than they are on more highly graded, synthesized research. Although research is generally considered the more highly regarded evidence and often possesses a higher level of quality and validity than expert opinion, in its absence expert opinion may be the best available evidence. Some feel that in the absence of rigorously derived research, it is not defensible to discount expert opinion as nonevidence (Pearson, Fields, & Jordan, 2007).

CHAPTER QUESTIONS

1. How do the steps of the nursing process and the evidence-based process align in this chapter's clinical story?

2. How did Adam judge the strength and quality of the evidence? Do you agree with his assessment?

CHAPTER QUESTIONS (continued)

3. Justify the position of using a guideline that was developed from the evidence of expert opinion.

4. Considering that you might want to narrow the focus of your search, what other PICO questions could you ask about prevention and/or management of workplace violence in health care?

5. Adam chose to focus on developing an education program as his first priority. Considering the best available evidence, do you agree with that decision?

6. Given Adam's recommendations from the evidence, how would you prioritize an implementation plan?

7. Develop a written implementation plan using the PARIHS framework.

8. Develop a plan to gain acceptance of your implementation plan from a diverse group of stakeholders.

References

AGREE Collaboration (2013). Appraisal of Guidelines for Research and Evaluation II. AGREE II Instrument. Retrieved from http://www.agreetrust.org

Arnetz, J., Hamblin, L., Ager, J., et al. (2015). Underreporting of workplace violence comparison of self-report and actual documentation of hospital incidents. *Workplace Health and Safety, 63*(5), 200–210.

Beech, B., & Leather, L. (2006). Workplace violence in the health care sector: A review of staff training and integration of training evaluation model. *Aggression and Violent Behavior, 11,* 27–43.

Critical Appraisal Skills Programme (CASP). (2018). CASP Checklist for Systematic Reviews. Retrieved from http://www.CASP-uk-net

Harvey, G., & Kitson, A. (2015). PARIHS revisited: From heuristic to integrated framework for the successful implementation of knowledge into practice. *Implementation Science, 11,* 33. doi:10.1186/s13012-016-0398-2

Kitson, A., Harvey, G., & McCormack, B. (1998). Enabling the implementation of evidence-based practice: A conceptual framework. *Quality Health Care, 7,* 149–158. doi:10.1136/qhsc.7.3.14.9

Kynoch, K., Wu, J., & Chang, A. M. (2009). The effectiveness of interventions in the prevention and management of aggressive behaviors in patients admitted to an acute hospital setting. A systematic review. *JBI Library of Systematic Reviews, 7*(6), 175–223.

McPaul, K., & Lipscomb, J. (2004). Workplace violence in healthcare: Recognized but not regulated. *Online Journal of Issues in Nursing, 3*(9), Manuscript 6.

Pearson, A., Fields, J., & Jordan, Z. (2004). *Evidence-based clinical practice in nursing and health care: Assimilating research, experience and expertise.* Oxford, United Kingdom.

The Joint Commission. (2012). Leadership standard clarified to address behaviors that undermine a safety culture. Retrieved from https://www.jointcommission.org/-/media/tjc/documents/standards/jc-requirements/leadership_standard_behaviorspdf.pdf?db=web&hash=40E293B4C6412D1A4C6D63DFDF709F1F

U.S. Department of Labor and Occupational Safety and Health Administration. (2016). *Guidelines for preventing workplace violence for healthcare and social service workers* (No. OSHA 3148-06R). Washington, DC: Author. Retrieved from http://www.OSHA.gov/

CHAPTER 21

Nursing Care of the Older Adult

Manisa Baker, Jane Walker

- Apply the evidence-based practice process to identify suitable printed medication information materials to use with elderly patients.

- Analyze the role of an evidence-based practice committee in using the evidence-based practice process to address an identified clinical problem.

- Develop strategies to improve the readability of written patient information material using recommended evidence.

Critical Appraisal Skills
 Program (CASP)
Easy-to-read
Health literacy
Integrated Promoting Action on
 Research Implementation in

Health Services (i-PARIHS)
 framework
Patient education
Printed medication information
 sheets
Readability

Clinical Story

Susan, an advanced practice nurse in a congestive heart failure (CHF) clinic is reviewing medication lists with patients after discharge from the hospital. She finds that many of the elderly patients are asking questions about what medications they should be currently taking and how to take their medications. Although patients tell her they received a written medication instruction sheet at discharge, they are having trouble reading and understanding the information.

After compiling the feedback from several visits, Susan presents her findings to the nurse manager of the telemetry unit. The unit manager brings Susan's concerns to the unit shared governance meeting for the staff's feedback. Ainsley, one of the more experienced nurses, voices a concern about the way the information on the medication instruction sheets is formatted and written. The standard hospital medication information sheets are formatted using single spacing and small fonts. In addition, the instruction sheets use generic terms for the medications and include complicated medical terminology. Sentences are long, and many of the terms are multisyllabic. The shared governance committee questions whether elderly patients are able to read and understand the information. Because taking the correct dose of medications on the right schedule is important, the manager asks Kristin, the unit's representative to the hospital's evidence-based practice committee, to take this problem to the next committee meeting. By doing so, the committee members can review the scope and scale of the problem and explore current evidence related to the readability of instruction material written for elderly patients.

Think Before You Read

- What are the steps of the EBP process?
- What PICO or PICo questions can you imagine that are relevant to the clinical story?
- What model can you use to structure how you approach implementing the evidence?
- What might be some key issues to consider as you search for and appraise the evidence?
- What might be some candidate implementation strategies?
- What do you need to consider to judge the success or failure of a project like the one in the clinical story?

Introduction

Nurses working in acute care settings are responsible for teaching patients about medications and providing printed information sheets describing their medications before the patients go home. This information typically includes the purpose of each medication, major side effects, drug–food interactions, schedule for taking the medications, and dosage instructions. The goal of giving **printed medication information sheets** to patients is to help them safely take their medications independently when they are home. However, if patients are not able to read and understand the written material, they might not take their medications correctly, which may place them at risk for serious adverse effects. Polypharmacy is a common occurrence in the care of elderly patients. Patients with five to ten medication prescriptions may be at higher risk for adverse outcomes, increased cost of care, or confusion taking medication as prescribed (Golchin, Frank, Vince, et al, 2015). The risk is even greater for elderly patients who have difficulty reading and understanding printed medication instructions.

This chapter helps you apply the evidence-based practice process to identifying suitable printed materials for medications for elderly patients. This process includes exploring the scope and scale of the problem, generating a PICO question, searching for and evaluating the evidence, and translating the evidence into practice. You will also learn more about health literacy and the elderly.

What Are the Key Issues?

Patients' ability to read and understand the printed materials you give them is influenced by their **health literacy** level as well as the readability of the information. The most widely used definition of health literacy is the one developed by Ratzan and Parker (2000) for the National Library of Medicine. According to this definition, health literacy is "the degree to which an individual has the capacity to obtain, process and understand basic health information and services needed to make appropriate health decisions" (Introduction section, para. 7). Health literacy affects patients' ability to perform a number of health-related tasks, including how to monitor their health conditions, schedule appointments with their doctors and other health-care providers, and understand why each medication is being used as well as when and how to take the medications (Box 21■1).

A National Assessment of Adult Literacy (NAAL) study, published in 2003, assessed the literacy levels of adults in the United States and included an assessment of health literacy. Findings demonstrated that 35% of the population has health literacy abilities that are in the *below basic* and *basic* ranges. Among those age 65 years and older, 59% read at *below basic* and *basic* levels (Kutner Greenberg, Jin, et al, 2006). At *below basic* and *basic* levels of ability, individuals are able to read and understand simple health information only. For example, individuals who read *below basic* level can understand how often they should have a medical exam from reading clearly written material. They can also circle dates for medical follow-up on an appointment slip (Kutner et al, 2006). At the *basic* level, when individuals read a clearly written pamphlet, they can identify at least two reasons for obtaining screening related to a specific disease. However, individuals who read at *basic* and *below basic* levels cannot read and follow instructions on a prescription drug label that relate to timing medication doses in relation to eating. They also cannot identify

---

BOX 21■1 **Significance of Health Literacy**

- Thirty-six percent of the population has health literacy abilities that are in the *Below Basic* and *Basic* ranges (Kutner, Greenberg, Jin, et al, 2006).
- Adults over age 65 have literacy abilities lower than do younger adults (Kutner et al, 2006).
- Adults living below the poverty level have lower health literacy than do those living above the poverty level (Kutner et al, 2006).
- The cost of low health literacy on the health-care system ranges from 3% to 5% of total health-care costs (Eichler, Wieser, & Brugger, 2009).
- In 2007, the cost of low health literacy to the U.S. economy was estimated to range between $106 and $238 billion annually (Vernon, Trujillo, Rosenbaum, et al, 2007).
- Adults with limited health literacy reported poorer health status and lower use of preventive health services (Institute of Medicine [IOM] of the National Academies, 2004).
- Elderly patients with low health literacy were associated with higher mortality rates. (Berkman, Sheridan, Donahue, et al, 2011).
- Adults with low health literacy are less likely to follow prescribed treatment and self-care regimens, more likely to make more medication errors, make increased use of emergency rooms, and lack the skills needed to effectively use the health-care system (Berkman et al, 2011).

---

drug interactions based on over-the-counter drug labels (Kutner et al, 2006). This means many patients in these two health literacy categories may have difficulty understanding and acting on printed medication information.

There have been no assessments focused specifically on health literacy since 2003. However, the National Center for Health Statistics continues to study adult literacy skills through the Program for the International Assessment of Adult Competencies (PIAAC, 2017). Although this assessment did not include adults over the age of 65, data demonstrated that as self-reported health decreases, literacy levels also decreased. When self-reported health was fair or poor, 69% of the population had a literacy level of 2 or below on a scale of 1 to 5, with 1 representing the lowest level. In comparison, when self-reported health was excellent or very good, 44% of the population had a literacy level of 2 or below (PIAAC, 2017). Therefore, it is possible that older adults who also experience a number of adverse health conditions may be at risk for lower literacy levels.

In addition to health-related problems, aging can affect literacy abilities for a variety of other reasons. These reasons can be related to decreases in visual ability, limiting the ability to read; slower processing of information; decreases in working memory; and increased difficulty interpreting information and drawing conclusions (Centers for Medicare & Medicaid Services [CMS], 2010).

The readability, or usability, of written communication materials is another piece of the equation related to a person's ability to comprehend information they are attempting to read (Office of Disease Prevention and Health Promotion [ODPHP], n.d.). Written materials that are unclear, use medical jargon, contain too much information, and ignore **easy-to-read** design principles may make it difficult to actually use the information provided (Centers for Disease Control and Prevention [CDC], 2010). Therefore, one way to help your patients understand printed medication information may be to use educational materials printed in plain language that follow evidence-based guidelines.

Ask/Assess

At the hospital evidence-based practice committee meeting in this chapter's clinical story, Susan describes the problem she is experiencing with elderly patients who do not understand their medications or how to take them after going home. She also shares the nurses' suspicion that the cause of the problem could be the format and reading level of the medication instruction sheets. She works with Kristin to distribute samples of the unit's medication instruction sheets to the committee members. After reviewing the sample instruction sheets, the members of the evidence-based practice committee question whether there is a mismatch between the format of the hospital's current medication information sheets and the health literacy ability of many elderly patients. The committee decides the next step is to determine the scope and scale of this potential problem. The members establish a task force to work with Susan to continue the investigation into this issue.

To describe the scope of the potential problem (difficulty using and understanding printed health information), the task force searches the Internet to locate information from national institutes and organizations that addresses issues related to health literacy and readability of written health materials. They discover the Institute of Medicine (IOM) of the National Academies (now called the National Academy of Medicine) (2004) reported that more than 90 million people in the United States have difficulty reading and understanding health information. The NAAL data also include statistics addressing the relationship between age and health literacy abilities, which show that adults older than age 65 years have lower average health literacy abilities than do younger adults (Kutner et al, 2006). In addition to national statistics, the committee members are also able to locate state information pertaining to general literacy levels for their locale. They find approximately 60% of their local population reads at a level below that of the eighth grade.

The task force also identifies several Web sites that provide background information related to the problem of health literacy and readability. These include the National Institutes of Health's Clear Communication Web site; the Office of Disease Prevention and Health Promotion's Web site related to health communication, literacy, and older adults; and the CDC information related to health literacy and older adults. You can find a listing of these helpful Web sites and others in Box 21■2.

To determine the scale of the problem, Kristin conducts an audit on her unit to assess how well the recently discharged elderly patients understood their medication regimen. The nurses indicate that the majority of the discharged patients were older

---

BOX 21■2 **Selected Web Sites Containing Health Literacy and Readability Information**

- Agency for Healthcare Research and Quality: AHRQ Health Literacy Universal Precautions Toolkit (https://www.ahrq.gov/health-literacy/quality-resources/tools/literacy-toolkit/index.html)
- Centers for Disease Control and Prevention: CDC's Health Literacy Action Plan (https://www.cdc.gov/healthliteracy/planact/cdcplan.html)
- Centers for Disease Control and Prevention: Health Literacy—Older Adults (https://www.cdc.gov/healthliteracy/developmaterials/audiences/olderadults/index.html)
- Centers for Disease Control and Prevention: Health Literacy (https://www.cdc.gov/healthliteracy/index.html)
- Centers for Medicare & Medicaid Services Toolkit for Making Written Material Clear and Effective (https://www.cms.gov/Outreach-and-Education/Outreach/WrittenMaterialsToolkit/index)
- Harvard T.H. Chan School of Public Health: Health Literacy Studies (https://www.hsph.harvard.edu/healthliteracy/)
- Healthy People 2020—Health Literacy (https://www.healthypeople.gov/2020/topics-objectives/topic/social-determinants-health/interventions-resources/health-literacy)
- IHA: The Health Literacy Solutions Center (https://www.healthliteracysolutions.org/home)
- National Center for Education Statistics Program for the International Assessment of Adult Competencies (PIAAC) (https://nces.ed.gov/surveys/piaac/)
- National Network of Libraries and Medicine (http://nnlm.gov/outreach/consumer/hlthlit.html)
- National Institutes of Health: Clear Communication: An NIH Health Literacy Initiative (https://www.nih.gov/institutes-nih/nih-office-director/office-communications-public-liaison/clear-communication)
- plainlanguage.gov (https://plainlanguage.gov/resources/content-types/healthcare/)
- U.S. Department of Health and Human Services, Office of Disease Prevention and Health Promotion: Health Communication Activities (http://www.health.gov/communication/literacy/)

---

than 65 years, and 80% of them were not able to answer simple questions about their medications after leaving the hospital, despite the answers to these questions being readily available in the printed medication information material the patients were given. Meanwhile, the task force finds that the majority of patients admitted to the hospital are also over the age of 65 years and that this problem of lack of understanding of printed medication information could be widespread. Although the Joint Commission does not specifically use the term *health literacy*, requirements pertaining to health literacy issues are embedded into several requirements addressing communication. According to these requirements, information provided must be understandable and written in plain language (Cordero, 2018). In addition, the IOM (2004) recommended that health-care institutions develop strategies to address problems with health literacy. Based on all of this information, the task force recognizes the need for further action related to printed medication information.

To more fully assess the scale of the problem, the task force members test the readability of the most frequently used medication instruction sheets. Testing readability involves assessing the reading level as well as the overall understandability of the printed materials. To assess the reading level of the instruction forms, the task force uses the Fry formula (1977), which is a widely accepted and easy-to-use method. The Fry method involves testing sample text from three sections of a document. Sentences and syllables are counted in these samples and averaged. Users then plot the results on a graph to identify a readability level, which reflects a grade level from first grade to a post-college grade of 17 (Readability Formulas, n.d.). To assess understandability of the medication sheets, they chose the frequently used Suitability Assessment of Materials (SAM) tool, which is also considered reliable and valid (Doak, Doak, & Root, 1996) and recommended by Brega, Barnard, Mabachi, et al (2015). Suitability factors addressed by the SAM tool include content, literacy demand (e.g., grade level, writing style, learning aids), graphics, layout, learning stimulation through the use of interaction and self-efficacy, and cultural appropriateness (Doak et al, 1996). Reviewers use criteria related to each factor to assign points related to an assessment of written material, and the final suitability assessment results are reported as percentages. Superior ratings range from 70% to 100%, adequate ratings range from 40% to 69%, and materials that receive scores lower than 40% are considered not suitable (Doak et al, 1996). Based on members' evaluation of the printed medication sheets, the task force finds the average reading level of the medication sheets was grade 13 and the average suitability score was 34%, indicating the materials are not suitable for patients as written.

As a result of this assessment, the task force determines the scale of the problem is quite large, and the members need to find a way to provide elderly patients with printed medication information that is easy to read. The task force's broad background question initially focuses on identifying the best types of printed medication information materials to use with elderly patients. After further discussion, they identify a narrower question to better focus their search for best evidence. This narrower question addresses the best way to format written medication information material so elderly patients can understand it more easily. This question is then further refined into a PICO format to guide the search for evidence (Table 21■1).

Acquire/Diagnose

At the next evidence-based practice committee meeting, the task force presents its recommendations. First, members discuss the information they have collected regarding

TABLE 21■1 **Narrowing the Focus and Generating the PICO Question**

Broad	What are the best types of printed medication information materials to use with elderly patients?	
Narrow	What is the best way to format written medication information material that can best be understood by elderly patients?	
Searchable PICO	What is the effectiveness of using easy-to-read written medication information material compared with standard written medication information material on knowledge and understanding among elderly hospitalized patients?	P = elderly hospitalized patients I = easy-to-read written medication information material C = standard written medication information material O = knowledge, understandability

the scope and scale of the problem. Based on this information, they suspect the lack of understanding of the medication regimen by elderly patients is likely the result of a mismatch between the readability and suitability of the medication information sheets and the health literacy abilities of their elderly patient population. Second, the task force recommends conducting a search of the literature to identify the most appropriate strategies for writing and formatting written medication information materials for elderly patients. The task force also presents its PICO question to the committee. The evidence-based practice committee agrees with the task force's assessment of scope and scale, their PICO question, and the plan to search the literature for best evidence.

After receiving support from the evidence-based practice committee to proceed, the task force meets with the hospital's medical librarian to develop a plan to search for the evidence. Their goal is to identify the best evidence-based methods for selecting written medication information that can be easily read and understood by elderly hospitalized patients. The librarian helps the group use its PICO question to create a list of search terms (Table 21■2) and to decide on a strategy to locate the best sources of evidence.

Using the hierarchy of evidence (see Chapter 11), the task force begins searching for evidence that is already pre-appraised and synthesized. The task force begins its search by looking for practice guidelines. If the search for practice guidelines is unsuccessful, the task force will search for systematic reviews in the JBI Database of Systematic Reviews and the Cochrane Library of Systematic Reviews as well as in CINAHL and MEDLINE. If systematic reviews are not available, controlled trials in CINAHL and MEDLINE will be sought. If adequate controlled trials are not present, the task force plans to seek expert opinion by searching the Web sites of government agencies and health literacy organizations, associations, and foundations.

To locate guidelines, the task force searches the Web sites of government groups such as the Agency for Healthcare Research and Quality (AHRQ), CDC, national associations, and literacy organizations. With this strategy, the task force

TABLE 21■2   **Key Search Terms and Search Strategies for Medical/Nursing Databases**

PICO*	Synonyms	Search Strategy
What is the effectiveness of using easy-to-read written medication information material compared with standard written medication information material on knowledge and understanding among elderly hospitalized patients?		
P = elderly hospitalized patients	1. elder* 2. aged 3. hospitali*	Link 1 through 3 with OR
I = easy to read written medication information material	4. easy-to-read 5. plain language 6. teaching material* 7. print material* 8. written information 9. written medication information 10. pamphlet 11. brochure	Link 4 through 11 with OR
O = knowledge, understandability	12. knowledge 13. medication knowledge 14. suitab* 15. comprehen* 16. understand*	Link 12 through 16 with OR
P + I + O		Link with AND

* Note that there was no need to include the comparison (C) in the search because the process of searching on standard materials would not yield additional information.

locates an AHRQ health literacy universal precautions toolkit (Brega, Barnard, Mabachi, et al, 2015). This toolkit is comprehensive and includes tools to improve written information, resources to improve the system's approach to health literacy, a quick start guide, and numerous resources and supporting information. However, the committee notices there is no research-based evidence associated with the various strategies. They do find that the toolkit references a publication describing the process of the toolkit's development (DeWalt, Broucksou, Hawk, et al, 2011). Within the toolkit, they also locate a publication demonstrating how using the toolkit might improve the quality of patient materials (Brega, Freedman, LeBlanc, et al, 2015). The committee downloads these publications and decides to continue to search for additional sources of synthesized evidence.

In order to search for synthesized evidence, the task force then searches the JBI Evidence Synthesis along with its best practice information sheets, evidence summaries, and evidence based recommended practices as well as the Cochrane Database of Systematic Reviews. They use the keywords *written information, easy-to-read,* and *health literacy.* Using this strategy, the task force is not able to locate a systematic review in the JBI Library. However, the Cochrane Database has a systematic review completed by Nicolson, Knapp, Raynor, et al (2009) that addresses the impact of written information about medications. But the focus of this review does not fully address the task force's question. The task force is not able to locate any additional systematic reviews in Cochrane that is focused on their question.

The task force meets again with the librarian to ask for help with the MEDLINE and CINAHL search. Seeking help from your librarian is a strategy you may also find useful due to the expertise and time required to perform a thorough search. The librarian performs a search using the search terms in Table 21■2. Within both databases, she continues to refine the search. When she is satisfied that the search is complete, she gives a list of publication titles and accompanying abstracts to the evidence-based practice committee task force.

After reviewing the abstracts, the task force asks the librarian to retrieve full-text versions of several articles. Next, the task force identifies publications that relate to the PICO question and decides to focus on the toolkit, along with a systematic review, and two primary research articles published after the systematic review was published.

Appraise/Plan

Based on what you have learned, you know that the task force will need to examine the quality of the evidence they locate before they can confidently rely on findings and recommendations. Although there is no formal tool to evaluate the quality of a toolkit, a good tool to use to evaluate systematic reviews is the **Critical Appraisal Skills Program (CASP)** evaluation checklist for systematic reviews (Public Health Research Unit [PHRU], 2007). This tool is reliable, concise, and easy to use.

Since no tool exists to evaluate the toolkit's quality, the task force decides to find out the following: what population the toolkit was focused on; how the toolkit authors developed the toolkit; and how much of an impact the toolkit had on the quality of health education materials. First, they evaluate the development of the toolkit as described by DeWalt and colleagues (2011). Their review of the publication reveals that the toolkit targeted primary care practices as opposed to hospitals. They also found that developers relied primarily on Internet searches and expert opinion, as opposed to research-based evidence, to develop their recommendations and sample forms and documents. However, the task force recognizes that the purpose was clear, stakeholders were involved, the toolkit was user friendly, and the developers pilot-tested it with the stakeholders who provided positive feedback.

The task force also reviews a publication describing a trial of the toolkit with respect to its impact on designing easy-to-read **patient education** material to improve their knowledge (Brega, Freedman, et al, 2015). After several primary care practices used the toolkit to make patient education easier to read, the investigators found some improvement in **readability** (how easy it is to read the material), understandability, and actionability, but the improvement was not statistically significant. Potential reasons for not seeing a larger improvement may have been due to wide use of externally sourced material and the relatively short study timeline (Brega, Freedman, et al, 2015).

The systematic review that the task force has located focuses on the effectiveness of written medication information to convey knowledge and understanding (Raynor, Blenkinsopp, Knapp, et al, 2007). The task force uses the CASP tool to evaluate the quality of the systematic review conducted by Raynor et al (2007). The purpose of the review by Raynor et al (2007) was to determine to what extent patients, caregivers, and health professionals rated the role and value of written information pertaining to medications. Findings most closely related to the evidence-based practice task force's area of interest include patient concerns about the use of complex language and the poor appearance of written materials. The authors conclude that a gap exists between provided print information and the type of information patients would like to have (Raynor et al, 2007).

When the task force evaluates this systematic review using the CASP criteria, members conclude that the quality of this systematic review is high. The review's questions were clearly written, appropriate types of studies were included, the search was exhaustive, and there was a clear method for evaluating the quality of each included study. Because of the nature of the evidence included in this systematic review, the authors appropriately performed a narrative analysis of the evidence. They carefully considered all important outcomes, and the results can be applied in the local setting.

In addition to the high quality of this systematic review, the task force finds that the review by Raynor et al (2007) contains a synthesis of texts devoted to information design. These texts were nominated by a panel of six experts from the information design field who agreed on a final selection of six texts. The panel of experts then synthesized key information design strategies from these texts and presented them in tabular and narrative form in the review. Based on this information, the task force is able to identify many elements, although not all are focused specifically on the elderly, that may make patient information easier to read and understand (Raynor et al, 2007). Following is a list of key design elements mentioned by at least four of the six texts (Raynor et al, 2007):

- Use words that are short and familiar, preferably no more than two syllables.
- Use as little jargon as possible; if it must be used, include a glossary.
- Write using the active as opposed to passive voice.
- Keep sentences short, with an average of 15 to 20 words.
- Use plenty of white space.
- Use bullet points to break up and organize information.
- Use boldface text when you want to emphasize a point. Avoid capital letters, italics, and underlining.
- Use a writing style that is relaxed and positive.

In addition to these most frequently agreed on design aspects, the systematic review gives the task force recommendations regarding typeface, line length, and spacing, and the use of pictures. Therefore, the task force finds this systematic review to be extremely helpful in the search for evidence related to readability.

There were two recent studies addressing the topic of understanding medications. Oliffe, Thompson, Johnston, et al (2019) conducted a study to determine the readability of rheumatology medicine information sheets and assessed how well patients comprehended them. They found that the reading level of the information sheets exceeded the eighth grade, and in most cases was much higher. Patient understanding of the information was poor (Oliffe et al, 2019).

In the second study, Send, Peters-Klimm, Bruckner, et al (2016) conducted a randomized controlled trial to test the effect of a written medication plan that included graphics and additional information about how to take medications on medication knowledge (enhanced plan) compared to the usual medication plan. The researchers found that medication knowledge scores were statistically significantly higher among outpatients (average age was greater than 65) who received the enhanced medication plan. There was no difference in confidence or satisfaction between groups (Send et al, 2016). The task force decides that the Oliffe et al (2019) study gave them an additional rationale for moving forward with their plan and the Send et al (2016) study provided an example for formatting medication information that was consistent with information provided in the systematic review.

The task force is not able to locate systematic reviews of primary research focused specifically on the effectiveness of using easy-to-read instructional materials with the elderly. Nonetheless, in spite of this lack of ideal evidence of effectiveness, the task force knows it needs to change the format of the medication instruction sheets to meet national calls for using clear writing and plain language with patients (IOM, 2004). The task force decides to use the health information design recommendations published in the AHRQ toolkit (Brega, Barnard, et al, 2015), and the CMS toolkit (n.d.) for making material clear and effective. After further analyzing these sources, the task force finds they contain similar recommendations. The task force also finds these design recommendations are very similar to those published in the systematic review by Raynor et al (2007). Therefore, in spite of the lack of high-level evidence, task force members are comfortable that the information contained in these publications is the best available evidence at this point in time. The task force also takes into consideration the various calls for using plain language (plain-language.gov, n.d.) as another rationale for moving forward with providing easy-to-read medication information material to patients.

As you begin to question nursing practices, you may encounter similar situations in which practice guidelines and/or systematic reviews are not available to fully inform your practice. Therefore, expert opinion and published practice standards might be the best available evidence to support a practice change.

As a result of this evidence review, the task force decides to make the following recommendations to the evidence-based practice committee. They pair these recommendations with the levels of evidence corresponding with the JBI (2014) evidence rating system for studies of effectiveness. According to this system, Level 1 refers to experimental designs including systematic reviews and randomized controlled trials; Level 2 refers to quasi-experimental designs including systematic reviews, quasi-experimental primary studies, or control group designs; Level 3 refers to observational, analytical designs including systematic reviews, cohort, case-controlled, or observational studies; Level 4 refers to observational/descriptive studies including systematic review of descriptive studies and cross-sectional or case studies; and Level 5 refers to expert opinion, consensus, or bench research. The specific recommendations of the task force are as follows:

- Ensure that written patient information materials are written at an appropriate level. (Level 5)
- Ensure that written patient information materials incorporate design characteristics that are recognized as being easy-to-read. (Level 5)
- Always give patients a verbal explanation of the topic of instruction in addition to written information. (Level 4)

Apply/Implement

Kristin and her task force take their recommendations to the next evidence-based practice committee. Along with their recommendations, they prepare a slide presentation that outlines the easy-to-read design characteristics they have learned from the literature. The evidence-based practice committee is quite interested in this material and discusses it at length. As a result, the committee decides it is important to redesign the current written medication information materials to make them easy-to-read and usable.

Before moving forward with implementation, the committee discusses the best way to put their recommendations into practice. The committee uses the **integrated Promoting Action on Research Implementation in Health Services (i-PARIHS) framework** (see Chapter 5) to guide the evidence implementation activities (Harvey & Kitson, 2016). This model addresses the need to consider four main elements as components of successful implementation. These elements include innovation, recipients, context, and facilitation.

With respect to innovation, the model recommends considering evidence with respect to its fit with local priorities, potential advantages and potential for application in the practice setting. This conceptualization of innovation provides support for the committee's work. The committee looked broadly at the evidence, determined the evidence aligned with the problem and priorities related to patient understanding of medication information, it has potential for improving care, and it has excellent implementation potential.

Harvey and Kitson (2016) define recipients as individuals in addition to collective groups who may be impacted by the innovation. They propose that successful implementation depends not only on the beliefs and motivations of individuals, but also on the beliefs and motivations of the affected group. Other important characteristics of recipients include time, power and authority, and the presence or absence of collaboration and teamwork (Harvey & Kitson, 2016). In the case of the task force, they have obtained a buy-in from the larger committee. However, to be successful, they will need to seek broader consensus from key stakeholders, including bedside nurses and physicians.

Regarding context, the i-PARIHS framework refers to the setting in which the evidence will be implemented and also includes implications beyond the immediate setting. Harvey and Kitson (2016) refer to varying layers of context that include the micro (e.g., unit), meso (e.g., organization) and macro (e.g. societal) levels. Some characteristics of context include culture, local formal and informal leadership support, and past experience with change and evaluation (Harvey & Kitson, 2016). Therefore, the task force will need to evaluate the context at the unit level to determine if the innovation might succeed. They will need to consider the unit's culture, formal and informal leadership support, and past experience managing and responding to change. At the organizational level, they will need to consider top-level support from leadership as well as organizational priorities. Finally, at the external level, the task force will need to assess regulatory requirements, external incentives, and health policy. As a result of their assessment, the task force has reason to believe the practice change will be supported in the current context. The culture in this hospital at the local and organizational level is quite supportive of changing practice based on evidence and provides multiple opportunities for the staff to try new ways of doing things. The top leadership is also visible on the patient care areas and promotes autonomy of staff. Finally, external accreditation requirements and government recommendations reinforce the need to make this practice change.

The final component of the model is facilitation. As a core concept, facilitation is key to introducing, enabling, and sustaining the innovation among recipients and in the setting or context (Harvey & Kitson, 2016). Facilitators use best evidence to guide implementation strategies and tailor these strategies to align with recipient and context characteristics. In this case, the committee decides the best way to facilitate this practice change is to establish a multidisciplinary task force that includes current evidence-based practice task force members as well as the adult health clinical nurse specialist, a pharmacist, a physician, and a patient educator (Box 21■3). The clinical nurse specialist is assigned to chair the task force. They also plan to use audit and feedback as an implementation strategy (Harvey & Kitson, 2016). The committee is confident that the implementation process for this practice change will proceed smoothly based using the i-PARIHS model as a guide.

Assess/Evaluate

As part of the planning process for using easy-to-read medication information materials, the implementation task force needs to identify the best measures to assess the integration of the evidence into practice (the process) as well as measures to assess the impact of the change on knowledge and understanding (the outcome). It is important to evaluate the process to make sure that the practice change is actually taking place. Therefore, the task force needs to ensure that new medication sheets are actually available on each unit and that nurses explain the medication sheets when giving them to patients. Nurses can assess the implementation process by making rounds on the units, conducting audits, and giving feedback.

BOX 21■3 **Interdisciplinary Implementation Task Force**

It takes a team of health-care providers to implement easy-to-read medication instruction sheets in a hospital setting. Consider involving the following individuals:

- Bedside nurses
- Clinical nurse specialists
- Clinical pharmacists
- Nurse researcher
- Patient educators
- Physicians
- Quality/safety specialists
- Risk managers
- Patients
- Nursing leadership (unit manager, directors, chief nursing officer)

Because there was little research-based information in the literature, the task force decides to carry out a research project to examine the effect of easy-to-read medication instruction sheets on knowledge and understanding among elderly patients. Members prepare a research proposal and obtain approval through the hospital's human subjects committee. While collecting baseline data, they search for appropriate preprinted, easy-to-read materials. If they cannot find preprinted materials, the task force members are prepared to create their own instruction sheets using guidelines from their initial evidence search. After this phase is completed, the task force can then follow the steps outlined in the research protocol to implement the new forms and to evaluate the outcome of the change.

■ Summary

The process of applying evidence in daily nursing care occurs at many levels, ranging from individual nurses to an entire organization and beyond. In this chapter's clinical story, Kristin took the unit-based problem of lack of understanding of medication instructions to the hospital-wide evidence-based practice committee and found the problem actually applied to all units with elderly patients. Kristin worked with a task force and the hospital's librarian to assess the scope and scale of the situation, ask questions, and acquire evidence. They appraised the evidence and made recommendations based on this evidence. Although they were not able to locate clinical practice guidelines or systematic reviews specifically addressing the question they were exploring, they did locate consistent expert opinions. Therefore, they decided to change the hospital's practices related to printed medication information for the elderly. They also recognized the need for additional research testing the effectiveness of using easy-to-read methods. As a result, they decided to perform a study to test this intervention.

In nursing, you may find that clinical practice guidelines and systematic reviews are not available to answer all of your questions and that more research needs to be performed. In this chapter's clinical story, you can see how a team of nurses and other health-care professionals can make contributions to nursing practice and the larger community by exploring, applying, and creating evidence. For practice using the evidence-based practice process, refer to Box 21■4.

BOX 21■4 **Tools for Learning and Practice**

- Generate additional PICO questions related to patient education at discharge.
- Search for evidence using keywords in your PICO questions following the strategy supplied in this chapter's clinical story as an example.
- Develop one medication information sheet using the criteria identified in the chapter. Check the readability level using the FRY method and assess the suitability of the information sheet using the SAM format.
- Develop a simple audit tool that incorporates evidence-based recommendations for developing written health information.
- Conduct an audit of medication information sheets/materials, summarize data, and provide feedback to colleagues.
- Pilot the medication information sheet with elderly patients and obtain feedback. Reevaluate the medication information sheets based on patient feedback.
- Identify policies that address development of written patient education materials and evaluate the strength and currency of the supporting evidence. If warranted, recommend changes to policies based on best available evidence.

CHAPTER QUESTIONS

1. This chapter's clinical story presented the problem of elderly patients not understanding medication instructions. What steps of the evidence-based process were used to address the identified problem?

2. What were the strengths of the evidence that the medication information task force found?

3. Given the evidence that was implemented in the clinical story, construct a simple tool to evaluate whether nurses are using the easy-to-read medication information sheets. If the audit reveals that some nurses are not using the easy-to-read medication information sheets, suggest some strategies to implement their use.

(continues on page 336)

CHAPTER QUESTIONS (continued)

4. To evaluate the impact of the easy-to-read medication information sheets, it is necessary to identify some appropriate outcomes and measure them. What are some outcomes that you think would be applicable to measure the effectiveness of the easy-to-read medication sheets? What are some potential ways to go about doing this?

5. Patient education involves more than the use of printed materials. What is another PICO question that you could ask about teaching patients?

6. Using this alternative PICO question, search for a systematic review or practice guideline. Using an appropriate appraisal instrument, critique the evidence you found. Based on that critique, explain whether you would use this evidence and provide a rationale for your decision.

7. If you found more than one guideline or systematic review, compare them and identify the similarities and differences in the findings.

8. If you were to use the evidence-based recommendations you found in your search, explain how you would implement them using the i-PARIHS framework.

References

Berkman, N. D., Sheridan, S. L., Donahue, K. E., et al. (2011, July 19). Low health literacy and health outcomes: An updated systematic review. *Annals of Internal Medicine, 155,* 97–107. http://dx.doi.org/10.7326/0003-4819-155-2-201107190-00005

Brega, A. G., Barnard, J., Mabachi, N. M., et al. (2015). *AHRQ Health Literacy Universal Precautions Toolkit* (2nd ed., AHRQ Publication No. 15-0023-EF). Rockville, MD: Agency for Healthcare Research and Quality. https://www.ahrq.gov/health-literacy/quality-resources/tools/literacy-toolkit/index.html

Brega, A. G., Freedman, M. A. G., LeBlanc, W. G., et al. (2015). Using the health literacy universal precautions toolkit to improve the quality of patient materials. *Journal of Health Communication, 20*(Suppl. 2), 69–76. https://doi.org//10.1080/10810730.2015.1081997

Centers for Disease Control and Prevention. (2010). *Simply put* (3rd ed.). Retrieved from https://stacks.cdc.gov/view/cdc/11938

Centers for Medicare & Medicaid Services. (n.d.). Toolkit for making written material clear and effective. Retrieved from http://www.cms.gov/WrittenMaterialsToolkit/01_Overview.asp#TopOfPage

Centers for Medicare & Medicaid Services. (2010). *Part 9: Things to know if your written material is for older adults* (CMS Product No. 11476). Washington, DC: U.S. Department of Health and Human Services. https://www.cms.gov/Outreach-and-Education/Outreach/WrittenMaterialsToolkit/Downloads/ToolkitPart09.pdf

Cordero, C. (2018, November 13). Helping organizations address health literacy. *Dateline @ TJC.* https://www.jointcommission.org/dateline_tjc/helping_organizations_address_health_literacy/

DeWalt, D. A., Broucksou, K. A., Hawk, V., et al. (2011). Developing and testing the health literacy universal precautions toolkit. *Nursing Outlook, 59,* 85–94. https://doi.org/10.1016/j.outlook.2010.12.002

Doak, C. C., Doak, L. G., & Root, J. H. (1996). *Teaching patients with low literacy skills.* Philadelphia, PA: Lippincott.

Eichler, K., Wieser, S., & Brugger, U. (2009). The costs of limited health literacy: A systematic review. *International Journal of Public Health, 54,* 313–324. http://dx.doi.org/10.1007/s00038-009-0058-2

Golchin, N., Frank, S. H., Vince, A., et al. (2015). Polypharmacy in the elderly. *Journal of Research in Pharmacy Practice, 4,* 85–88. http://dx.doi.org/10.4103/2279-042X.155755

Harvey, G., & Kitson, A. (2016). PARIHS revisited: From heuristic to integrated framework for the successful implementation of knowledge into practice. *Implementation Science, 11*, Article 33. https://doi.org/10.1186/s13012-016-0398-2

Institute of Medicine of the National Academies. (2004). *Health literacy: A prescription to end confusion.* Washington, DC: National Academies Press.

Joanna Briggs Institute. (2014). JBI levels of evidence. Retrieved from https://joannabriggs.org/sites/default/files/2019-05/JBI-Levels-of-evidence_2014_0.pdf

Kutner, M., Greenberg E., Jin, Y., et al. (2006). *The health literacy of America's adults: Results from the 2003 National Assessment of Adult Literacy* (NCES 2006-483). Washington, DC: U.S. Department of Education, National Center for Education Statistics.

Nicolson, D., Knapp, P., Raynor, D. K., et al. (2009). Written information about individual medicines for consumers. *Cochrane Database of Systematic Reviews, 2009*(2). doi:10.1002/14651858. CD002194.pub3

Office of Disease Prevention and Health Promotion. (n.d.). *Quick guide to health literacy.* Washington, DC: U.S. Department of Health and Human Services. https://health.gov/communication/literacy/quickguide/Quickguide.pdf

Oliffe, M., Thompson, E., Johnston, J., et al. (2019). Assessing the readability and patient comprehension of rheumatology medicine information sheets: A cross-sectional health literacy study. *British Medical Journal Open, 9*, Article e024582. https://doi.org/10.1136/bmjopen-2018-024582

plainlanguage.gov. (n.d.). What is plain language? Retrieved from http://www.plainlanguage.gov/whatisPL/index.cfm

Program for the International Assessment of Adult Competencies. (2017). *Highlights of 2017 U.S. results.* Retrieved from https://nces.ed.gov/surveys/piaac/current_results.asp

Public Health Research Unit. (2007). Critical appraisal skills program. Retrieved from http://www.phru.nhs.uk/pages/phd/resources.htm

Ratzan, S. C., & Parker, R. M. (2000). Introduction. In *National Library of Medicine current bibliographies in medicine: Health literacy.* Retrieved from http://www.nlm.nih.gov/archive//20061214/pubs/cbm/hliteracy.html

Raynor, D. K., Blenkinsopp, A., Knapp, P., et al. (2007). A systematic review of quantitative and qualitative research on the role and effectiveness of written information available to patients about individual medicines. *Health Technology Assessment, 11*(5).

Readability Formulas. (n.d.). *The Fry graph readability formula.* Retrieved from http://www.readabilityformulas.com/fry-graph-readability-formula.php

Send, A.F.J., Peters-Klimm, F., Bruckner, T., et al. (2017). A randomized controlled trial to assess the effect of a medication plan containing drug administration recommendations on patients' drug knowledge after 2 months. *Journal of Clinical Pharmacology and Therapeutics, 42*, 69–74. https://doi.org/10.1111/jcpt.12476

Vernon, J. A., Trujillo, A., Rosenbaum, S., et al. (2007). *Low health literacy: Implications for national health policy.* Retrieved from http://npsf.org/askme3/pdfs/Case_Report_10_07.pdf

CHAPTER 22

Community Health Nursing

Janet Davis

LEARNING OBJECTIVES

- Given the ill-structured description of a community-based clinical case, apply all phases of the evidence-based practice process to guide decisions related to an area of community health.

- Analyze the challenges to making evidence-based decisions in a complex and community-based health-care environment.

- Generate next-step strategies to put better evidence into practice.

KEY TERMS

Qualifications

School health provider

School health services

School nurse

C linical Story

Leanna is the head school nurse in an urban public school system that serves a racially and ethnically diverse population. Most of the district's population is medically underserved. The school nurse's office in the district meets the needs of both students and families by providing day-to-day care, education, and consultations. In addition, through partnerships with the medical and business communities, a robust referral system allows students and families to access services that might otherwise be difficult to procure. In all locations across the district, the school nurse's office is seen as a valuable asset by the community.

Unfortunately, Leanna has just been informed by the superintendent that the school board is considering terminating the school nurse positions. The board is considering replacing the nurses with unlicensed assistive personnel (UAP) and parent volunteers, with one nurse supervisor for the entire school district. This potential action is meant as a cost-cutting measure and is legal in this particular state because registered nurse (RN) licensure is not required for the school nurse position. At the board's request, Leanna has 2 weeks to prepare data to justify keeping the current system in place.

Think Before You Read

- What are the steps of the EBP process?
- What PICO or PICo questions can you imagine that are relevant to the clinical story?
- What model can you use to structure how you approach implementing the evidence?
- What might be some key issues to consider as you search for and appraise the evidence?
- What might be some candidate implementation strategies?
- What do you need to consider to judge the success or failure of a project like the one in the clinical story?

Introduction

School nurses are an extension of the public health system and play a vital role in assisting children to successfully adapt to the school environment. On a daily basis, 56.6 million children attend school (National Center for Educational Statistics, 2019). There are approximately 95,776 Full Time Equivalent (FTE) nurses working in schools and caring for children with an array of health problems, chronic illnesses, and disabilities (Willgerodt, Brock, & Maughan, 2018). The responsibilities of school nurses are varied and challenging because a significant amount of health care is provided in the schools (National Association of School Nurses, 2018). Every day, school nurses handle emergencies, complete health screenings, identify outbreaks of communicable disease, administer medication, verify immunization records, and plan health-care strategy. In addition, the school nurse provides psychological support for the students, families, teachers, and administration while addressing the specific health-care needs of schoolchildren living with various disabilities and chronic illness. The National Association of School Nurses (NASN) defines school nursing as "a specialized practice of nursing that protects and promotes student health, facilitates optimal development, and advances academic success." To that end, school nurses "bridge health care and education, provide care coordination, advocate for quality student-centered care, and collaborate to design systems that allow individuals and communities to develop their full potential" (2017, p. 1).

Healthy People (HP) 2020, the federal initiative to improve America's health, recognizes the multifaceted and demanding role of the school nurse. HP 2020 has specifically identified objectives related to the suggested proportion of school nurses to students at all grade levels. Specifically, the HP objective for Educational and Community Based Program No. 5 proposes to "increase the proportion of the nation's elementary, middle, and senior high schools that have a full-time registered nurse-to-student ratio of at least 1:750" (Office of Disease Prevention and Health Promotion, n.d.). In addition, the NASN and the American Academy of Pediatrics (AAP) posit that students and staff are entitled to quality health services and that these services can be ensured when school nurses earn appropriate education, licensure, and certification. The AAP recommends that every school have a full-time school nurse, thereby ensuring a strong connection with each student's medical treatment (American Academy of Pediatrics, 2016). It is the position of the NASN that "every school-age child should have access to a registered professional school nurse (hereinafter referred to as the school nurse), who has a *minimum of* a baccalaureate degree in nursing from an accredited college or university and is licensed as a registered nurse through a board of nursing" (National Association of School Nurses, 2016, p. 1). According to both the NASN and the AAP, these requirements are the minimal preparation needed at the entry level of school nursing practice.

In this chapter's clinical story, as Leanna thinks about her response to the school board, she realizes she needs the best available evidence to make a convincing argument to support her belief that every school-age child in her community deserves and benefits from a baccalaureate prepared school nurse. She knows the school health issue is complex, and her community has unique health needs. It has been hit hard by an economic downturn and is experiencing high rates of unemployment. In addition, if her district succeeds in eliminating school nurses, the decision will set a precedent for eliminating the school nurse position and replacing that nurse with UAP, which could affect other schools. Leanna is aware that her arguments are vital not only to her school nurse colleagues but also to the children, families, teachers, staff, and administrators within her employing school district.

This chapter applies the evidence-based practice process to a community problem. In an attempt to keep this complicated problem controllable, the chapter focuses on the effectiveness of the school nurse in maintaining and promoting school health.

What Are the Key Issues?

Leanna needs credible resources that will support a solution to this grave community dilemma. She begins by asking a series of questions, both general and specific:

1. What is the role of the school nurse in meeting the health needs of school-age children in the United States?
2. How should she factor in the uniqueness of her local community when making this cogent argument to the school board?
3. What are the experiences of communities that do not currently employ RNs as school nurses?
4. What are the sources of support for her argument?
5. Are there established standards for school nurses' academic and professional qualifications—locally, by state, and nationally?
6. If there are established standards, what sources of evidence informed them?
7. Are there national, state, and/or local data to support the employment of school nurses?
8. Are there systematic reviews that focus specifically on the effectiveness of school nurses related to school health?
9. Are there primary studies that have investigated the effectiveness of school nurses?
10. Is there expert opinion about the need for school nurses in the U.S. kindergarten through twelfth grade educational system?
11. Are there any places in the United States that have achieved the Healthy People objective of one nurse to every 750 students?

The evidence-based practice process starts with a willingness to answer these questions by considering data that both support and contradict your position. Leanna approaches these questions by first searching the Internet for professional organizations devoted to school nursing and school health. Leanna is a member of her state's school nurses association, an affiliate of the NASN, so she starts her search on their Web sites. While reading their position, she finds the AAP supports the NASN position: schools should employ only RNs with at least a baccalaureate degree as school nurses. However, her state SNA *prefers* a baccalaureate but does not *require* even an RN for those who provide school health services. In her state, the exception is that school districts must employ an RN to supervise UAP providing school health services.

In addition, Leanna discovers that the American Nurses Association (ANA) has historically held to a policy supporting the employment of RNs in schools, based on the premise that those with RN competencies are better equipped to maintain the health of the schoolchildren (American Nurses Association & National Association of School Nurses, 2011). As she seeks data, Leanna knows she may benefit from a listing of national nursing organizations and specific state SNAs. She also wants to consult federal mandates regarding school health from the U.S. Department of

Education, Centers for Disease Control and Prevention (CDC), and HP 2020. She will also consider her state's department of education, which is directly responsible for school health services. She realizes that international sources and studies may be judged irrelevant to her school system because other nations differ in school policy and organizational structure. Because of this, she decides not to pursue global sources in this undertaking.

A next important step in developing a position is verifying the *scope* and *scale* of the problem. Leanna has identified many questions associated with this problem, and its complexity seems overwhelming. However, she knows she must be realistic. The scope means identifying the breadth of the problem. Scale is finding out, in this case, if the elimination of the school nurse position is just an isolated experience occurring only in her school system. In the school nurse dilemma, national data will outline the scope of the problem: Leanna can consult the CDC for the results of the Youth Risk Behavior Survey, which is conducted nationally every other year. The primary purpose of the Youth Risk Behavior Survey is to identify health-risk behaviors among youth ninth through twelfth grade and ascertain changes in risk behaviors over time (Centers for Disease Control and Prevention, 2017). The 2017 Youth Risk Behavior Survey results show that in her specific state, health-risk behaviors have increased in key areas: alcohol and drug use, obesity, sexual behaviors that contribute to unintended pregnancy and sexually transmitted infections, tobacco use, violence, and suicide.

To further define the scope of the problem Leanna searches the NASN, federal mandates regarding laws that affect school health practices, the American School Health Association (ASHA), the National Association of Elementary School Principals (NAESP), and the Robert Wood Johnson Foundation. The No Child Left Behind Act of 2001, Individuals with Disabilities Education Act (originally authored in 1975), and the Rehabilitation Act of 1973 are federal mandates that require children with disabilities to receive health-related services in school. However, none of these federal laws legislates that health-related services must be delivered by nurses, an important distinction for Leanna. The ASHA considers schools vital in assisting the physical, emotional, social, and environmental factors related to student health and indicates that student well-being can affect the learning process, although it does not address the **qualifications** (credentials, skills, and knowledge) for those providing **school health services** (American School Health Association, 2016). Those school health services can include acute emergency care, care coordination, and chronic disease management while engaging with families (Centers for Disease Control and Prevention, 2019). The NAESP states in its 2019–2020 platform, "Every school should have a certified school nurse to attend to students' medical, health and wellness needs (National Association of Elementary School Principals, 2019, p. 17).

The Robert Wood Johnson Foundation has shed light on entrenched issues around school nursing, and they identified too much variance in school health services. Over half of the nation's schools lack an RN, and they noted that this variance contributes to the vast health disparities among our school-age children. In addition, it has reported on a wide range of medical health problems as well as an increase in social issues, such as poverty and homelessness, affecting schoolchildren (Robert Wood Johnson Foundation, 2010).

The *scale* of the problem includes whether the elimination of school nurse positions is an isolated occurrence or a trend across the United States. National results indicate that 81.5% of schools in the United States offer health services. However, only 33.7% of schools required a full-time school nurse; 18.1% of schools required a part-time school nurse; and 10.9% of all schools required a maximum nurse-to-student ratio (Centers for Disease Control and Prevention, 2016). These data suggest the scale of the problem transcends this local community. Ultimately, Leanna views this problem of eliminating school nurse positions as being both large in scope and scale. After reviewing some of the data acquired from her initial search, she begins to think about how to best approach this problem. Her next step is to develop a PICO question that will assist her in searching for the best available evidence.

Ask/Assess

Both the nursing process and evidence-based practice processes start with assessment and asking questions that direct you to the best available evidence. In Leanna's case, the evidence will serve as a basis for her justification to the school board. Leanna starts her assessment by seeing if needed data concerning this problem are already available through her state department of education and or the state SNA, an affiliate of the NASN. The state department of education Web site provides definitions and laws relevant to health services provided in schools. She notes that it presents the state's nurse practice act as a source of information, but the act fails to address school nursing specifically. She discovers that state law allows for UAP to provide health services, and there must be an RN with a baccalaureate degree in nursing as a school district supervisor, although not necessarily on site. The state law specifically states that licensed personnel are preferred but not required to provide school health services.

On the SNA Web site, Leanna locates a district map and identifies the area representatives who are responsible for overseeing school nursing and school health services in public schools for all the counties in the state. She contacts these representatives and asks the following questions:

- How many schools are in their district?
- How many school nurses are employed in the district?
- How many school districts use the model of UAP who provides health services with an RN supervisor?
- Have these schools ever employed school nurses, and if yes, when and why did their policy change?
- What is the ratio of school nurses to children?

These *local data* are particularly important because they reveal trends across the state and allow Leanna to compare her state to the nation. She can obtain data

TABLE 22■1 **Narrowing the Focus and Generating Questions**

Broad	What are the best practices for providing school health services?
Narrow	What are the best practices for providing school health services in the United States?
Narrow	What are the best practices for providing school health services for urban school districts with a diverse student population?
Searchable PICO	What is the effectiveness of the school nurse in providing school health services versus the use of Unlicensed Assistive Personnel (UAP) to students, staff, faculty and administrators?

Intervention: school nurses.
Comparison: unlicensed assistive personnel (UAP).
Outcome: school health services.

from neighboring school districts that encounter the same or similar challenges as hers. According to the state SNA documents, out of 42 school systems in her district, only three school systems employ UAP with one supervising RN. Statewide there are 19 school systems using this model out of a total of 342 state school systems.

Based on this information, Leanna believes she has enough initial data to provide the basis for her response to the school board. To guide her in finding the best available evidence, she formulates the following two PICO questions:

1. What is the effectiveness of the school nurse in providing school health services to students, staff, faculty, and administrators?
2. What is the effectiveness of UAP in providing school health services to students, staff, faculty, and administrators?

See Table 22■1 for more guidelines for developing PICO questions.

Acquire/Diagnose

After assessing the local data and the apparent problem, you can proceed to the next step of the evidence-based practice process and determine how you will *acquire the best available evidence.* Depending on your experience with searching, this step may be challenging, and in some circumstances, it may be prudent to request the assistance of your local school, public, or academic librarians. However, prior to meeting with the librarian, you will need to take some steps to expedite this process. You may want to provide the librarian with your question(s) and a list of keywords. Look at the keywords used in related articles; frequently, you can locate these keywords on the first page of the article. For example, you may have been using the term "school nurse" but notice that other authors use "**school health providers**" (a broad term representing anyone who provides health services in a school or school system) as a keyword. In addition, you may want to access the U.S. National Library of Medicine, Medical Subject Headings Web site (https://www.nlm.nih.gov/mesh/meshhome.html). This site provides an online MeSH browser to assist you in identifying descriptors/keywords. For example, when you enter "school health services," the site will display a list of related descriptors such as "health services school," "school health," and "school-based health." This is a good method for adding to and verifying your list of keywords. Be sure to use words from your PICO question, and thinking of synonyms and alternate spellings will assist you in your search.

For the first PICO question (effectiveness of school nurses), Leanna searches for clinical practice guidelines that are based on systematic reviews of randomized clinical trials and tested health services outcomes in schools with RNs and in schools using UAP. If there is no guideline, she can search for systematic reviews or primary research using bibliographic databases such as CINAHL or MEDLINE. After developing a list of keywords, Leanna works with a local community college academic librarian and uses the search strategy and keywords listed in Table 22■2.

In an effort to find ideal sources first, Leanna and the academic librarian first search the ECRI database (https://guidelines.ecri.org—the new home for the former National Guideline Clearinghouse). Using a Boolean search strategy, Leanna uses the term "school nurse or school nursing" to start her search. This strategy reveals 25 recommended guidelines; however, on close review, the guidelines focus more

TABLE 22■2 **Keywords and Search Strategy for Bibliographic Databases**

PICO	Synonyms	Search Strategy
What is the effectiveness of the school nurse in providing school health services versus the use of UAP to students, staff, faculty, and administrators?		
I = school nurse	Nursing, School	Link with OR
C = UAP	UAP unlicensed assistive personnel Nurse Aide* "Nursing Assistant" Certified Nurses Assistant CNA Certified Nurse* Aide	Link with OR
O = school health services	Health services school School health School-based health services Services, school health	Link with OR
I + C + O		Link with AND

UAP = unlicensed assistive personnel

on management of chronic illnesses found in school-age children. No results yield guidelines focusing on the overall "effectiveness" of the school nurse. When she searches "school nurs*" and "school health" together, the results reveal two guidelines, but they are also not specific to her question.

Leanna and the librarian discuss expanding the search to find any pertinent synthesized evidence or primary research published within a 5-year window, using bibliographic databases such as CINAHL and MEDLINE. They use the same keywords plus the word "research" and limit the search for publications within the 5-year look back. That strategy results in 10 articles. However, on close review, two articles refer to school nursing in the United Kingdom, three are integrative reviews, and four do not specifically address the effectiveness of the school nurse.

One study, "Cost-Benefit Study of School Nursing Services" (Wang, Vernon-Smiley, Gapinski, et al, 2014), warrants further scrutiny. To widen her search, Leanna closely reviews the reference lists in the articles, seeking hitherto undiscovered but relevant research. This hand searching is an additional strategy that sometimes reveals pertinent literature. Then she searches using "Unlicensed Assistive Personnel" or "UAP" plus "school health services," and identifies one additional study. Unfortunately, the study examined an educational program for UAP and did not specifically address their effectiveness in providing school health services.

Finally, a search of the Cochrane Library and JBI Database of Systematic Reviews did not reveal any relevant systematic reviews pertinent to her question. Because Leanna has found only one research article for possible use, she decides to broaden her strategy to find studies relevant to nursing outcomes in other areas of nurse practice. She uses the following Boolean strategy: "quality nursing care" OR "nursing outcomes" OR "failure to rescue" AND "ped* nurs*" OR "nurs*" AND "research." Leanna selects Search All Text to find more results. Her search result identifies two research articles, but she discards both studies because they do not apply to her circumstances and locality.

Not discouraged by the absence of synthesized and limited primary research, Leanna decides the one study applies to her situation, and it warrants further appraisal in her quest for the best available evidence. In addition, she identifies the three national organizations or associations whose position or opinion statements regard qualifications and the need for school health services by school nurses. These statements are possible evidence for justifying the retention of school nurses in her district. The position papers and statements would constitute expert opinion narrative—not the strength of evidence she was hoping for but still evidence that warrants critical appraisal.

Appraise/Plan

You must critically appraise each research study to determine whether it is done well and is basically good enough to use in your argument. Leanna wants only solid research as she makes the case that the school board should retain the school nurse positions. The study she has found must be of high quality and apply to her question. There are various tools available for critical appraisal of primary research.

Standardized appraisal tools are important in evaluating research to answer the basic questions:

- What were the results of the study and what do they mean to my problem?
- Are the results valid?
- Can the findings of the study be applied locally to this situation?

The answers to these three questions are not a simple yes or no; many times, the answer is somewhere in the middle and ambiguous. Therefore, it is important for you to use a standardized appraisal tool that matches the type of evidence that you are considering. For example, in a study by Baisch, Lundeen, and Murphy (2011), the authors identify their research design as mixed method, but it is not the traditional mix of quantitative and qualitative methods. This study used two quantitative approaches: descriptive (survey) and quasi-experimental. Because of this, it requires two distinct critical appraisal tools, both applicable to quantitative research. First, Leanna appraises the study's cross-sectional descriptive approach; she uses the JBI Critical Appraisal Checklist for Analytical Cross-Sectional Studies (Fig. 22■1). Here is her evaluation of the descriptive design in the study by Baisch et al (2011):

- *The authors defined the criteria for inclusion in the sample clearly.* The study used only schools funded by Title I and all employed only baccalaureate-prepared RNs to provide school health services with a ratio of one nurse to 750 students. The authors excluded schools that served special education students, chronic disease programs, and school-based health centers.

JBI Critical Appraisal Checklist for Analytical Cross Sectional Studies

	Yes	No	Unclear	Not applicable
1. Were the criteria for inclusion in the sample clearly defined?	☐	☐	☐	☐
2. Were the study subjects and the setting described in detail?	☐	☐	☐	☐
3. Was the exposure measured in a valid and reliable way?	☐	☐	☐	☐
4. Were objective, standard criteria used for measurement of the condition?	☐	☐	☐	☐
5. Were confounding factors identified?	☐	☐	☐	☐
6. Were strategies to deal with confounding factors stated?	☐	☐	☐	☐
7. Were the outcomes measured in a valid and reliable way?	☐	☐	☐	☐
8. Was appropriate statistical analysis used?	☐	☐	☐	☐

Overall appraisal: ☐ Include ☐ Exclude ☐ Seek further info.

Comments (including reasons for exclusion):

FIGURE 22■1 The JBI Critical Appraisal Checklist for Analytical Cross Sectional Studies. (Courtesy of JBI, Adelaide, Australia.)

- *The authors described the study subjects and setting with some detail.* The authors provided a description the array of respondents (teachers, principals, and office clerical staff) from an urban district in the Midwest; 81% of the schools responded (a high response rate for a survey) and they included demographic data.
- *The exposure,* the presence of a baccalaureate-prepared professional nurse, *was measured in a valid and reliable way.*
- *Objective, standard criteria for measurement of the condition* was not applicable for the descriptive portion of the study.
- *The authors identified confounding factors* and the strategies they used to deal with them.
- The investigators *used objective, standard criteria* (a survey of perception) *to measure the outcomes* of satisfaction. They administered a survey using a Likert scale that measured the administrative and academic staff members' perceptions of their satisfaction with the school nurses' care of students. The researchers acknowledged the satisfaction survey was used with nurses in other settings. However, this area of the study would have been stronger if the investigators reported on the measurement quality of the survey, including internal consistency and measures of validity.
- *Appropriate statistical analysis* was used and appropriate for the level of measurement reflected in the survey.

In this appraisal process, Leanna's biggest challenge is her doubt that she understands the appropriateness of the statistical procedure in relationship to the data. To overcome that doubt, she calls on nursing faculty from her undergraduate program and consults them. She feels better after discussing the problem with more experienced nurses, and they confirm she is on the right track.

Next, Leanna appraises the study's second method: the quasi-experimental matched control design. Some methodologists would not call the study a quasi-experimental design because the investigators did not manipulate the independent variable of a professional nurse being present in the elementary school. For this method, Leanna selects the JBI Critical Appraisal Checklist for Comparable Case Control Studies (Fig. 22■2). She identifies the following strengths of the study by Baisch et al (2011):

- The *groups were not exactly comparable other than the presence or absence of the* nurse but they *were recruited from the same population.* While all of the schools were from the same district, nurses were assigned to schools with more lower income students. Because of the link between lower socioeconomic status and poorer health outcomes, those schools with nurses may have been biased toward worse outcomes. The outcomes showed the opposite.
- *The investigators matched the* cases (the schools with nurses) *and the controls* (those without nurses) using appropriate criteria like enrollment, location, ethnic background, numbers of students in special education, and numbers of students receiving free or reduced lunch.

JBI Critical Appraisal Checklist for Case Control Studies

	Yes	No	Unclear	Not applicable
1. Were the groups comparable other than the presence of disease in cases or the absence of disease in controls?	☐	☐	☐	☐
2. Were cases and controls matched appropriately?	☐	☐	☐	☐
3. Were the same criteria used for identification of cases and controls?	☐	☐	☐	☐
4. Was exposure measured in a standard, valid and reliable way?	☐	☐	☐	☐
5. Was exposure measured in the same way for cases and controls?	☐	☐	☐	☐
6. Were confounding factors identified?	☐	☐	☐	☐
7. Were strategies to deal with confounding factors stated?	☐	☐	☐	☐
8. Were outcomes assessed in a standard, valid and reliable way for cases and controls?	☐	☐	☐	☐
9. Was the exposure period of interest long enough to be meaningful?	☐	☐	☐	☐
10. Was appropriate statistical analysis used?	☐	☐	☐	☐

Overall appraisal: ☐ Include ☐ Exclude ☐ Seek further info.

Comments (including reasons for exclusion):

FIGURE 22 ■ 2 **The JBI Critical Appraisal Checklist for Comparable Cohort/Case Control Studies (Courtesy of JBI, Adelaide, Australia.)**

- *The investigators used the same criteria to identify the cases and controls* (see above).
- The investigators *measured the "exposure" using a standard, valid, and reliable way* because the exposure was the presence of a professional nurse.
- *The exposure was measured in the same way for the cases and controls.*
- *The authors identified confounding variables* such as the difference in socioeconomic status and an assumption of the accuracy of data entry for both the cases and the controls.
- *The authors addressed some strategies to deal with confounding variables* such as mentioning that the lower income students may have mitigated a larger effect size if the socioeconomic status of the cases impacted that group's outcome, and a larger sample size may have allowed for more precision if the outcomes were not measured with precision.
- *Outcomes were clearly assessed in a standard, valid, and reliable way:* the researchers reported completeness of health records and immunization rates between program and matched schools—data obtained from official school records.

- *The exposure period of interest was long enough to be meaningful* since they looked at 1 year of outcomes.
- Appropriate *statistical analysis* was used in analyzing health record data.

Beyond published research and systematic reviews, policy makers also base their decisions on expert opinion. As Craig and Smyth (2011) point out, expert opinion is an additional source of evidence for practice recommendations. For Leanna's question, three professional organizations explicitly support having a school nurse located in every school to provide school health services. The three organizations were the NASN, AAP, and NAESP. Leanna is curious about the origin of the NASN recommendation, as it was not evident on the organization's Web site. She makes a mental note of this issue and decides she will contact the organizations personally to obtain an explanation for the basis for their recommendations. Leanna contacts the NASN and discusses the association's recommendation regarding the use of registered nurses with baccalaureate degrees as providers of school health services; she wants to know how that specific position originated. Leanna finds that the decision was based on consensus opinion, and over the years several panels worked on the "Position Statement on Education, Licensure, and Certification of School Nurses" (National Association of School Nurses, 2016). In addition, Leanna requests information concerning gray literature sources related to her question.

From her previous search, Leanna has selected three expert opinion sources to critically appraise. Although expert opinion is not the level of evidence Leanna originally hoped to find, she acknowledges this is still important available evidence to justify her position to the school board. She chooses the position statements of NASN and the AAP, and the NAESP 2019–2020 platform document. The NASN asserts, "It is the position of the National Association of School Nurses (NASN) that every school-age child should have access to a registered professional school nurse (hereinafter referred to as the school nurse), who has a *minimum of* a baccalaureate degree in nursing from an accredited college or university and is licensed as a registered nurse through a board of nursing" (National Association of School Nurses, 2016, p. 1).

To assess these position statements, Leanna uses the JBI Critical Appraisal Checklist for Text and Opinion Papers (Fig. 22■3). Leanna identifies the following strengths of the expert opinion by the NASN:

- Although the statement is signed by the authors, it is unclear if other persons were involved in this opinion.
- The *source of opinion does have standing as an expert in the community.* The NASN is the recognized professional organization for school nurses; it currently has 50 affiliate state school nurses' organizations.
- The *interest* of the school nurse in providing health services to students is clearly the focus of the opinion.
- The opinion's *basis in logic/experience* is clearly argued. The authors describe the issue with relevant factors that impact children and support the need for a more comprehensive delivery of health-care services in schools.
- The argument is developed analytically: authors identify a detailed rationale about why they take their position.

JBI Critical Appraisal Checklist for Text and Opinion Papers

	Yes	No	Unclear	Not applicable
1. Is the source of the opinion clearly identified?	☐	☐	☐	☐
2. Does the source of opinion have standing in the field of expertise?	☐	☐	☐	☐
3. Are the interests of the relevant population the central focus of the opinion?	☐	☐	☐	☐
4. Is the stated position the result of an analytical process, and is there logic in the opinion expressed?	☐	☐	☐	☐
5. Is there reference to the extant literature?	☐	☐	☐	☐
6. Is any incongruence with the literature/sources logically defended?	☐	☐	☐	☐

Overall appraisal: ☐ Include ☐ Exclude ☐ Seek further info.

Comments (including reasons for exclusion):

FIGURE 22■3 The JBI Critical Appraisal Checklist for Text and Opinion Papers (Courtesy of JBI, Adelaide, Australia.)

- An *extensive reference list* is provided, incorporating many other associated professional organizations' statements.
- *Overall appraisal:* Use this evidence when developing justification for retaining school nurses as the provider of school health services.

Leanna appraises her second expert opinion, the AAP's position statement on the role of the school nurse in providing school health services. Again using the JBI Critical Appraisal Checklist for Text and Opinion Papers (see Fig. 22■3), Leanna identifies the following strengths of the expert opinion by the AAP's Council on School Health:

- An extensive list of members of the Council on School Health is provided.
- The source of opinion does have standing as an expert in the community. The AAP is a recognized national professional organization of pediatricians; in addition, the association has a council specifically focusing on school health.
- The interest of the students/children is clearly the focus identified in the background discussion supporting their position.
- The opinion's basis in logic/experience is clearly argued through a detailed discussion of the crucial role of the school nurse in providing school health services.
- The argument is developed analytically, identifying a detailed rationale for the AAP's position and focusing on the importance of a working relationship between school nurse and pediatrician to promote the health of children.
- The AAP authors provide an extensive list of research references that serves as a basis for its position.
- The position statement indicates the participation of the NASN.

Overall appraisal: Use this evidence when developing justification for retaining school nurses as the provider of school health services.

As her third expert opinion, Leanna identifies the 2019–2020 NAESP platform (National Association of Elementary School Principals, 2019). The JBI Critical Appraisal Checklist for Text and Opinion Papers (see Fig. 22■3) will serve as the appraisal guide. Appraising this expert opinion, Leanna identifies the following strengths and weaknesses:

■ The source of the opinion is clearly identified as the Board of Directors; however, the opinion does not list names of the members.
■ The source of opinion does have standing as an expert in the community. The NAESP is a recognized professional organization that has both state and international affiliates; it sponsors conferences and offers considerable opportunities for professional development for members.
■ The interest of the students/children and the need for school nurses are clearly two of the many focuses of their platform document.
■ The opinion's basis in logic/experience is clearly presented; the organization discusses meeting the health needs of children by providing every elementary school with a full-time school nurse.
■ The argument is developed analytically, identifying the many health problems to which elementary children may be exposed.
■ An extensive reference list is *not* provided in the platform document.
■ There was *no* specific evidence that the opinion was supported by peers or other similar professional groups.

Overall appraisal: Include this study when developing justification for retaining school nurses as the provider of school health services.

After careful appraisal and recommendations of her sources, Leanna selects the levels of evidence and the strength of each recommendation. Levels of evidence are usually related to how much confidence you can have in the appraised sources. To rank the sources, Leanna uses the following A to D scale:

■ Grade A = strong support that merits application; evidence from a systematic review or from a precise, randomized controlled trial
■ Grade B = moderate support that merits consideration; evidence from single well-defined studies
■ Grade C = moderate support that merits consideration; evidence from case series or expert consensus
■ Grade D = evidence that does not support the adoption of the practice

Apply/Implement

Although Leanna would have preferred finding stronger evidence regarding the effectiveness of school nurses in providing school health services, she is feeling confident she has the best available evidence at this point in her search. She is pleased the appraised documents are unmistakably consistent regarding the necessity for school nurses to assume direct responsibility for school health services. Reflecting on her college courses, she now understands why her professors stressed that nursing needs research evidence as a catalyst for change. However, she also acknowledges the complexity of her current situation.

As a guiding implementation framework for evidence-based decisions, she selects the long-recognized PARIHS model (Promoting Action on Research Implementation in Health Service) (Kitson, Rycroft-Malone, Harvey, et al, 2008). This model asserts that successful implementation of the evidence is based on the type of evidence, the context in which the evidence is implemented, and the facilitation of the process. As a facilitator for changing minds and policies in this chapter's clinical story, Leanna realizes she cannot reach that goal merely by presenting the evidence. She also needs to examine the context of the situation (school, school board, and community). Ultimately, she will need to include her colleagues and vested stakeholders related to retaining school nurse positions in every school.

Leanna arranges a meeting with all the school nurses in her district and informs them of evidence findings. In the course of their meeting, they identify key stakeholders who need to be involved: parents, administrators, teachers, staff, local pediatricians, and community clinic health-care personnel. Leanna arranges another meeting to discuss the situation and evidence with them.

In addition, Leanna turns to her state SNA to assist her through this process by identifying the strength of the context and illustrating how to use the best evidence to change thinking and policy. Providing a classic view, Mallory (2010) points out, "Although implementing evidence based practice changes in the practice setting is usually seen as a major responsibility of the practice environment, nursing societies are ideally positioned to provide expert knowledge about the best evidence for practice and readily available resources for facilitating practice changes" (p. 283).

In this situation, leaders from the state SNA can best serve and support Leanna by helping her gain a clearer perspective on the organizational culture that surrounds the school district and school board. She turns to them for their expertise and assistance in convincing the school board to implement the evidence. Here are some strategies Leanna can use to include key resources in her platform for change (Kostas-Polston, Thanavaro, Aridson, et al, 2015):

- Assess if the professional societies related to school health services and school nurses have established toolkits to address this issue, including identified leaders who have expertise in this area.
- Identify a core group and/or change champions to support the policy of retaining school nurses as the providers of school health services.
- Provide the school board with quality-evaluation evidence that school nurses positively influence immunization rates, absenteeism, the accuracy of student health records, and efficient management of student health concerns.
- Provide the school board with quality data that show the relationship/impact between nurses as the health service providers and the child's school performance and satisfaction of parents and staff.

Assess/Evaluate

Part of the evidence-based process is evaluating the effectiveness of a combined strategy to change policy. Leanna assesses all components of her strategy to persuade the school board to uphold the recommendations of professional associations and organizations that every school should have an RN. She knows the outcome of the school board's decision will have a profound effect on the community. In an effort to enhance the recognition of the school nurses, she is going to study for school nurse certification and encourage her colleagues to follow her example.

The health-care services provided for the students are the main concern for the school nurses. However, the process of implementing those services is an important assessment. Leanna will continue to work with her state SNA to enhance the practice of school nursing and to implement established evidence-based practices relevant to her role (Box 22■1).

■ Summary

As Leanna continues functioning as head nurse in her school district, she realizes that the field of school nursing needs both more primary research and systematic reviews. She feels fortunate to have congruent expert opinion evidence to support her position, as it enhances her confidence in attempting to sway the school board. The *asking of the question* was paramount in proceeding to *acquiring data*—that is, her search for the best available evidence. Her *appraisal of the evidence* was challenging, and she learned to rely not only on expert opinion but the expertise

---

BOX 22■1 **Tools for Learning and Practice**

- Generate your own list of keywords and then access the National Library of Medicine Web site (http://www.nlm.nih.gov/nlmhome.html) and click on MeSH. Type in one of your keywords and then click on Find Exact Words to see what other terms are identified. Compare your list to those identified.
- Search the Internet for the term "gray literature." What is the relevance of gray literature to evidence-based practice?
- Search the Internet for the relevance of hand searching to evidence-based practice.
- Search for additional organizations with opinions concerning school nurses providing health-care services.
- Search the Internet for the states that require specific student-to-nurse and school-to-nurse ratios meeting Healthy People guidelines.
- Search the Internet to find states that require newly hired school nurses to have specific educational, licensure, and certification status.

of others such as the librarian, nursing faculty, and professional organizational leaders. In the *application* of the evidence, she realizes this process is best done in collaboration with others. As she *evaluates* retrospectively, Leanna knows she has learned a great deal through this endeavor. Most important, she now sees the evidence-based process along with the nursing process as co-contributors to her role as a school nurse.

CHAPTER QUESTIONS

1. In this example chapter's clinical story of justifying the effectiveness of the school nurse, how would you compare and contrast the steps of the evidence-based process and the nursing process?

2. In this example, Leanna uses three professional organizations' position statements or platforms as expert opinion evidence. What are your thoughts regarding the selection of these organizations to justify her position? Were they appropriate? Should she have used only the two organizations (NASN and AAP) whose priorities directly relate to health needs of children as sources of evidence? Was it suitable to use the NAESP's platform as a source of evidence?

3. Knowing that there are many other factors that can affect this situation, what other PICO questions could Leanna have asked?

4. Reflecting on some of the implementation strategies offered, what other strategies would you suggest? What evidence do you have to support your proposed strategies?

5. What challenges did Leanna encounter in applying the PARIHS framework to this situation? What are the nature and type of evidence? What are the qualities of the context? How is the process facilitated?

6. Develop a plan for how Leanna and her colleagues could achieve stakeholder support to back up their position. Would you identify additional stakeholders?

7. When questioned on her sources, how would Leanna defend including expert opinion in place of rigorously derived research?

8. What do you think will be the school board's response to Leanna's arguments? What additional questions do you think the board might have for Leanna? What do you think board members will identify as strengths in her arguments? What weaknesses might be apparent to the board?

References

American Academy of Pediatrics. (2016). AAP policy statement recommends full time nurse in every school. Retrieved from https://www.aap.org/en-us/about-the-aap/aap-press-room/pages/AAP-Policy-Statement-Recommends-Full-Time-Nurse-in-Every-School.aspx

American Nurses Association & National Association of School Nurses. (2011). *Scope and standards of practice: School Nursing* (2nd ed.). Silver Spring, MD: Nursesbooks.org.

American School Health Association. (2016). ASHA position statement: School administrators enhance student achievement by supporting the whole child. Retrieved from http://www.ashaweb.org/wp-content/uploads/2016/11/ASHA-Position-Paper-Administrators-WSCC-FINAL.pdf

Baisch, M. J., Lundeen, S. P., & Murphy, M. K. (2011). Evidence-based research on the value of school nurses in an urban school system. *Journal of School Health, 81,* 74–80. doi:10.1111/j.1746-1561.2010.00563.x

Centers for Disease Control and Prevention. (2019). School health services. Retrieved from https://www.cdc.gov/healthyschools/schoolhealthservices.htm

Centers for Disease Control and Prevention. (2016). Results from the school health policies and practices study. Retrieved from https://www.cdc.gov/healthyyouth/data/shpps/pdf/shpps-results_2016.pdf

Centers for Disease Control and Prevention. (2017). YRBSS results. Retrieved from https://www.cdc.gov/healthyyouth/data/yrbs/results.htm

Craig, J. V., & Smyth, R. L. (Eds.). (2011). *The evidence-based practice manual for nurses* (3rd ed.). New York, NY: Elsevier.

Kitson, A., Rycroft-Malone, J., Harvey, G., et al. (2008). Evaluating the successful implementation of evidence into practice using the PARIHS framework: Theoretical and practical challenges. *Implementation Science, 3.* https://doi.org/10.1186/1748-5908-3-1

Kostas-Polston, E., Thanavaro, J., Arvidson, C. R., et al. (2015). Advanced practice nursing: Shaping health through policy. *Journal of the American Association of Nurse Practitioners, 27*(1), 11–20. doi.org/10.1002/2327-6924.12192

Mallory, G. A. (2010). Professional nursing societies and evidence-based practice: Strategies to cross the quality chasm. *Nursing Outlook, 58,* 279–286. doi:10.1016/j.outlook.2010.06.005

National Association of Elementary School Principals. (2019). NAESP platform, 2019–2020. Retrieved from https://www.naesp.org/sites/default/files/NAESP%20Platform2019-20(NEW).pdf

National Association of School Nurses. (2016). Position statement on education, licensure, and certification of school nurses. Retrieved from https://www.nasn.org/advocacy/professional-practice-documents/position-statements/ps-education

National Association of School Nurses. (2017). Definition of school nursing. Retrieved from https://www.nasn.org/about-nasn/about

National Association of School Nurses. (2018). The role of the 21st century school nurse. Retrieved from https://www.nasn.org/advocacy/professional-practice-documents/position-statements/ps-role

National Center for Educational Statistics. (2019). Fast facts: Back to school statistics, 2019. Retrieved from https://nces.ed.gov/fastfacts/display.asp?id=372#PK12_enrollment

Office of Disease Prevention and Health Promotion. (n.d.). Healthy People 2020 topics and objectives. Retrieved from https://www.healthypeople.gov/2020/topics-objectives/topic/educational-and-community-based-programs/objectives

Robert Wood Johnson Foundation. (2010). Charting nursing's future: Unlocking the potential of school nursing: Keeping children healthy, in school, and ready to learn. Retrieved from http://www.rwjf.org/files/research/cnf14.pdf

Wang, L. Y., Vernon-Smiley, M., Gapinski, M. A., et al. (2014). Cost-benefit study of school nursing services. *JAMA Pediatrics, 168*(7), 642–648. doi:10.1001/jamapediatrics.2013.5441

Willgerodt, M. A., Brock, D. M., & Maughan, E. M. (2018). Public school nursing practice in the United States. *The Journal of School Nursing, 34*(3), 232–244. doi:10.1177/1059840517752456

Glossary

Academic detailing — An expert, usually from an academic organization, who works closely with staff to develop evidence-based interventions.

Accidental suffocation or strangulation in bed (ASSB) — unintentional death of an infant caused by anything that limits the baby's breathing such as soft bedding or blankets obstructing breath or becoming trapped between objects like a mattress and wall.

Accountability — An assumption of responsibility for one's actions and decisions.

Acquire — Using your question to determine how to search for the evidence and find the best information that links the question related to the patient problem with potential solutions.

Acute care setting — An entity that provides services to patients with acute care needs as opposed to chronic rehabilitative or palliative needs, such as a medical-surgical hospital unit.

Ad hoc committees — Committees that spawn from the original group, allowing key stakeholders to work with nurses to support implementation of evidence-based practice innovations.

Advocate — To champion or support the patient to meet her needs and wishes.

Agency for Healthcare Research and Quality (AHRQ) — A U.S. federal-level agency that supports research and policies to help people make more informed decisions and improves the quality of health-care services.

AGREE tool — A standardized appraisal tool for practice guidelines, rigorously developed by an international group of experts.

American Academy of Pediatrics (AAP) — A society of pediatricians who are committed to the optimal physical, mental and social health and well-being from infancy to young adulthood.

American Health Policy Institute — An association whose mission is to advance quality of care and patient safety nationwide.

American Health Quality Association — An association whose mission is to advance quality of care and patient safety nationwide.

ANCC Magnet Recognition® — A program, offered by the credentialing arm of the American Nurses Association, that recognizes health-care organizations for quality patient care, nursing excellence, and innovations in professional nursing practice. Consumers rely on the designation as the ultimate credential for high-quality nursing.

Animal-assisted therapy — The use of animals as a tool to achieve a therapeutic effect.

Apply — Putting evidence into action and practice.

Appraise — To critically evaluate the evidence for its quality and applicability.

Ask — To state a clear question that will lead to the right evidence for your problem.

Assess — To gather data from physical assessment, laboratory data, and from what the patient says in order to make a judgment about a patient's condition. In the 5 As of evidence-based practice, assess means to evaluate outcomes using the same methods that could be used to assess a patient's condition.

Attitude of inquiry — Being curious, somewhat skeptical, and willing to pursue the evidence.

Audit and feedback — The process of making clinical observations of behaviors against specific criteria and feeding back the findings of the audit to the stakeholders.

Authority to change practice — Ability to have control over or influence practice.

Autonomy — Independence or free will to make choices.

Available resources — In the context of evidence-based practice, the resources available to implement evidence including the right people (human resource), technology, equipment, and money.

Baby Box — a sustainable box (often cardboard) that provides a safe environment for infant sleep without items that can obstruct the baby's breathing.

Barriers — Any organizational, person, or resource gap or impediment that will challenge change.

Benchmarking — A standard, based on either an average performance among agencies or other means of setting a standard. The purpose is to establish a level of quality that can then be used to judge the quality of care.

Beneficence — A moral obligation to help another.

Best available research evidence — Best available represents two principles, available and best. *Available* implies the evidence that is accessible but only after an exhaustive and transparent search of multiple databases of published and unpublished literature. *Best* means that the investigator has rigorously appraised the evidence and determined it to be the highest, although often less than ideal, evidence.

Best practice — Generally accepted, informally standardized techniques, methods, or processes that seem to accomplish given tasks. Some best practices reflect the best available evidence, whereas others represent consensus opinion.

Beveridge model — A single-payer system in which health care is provided and financed by the government through a system of tax payments.

Bias — When a study is conducted in a way that might lead to an erroneous conclusion.

Bibliographic database — Searchable index of published literature that contains abstracts, a synopsis of articles, and (sometimes) the full text of articles. It is organized by taxonomy of keywords. Examples include the Cumulative Index of Nursing and Allied Health Literature (CINAHL) and MEDLINE.

Big data — Data sets of greater variety arriving in increasing volumes and with ever-higher velocity (known as the "three Vs") that are too large and complex to be analyzed with traditional software.

Bismark model — A model that uses an insurance system jointly financed by employers and employees. Bismark-type health insurance plans are mandated to cover all citizens, and they do not make a profit. Although this is a multipayer system, tight regulations give government as much cost control clout as in the single-payer system.

Boolean operators — Logical connectors including OR, AND, and NOT combined with keywords and phrases to structure a search in a bibliographic database.

"Borderless" evidence/knowledge — External, global evidence that crosses the boundaries of countries or disciplines.

Care Quality Commission (CQC) — an independent regulator of health and adult social care in England, ensuring that people receive safe, effective, compassionate, high-quality care.

Case-controlled study — Study in which researchers select cases (those with a particular condition) and the control group (those without the condition) and compare the two groups' outcomes.

Centers for Disease Control and Prevention (CDC) — A U.S. federal agency providing expertise, information, and tools to protect the public's health—through health promotion; prevention of disease, injury, and disability; and preparedness for new health threats.

Centers for Medicare & Medicaid Services (CMS) — A U.S. federal agency that administers the Medicare program, providing health-care security and choice for aged and disabled people. Jointly with the state governments, CMS administers the Medicaid program and the State Children's Health Insurance Program (SCHIP)

Centre for Reviews and Dissemination (CRD) — An online source of internationally developed systematic reviews. The CRD is made available from the National Institute for Health Research (NIHR) and the University of York.

Chief nursing officer (CNO) or chief nursing executive (CNE) — The most senior nursing leader in the organization who is administratively responsible for all aspects of the nursing care, including budget, patient care services, and so on. Sometimes the CNO or CNE carries the title of vice president.

Citation chasing — The process of using references or a bibliography to identify other relevant evidence.

Clinical decision making — When health-care providers choose among alternatives to affect a health outcome of individuals or groups.

Clinical expertise — Practical know-how that comes from professional experience. It is often integrated automatically when making decisions; it is tacit and intuitive but is strongest when exposed for critique and analysis.

Clinical nurse specialist (CNS) — An advanced practice nurse with graduate preparation (master's or doctoral degree); a clinical expert in a specialized area of nursing practice and in the delivery of evidence-based nursing interventions. The CNS provides direct and indirect care to patients and families as well as influences nursing personnel and organizations.

Clinical practice guidelines — When well constructed, they are a form of synthesized evidence designed to provide comprehensive recommendations about the diagnosis, management, or treatment of a particular condition or clinical question. The best guidelines are built upon systematic reviews.

Cochrane Collaboration — An international network of people founded in 1993. Multiple disciplines write systematic reviews and publish them in the Cochrane Library. The collaboration provides access to the reviews and other resources to help health-care providers, policy makers, patients, and their advocates make well-informed decisions about health care.

Cochrane Library — One of the most comprehensive collections of systematic reviews, controlled trials, and evidence-based health-care sources. It is composed of six databases: the Cochrane Database of Systematic Reviews (CDSR), Cochrane Central Register of Controlled Trials (CENTRAL), Cochrane Methodology Register (CMR), Database of Abstracts of Reviews and Effects (DARE), Health Technology Assessment (HTA) Database, and NHS Economic Evaluation Database (EED)

Cohort study — A study with a control group and a cohort group in which the cohorts share a characteristic (e.g., having a condition or having an occupation) and the control group is alike in all respects except the unique cohort characteristic.

Common cause variation — is variation inherent in the design of a process and is due to regular, natural or ordinary causes, also known as random variation.

Comparison — In a PICO question, the C stands for comparison. When comparing one intervention against another, one may include a comparison intervention in the question. The comparison may be another nursing intervention or taking no action at all.

Complex problems — Tend to be unique, are associated with a great deal of uncertainty, and are less predictable than other problems.

Complicated problems — Usually made up of a series of simple problems.

Conceptual framework — An abstract, theoretical approach that describes, explains, or predicts a set of variables and relationships to explain a phenomenon.

Conceptual research utilization — One thinks differently after understanding research but does not change his or her behavior.

Conduct and Utilization of Research in Nursing (CURN) Project — One of two large national projects aimed at improving how nurses evaluate and use research.

Context — The practice environment, including the subelements of organizational culture, leadership, and evaluation practices; the surroundings of the phenomenon or person.

Context of care — The environment or setting in which the proposed change is to be implemented.

Core measures — A set of care processes that helps institutions improve quality of patient care by focusing on outcomes.

Cost sharing — Employers require individuals to pay a portion of their health-care premium.

Credibility — In appraisal of qualitative research, it refers to how well the researcher made every effort to report an honest representation of the true voices of the participants.

Critical appraisal — Judging the quality of information in terms of its validity and degree of bias (quantitative research) and credibility and dependability (qualitative research). This is a critical step in the evidence-based practice process.

Critical Appraisal Skills Program (CASP) — Provides a set of tools appropriate for critical appraisal of both quantitative and qualitative methodologies.

Cumulative Index to Nursing and Allied Health Literature (CINAHL) — Bibliographic database that contains over 2 million abstracts from nearly 3,000 English-language journals and full-text English-language journal articles from over 600 journals published since 1981

Data — Observations, narrative, or measurements produced through the conduct of either qualitative or quantitative research.

Deductible — The amount of out-of-pocket expenses before the insurance company will cover remaining costs.

Dependability — In qualitative research, it refers to whether the results are logical, transparent, and clearly documented.

Descriptive framework or model — A framework or model that describes the nature of the elements of a phenomenon or process without making claims about the nature or direction of relationships among phenomena or concepts.

Easy to read — See Readability. Sometimes "easy to read" is used instead of readability, meaning that a piece is written so it can be read by people with lower literacy skills.

Effectiveness — The extent to which an intervention, when used appropriately, achieves the intended effect. Clinical effectiveness is about the relationship between an intervention and clinical or health outcomes.

Embase — Bibliographic database that contains over 20 million abstracts and full-text articles from over 7,000 peer-reviewed global journals published since 1974. Viewed as one of the most global sources of abstracts and full-text articles, Embase may have limited availability in U.S. nursing schools and hospital libraries.

Embedded evidence — When policies, protocols, and pathways transparently use evidence.

Empirical quality outcome — A measurement of patient-centered and organizational health outcomes that is the result of an organizational commitment of excellent nursing care.

Empowerment — Increasing the spiritual, political, social, or economic strength of individuals and communities.

Enculturation — The process by which a person learns the requirements of the surrounding culture, and acquires values and behaviors appropriate or necessary in that culture.

Environment — Immediate surroundings or sociopolitical or economical context of the person.

Epistemology — Foundations of knowledge or ways of knowing.

Evaluation plan — a plan to measure structure, process and outcome parameters of an improvement process.

Evidence-based health care — Clinical decision making that considers the best available evidence, the context in which the care is delivered, client preference, and the professional judgment of the health professional.

Evidence-based medicine movement — An approach to clinical decision making in medicine that uses research evidence instead of pathophysiological rationales, intuition, previous clinical experience, and expert opinion to determine appropriate interventions for patient care.

Evidence-based practice (EBP) — The conscientious, explicit, and judicious use of current best evidence in making decisions about the care of individual patients. It means integrating individual clinical expertise and patient preferences with the best available external clinical evidence from systematic research in a context of limited resources.

Evidence-based practice movement — A global initiative aimed at using an evidence-based approach to clinical decision making.

Evidence-based practice process — Problem solving that includes the following steps: identifying a problem, asking specific questions, acquiring evidence, appraising the evidence for its quality, applying the evidence, and assessing the outcomes of the intervention.

Evidence generation — Process of conducting primary research.

Evidence hierarchies — Systems used to rank evidence statements according to certain criteria.

Evidence/knowledge transfer — The act of transferring knowledge to individual health professionals, health facilities, health systems, and consumers by means of journals, other publications, electronic media, education, training, and decision support systems so that practitioners and patients can understand and use it in decision making.

Evidence synthesis — A pooling of available research findings through the process of systematic review.

Evidence utilization — The use of evidence to bring about practice or system change at point of care.

Experience — Knowledge and skill acquired through being involved in or exposed to practice over a period of time.

Expert consensus opinion — Occurs when experts in an area of science discuss and come to an agreement about the best approach to a problem. The best expert consensus opinion would involve a systematic and rigorous method to determine a conclusion that is then exposed to public opinion or external critique.

Expertise — See Clinical expertise.

Expert opinion — Presentation of pertinent data by one with special skill or knowledge representing a mastery of a particular subject. Evidence that draws on the expert knowledge of individuals or group; it is not research-based evidence.

Explanatory framework or model — A framework or model that specifies cause-and-effect relationships and mechanisms.

External evidence — Evidence from rigorous research, external to a local setting.

Facilitation — The process of enabling or making easier the implementation of evidence into practice.

Facilitators — Those who enable others to bring about an outcome or change in behavior through skillful negotiation, coaching, teaching, etc.

Forces of Magnetism — A term associated with the Magnet® recognition program, it refers to the attributes or outcomes that exemplify excellence in nursing. Organizations must fully operationalize these 14 attributes in order to be considered for recognition. The new model of the program consolidates these 14 attributes into 5 components: transformational leadership, structural empowerment, exemplary professional practice, new knowledge, innovation and improvements and empirical quality results.

Google Scholar — Internet search engine in which results include only information that is freely available from the Internet; therefore, the results do not include abstracts or articles found only within subscription-based bibliographic databases. Use caution and understand that results will not be comprehensive and often do not freely link to the full-text journal articles.

Grading of Recommendations Assessment, Development, and Evaluation (GRADE) Working Group — The GRADE Working Group is an international group of evidence-based medicine experts who aim to provide a standard system that guideline developers can use to grade the quality of the evidence and the strength of recommendations, and clinicians can understand without deep backgrounds in critical appraisal.

Hand searching — Looking through the references cited or a bibliography.

Health — How a person experiences wellness and illness along a continuum.

Health Care Commission — An agency that regulates care provided by the NHS, local authorities, private companies, and voluntary organizations. It aims to make sure better care is provided for everyone—in hospitals, care centers, and people's own homes. It seeks to protect the interests of people whose rights are restricted under the Mental Health Act.

Health literacy — The degree to which individuals have the capacity to obtain, process, and understand basic health information and services needed to make appropriate health decisions.

Heuristic — A "rule of thumb" or structure for problem-solving.

High-alert medications — Those medications that can cause significant harm if administered incorrectly.

Homogeneity — The degree that different studies measure the effects of interventions in the same way with limited variability to enable them to be combined in a meta-analysis.

Hospital-acquired conditions (HACs) — Conditions that are (a) high cost or high volume or both, (b) result in the assignment of a case to a diagnostic-related group (DRG) that has a higher payment when present as a secondary diagnosis, and (c) could reasonably have been prevented through the application of evidence-based guidelines.

Implementation science — The scientific study of methods to promote the systematic uptake of clinical research findings and other evidence-based practices into routine practice, and hence to improve the quality and effectiveness of health care. It includes the study of influences on health-care professional and organizational behavior.

Incidence — The occurrence rate of new conditions.

Infant mortality — The death of an infant who is alive at birth but dies before his/her first birthday.

Infant mortality rate (IMR) — The number of infant deaths before age of 1 per 1,000 live births.

Indian Health Services (IHS) — An operating division within the U.S. Department of Health and Human Services that provides medical and public health services to members of federally recognized Native American tribes and Alaskan tribes.

Innovation — The creation or improvement of interventions, products, technologies, or ideas.

Institute for Healthcare Improvement (IHI) — An independent, not-for-profit organization based in Cambridge, Massachusetts, IHI focuses on motivating and building the will for change; identifying and testing new models of care in partnership with both patients and health-care professionals; and ensuring the broadest possible adoption of best practices and effective innovations.

Instrumental research utilization — Application of research in some concrete way.

Interlibrary loan — A system where university libraries, public libraries, and hospital libraries share the full-text of articles, books, and other sources of information with one another.

Intervention — The nursing treatment or action that is the *I* part of a PICO question.

Iowa model — Developed at the University of Iowa Hospital, the purpose of this evidence-based practice model is to guide practitioners through a series of decision points as they move through the evidence implementation process.

i-PARIHS — Integrated Promoting Action on Research Implementation in Health Services framework is the 2015 modification of the original PARIHS framework. The formula for the revision is: $SI = Fac^n(I + R + C)$ where SI is successful implementation, Fac^n is facilitation, I is innovation, R is recipients, and C is context and includes inner and outer contexts. In this update, facilitation is the active ingredient.

Iterative — Dynamic, back-and-forth way of considering information.

JBI (previously known as Joanna Briggs Institute) — Founded in 1996 by Alan Pearson PhD, RN. It is a research center within the University of Adelaide and includes a multidisciplinary international collaboration of centers and groups. They engage in all aspects of evidence-based practice including evidence synthesis, evidence transfer, and implementation. JBI provides many different resources for health-care providers.

JBI Evidence Synthesis — A subscription-based library of rigorous, peer-reviewed systematic reviews. Protocols, another term for systematic review proposals, can also be found in the library.

JBI model — Describes the role of evidence generation, synthesis, transfer, and utilization in improving global health with an emphasis on tools and strategies to make each phase operational for local providers.

Joint Commission (JC) — An independent, not-for-profit organization that accredits and certifies more than 18,000 health-care organizations and programs in the United States.

Joint Commission National Patient Safety Goals (NPSGs) — Established to help accredited organizations address specific areas of concern regarding patient safety.

Joint Commission Performance Standard — A health-care leadership standard used to judge the eligibility of health-care agencies (such as hospitals) to become accredited.

Journal clubs — Clinician or student groups that meet to discuss research, systematic reviews, and evidence-based practice protocols to generate an awareness of evidence-based practice.

Keyword — A significant or descriptive word used as a reference point for finding other words or information.

Knowledge translation (KT) — The transmission of knowledge from research and other sources into everyday practice.

Levels of evidence — A system to rank confidence in research designs to control extraneous variables (questions of effectiveness) or offer credibility (questions of meaning)

Levels of recommendations — A system to rank recommendations based on the quality of the evidence, the magnitude of the effect, and the balance of harm and effectiveness. Some systems such as GRADE (the Grading of Recommendations, Assessment, Development, and Evaluation) incorporate both quality of the evidence and the strength of the recommendations.

Literature review — Often the first step in writing a paper or developing a research proposal. Its purpose is to summarize information from various authors and sources. Literature reviews help in the understanding of background issues and determining the scope of an area of literature. However, because they lack the rigor of other types of reviews, you should not directly inform your clinical decisions using casual literature reviews.

Lobbyists — Persons who attempt to influence legislation on behalf of special interests.

Local context — The environment in which the evidence is used and that affects the uptake of the evidence. The local context can be as narrow as a unit or as broad as a country.

Local data — Internal evidence that is obtained systematically from local sources and may include audit data, performance evaluations, feedback from a wide range of stakeholders, knowledge about the culture of an organization, and patient stories and narratives.

Local evidence — See Local data.

Magnet® recognition — The American Nurses Credentialing Center program that designates organizations worldwide when nursing leaders successfully align their nursing strategic goals to improve the organization's patient outcomes. It provides a roadmap to nursing excellence through education and development at every career stage and leads to best care for patients.

Magnet® model — Now in its second generation, the model illustrates a framework for nursing practice and research that serves as a road map for organizations pursuing Magnet recognition. It describes five components encompassed by the global issues in nursing and health care and encompasses the previous 14 forces of magnetism conceived in the first-generation model.

Magnitude — Refers to the "so-what" factor, or how big an effect the intervention makes on the outcome.

Meaning — The subjective interpretation that an individual places on something.

Meaningfulness — The extent to which someone experiences an intervention, activity, or phenomena.

Medicaid — Funded by both the federal government and the states. It is administered at the state level. It covers low-income children and their families.

Medical Literature Analysis and Retrieval System (MEDLINE) — The National Library of Medicine's bibliographic database, available by subscription through most nursing school libraries. It contains over 18 million abstracts and full-text journal articles from over 5400 global journals published since 1947

Medicare — A U.S., federally funded program that insures persons 65 years and older and some individuals with disabilities. Part A pays for hospital care, Part B, for physician services, and Part D, for prescription benefits.

MeSH — Medical subject headings (MeSH) were designed as a controlled vocabulary for medicine by the U.S. National Library of Medicine. Arranged in alphabetical and hierarchical structure, MeSH allows for more organized and accurate searching.

Meta-aggregation — A process of combining findings of individual qualitative studies (cases) to create summary statements that authentically describe the meaning of themes.

Meta-analysis — A statistical method that allows for the combination of the results of many studies to aggregate the conclusions into data that is stronger than that of just one study.

Meta-synthesis — A process of combining findings of individual qualitative studies (cases) to create summary statements that authentically describe the meaning of themes.

Meta-paradigm — Meta-paradigm is the broadest perspective of a discipline. The nursing meta-paradigm describes the concepts that are essential to the nursing domain. The four concepts in the nursing meta-paradigm are person, health, environment, and nursing.

Model — Representations of a real phenomenon that are narrower than theories or frameworks. They usually represent a specific situation, and are made of more precise assumptions.

Moral decision making — A step-by-step guide to decision making that includes the following steps: recognizing the moral issue, identifying the participants/stakeholders, distinguishing the values involved, weighing the benefits and burdens, looking for analogous situations, discussing with appropriate people, ascertaining organizational rules and legal codes, and examining one's own comfort with the decision.

Multipayer system — System in which more than one party is responsible for payment of health care.

Narrative data — Narrative data are data elicited through stories and verbal communications, often gathered through qualitative research methods.

Narrow confidence intervals — A statistical term that means how precisely the statistic estimates the true population value and to what degree of probability you can be sure of the estimate.

Nasogastric/orogastric (NG/OG) tube — A tube inserted either through the nostrils or mouth into the esophagus and advanced to the stomach.

National Academy of Medicine — (formerly Institute of Medicine or IOM) A nongovernmental organization within the National Academies of Science. It is highly regarded for its reports, as it recruits the highest level of experts to study and advise the decision makers on scientific matters including health.

National Association of Elementary School Principals (NAESP) — An organization whose mission is to advocate for every child to receive the world's best elementary education.

National Association of School Nurses (NASN) — A nonprofit specialty nursing organization that represents school nurses and is dedicated to improving the health and educational success of children.

National Guideline Clearinghouse (NGC) — An online collection of clinical practice guidelines formerly hosted by the Agency for Healthcare Research and Quality. The guidelines continue to exist but are no longer hosted by the Agency.

National Health Insurance model — Contains elements of both the Beveridge and Bismark models. It uses providers from the private sector, but reimbursement comes from a government-run insurance company that is funded by all residents.

National Health Service (NHS) — Manages the publicly funded health-care system in the United Kingdom. It was designed by William Beveridge.

National Hospital Quality Measures — Efforts by the Centers for Medicare & Medicaid Services and the Joint Commission to establish common national hospital performance measures and to share a single set of common documentation.

National Institute for Health and Care Excellence (NICE) — In the United Kingdom, an independent organization responsible for providing national guidance on promoting good health and preventing and treating ill health. NICE develops and defines the standards of health care that people can expect to receive. These standards indicate when a clinical treatment (or set of clinical procedures) is considered highly effective, cost effective, and safe as well as being viewed as a positive experience by patients.

National Quality Forum (NQF) — A U.S. nongovernmental organization that operates under a three-part mission to improve the quality of American health care by building consensus on national priorities and goals for performance improvement and working in partnership to achieve them; endorsing national consensus standards for measuring and publicly reporting on performance; and promoting the attainment of national goals through education and outreach programs.

National Service Framework (NSF) — Strategies that set clear quality requirements for care. These are based on the best available evidence of what treatments and services work most effectively for patients.

Nature of evidence — Fundamental characteristics of evidence and knowledge such as its purpose, type, quality, and usefulness.

Never events — Extremely serious, preventable, patient safety incidents that should not occur if the relevant evidence-based practice measures are in place.

Nonmaleficence — A moral obligation to not harm.

Nursing — The protection, promotion, and optimization of health and abilities; prevention of illness and injury; alleviation of suffering through the diagnosis and treatment of human response; and advocacy in the care of individuals, families, communities, and populations.

Nursing actions — How nurses intervene to protect, promote, and optimize health and abilities. Nurses act to prevent illness and injury; alleviate suffering; and advocate for individuals, families, communities, and populations to produce beneficial outcomes.

Nursing process — The nursing process serves as an organizational framework for practicing nursing. It includes assessment, nursing diagnosis, planning, implementation, and evaluation.

Nursing-sensitive indicators — Reflect the structure, process, and outcomes of nursing care. Patient outcomes that are determined to be nursing sensitive are those that change based on the quantity or quality of nursing care (e.g., pressure ulcers, falls, and intravenous infiltrations)

Nursing-sensitive patient outcomes (NSPOs) — Confirm nurses' contributions to patient care in areas such as quality of life, symptom management, safety, functional status, and utilization of nursing resources.

Nursing standard — An authoritative statement by which the nursing profession describes the responsibilities for which its practitioners are accountable; the outcomes for which registered nurses are responsible; and by which the quality of practice, service, or education can be evaluated.

Nursing theory — Aims to describe, predict, and explain the phenomena important to nursing.

Nursing traditions — Nurses performing as they do for no other reason than habit.

Observational study — A study that draws inferences about the possible effect of a treatment on subjects, in which the assignment of subjects into a treated group versus a control group is outside of the control of the investigator.

Occupational hazard — A working condition that places a person at increased risk for harm as a result of his or her job.

Occupational Safety and Health Act (OSHA) of 1970 — An act that mandates that, in addition to compliance with hazard-specific standards, all employers have a general duty to provide their employees with a hazard-free workplace.

Operational definitions — describe in detail what is being measured, how it is being measured, who is measuring it, and when the measurement should occur. Operational definitions are clear and unambiguous and help to ensure that everyone is measuring the same thing.

Opinion leaders — Well-respected colleagues who can influence others in the setting.

Organizational culture — The psychology, attitudes, experiences, beliefs, and values of an organization. It depends on the type of leadership, available resources, enculturation of value for evidence-based practice, expectation of nurses, and the individual nurse.

Ottawa Model of Research Use (OMRU) — A model focused on three phases that prescribe how to assess, monitor, and evaluate the evidence implementation process. It focuses on the innovation, the adopters, the practice environment, implementation strategies, and the outcomes.

Outcome — The specific effect(s) of an intervention or what matters to the nurse, patient and/or the health-care system. It is what the nurse would use to evaluate whether the intervention had a beneficial or harmful effect on the patient, nurse, or organization.

Outcome measures — a metric of the results of an intervention or change process.

Out-of-pocket model — In nations that are too poor to have any formalized health care, rich citizens pay out of pocket for health care, whereas the poor citizens cannot afford care and usually stay sick or die.

PARIHS (Promoting Action on Research Implementation in Health Services) framework — A framework describing the factors that contribute to successful implementation of evidence. It can be described as SI = f(E, C, F), where SI is successful implementation of evidence, f = function of, E is evidence, C is context, and F is facilitation.

Patient education — The process by which health professionals and others impart information to patients for the purpose of empowering them to make decisions that will improve their health status.

Patient preference — The right of an individual to be involved in the planning of his or her own care and ultimately having the final say about which interventions he or she chooses to accept or not accept. A patient's values, desires, and contributions to clinical decision making in the evidence-based practice process.

Patient Protection and Affordable Care Act (PPACA) — A recently enacted, large bill in the United States with many provisions that may change over time. Although the law is currently being challenged in the courts, and it is difficult to predict what will be the final outcome, it includes provisions to enhance effective health practices in the United States.

Patient-mediated strategies — Strategies to actively engage patients to improve their knowledge, experience, service use, health behavior, and health status.

Pay-for-performance — Reimbursement based on outcomes.

Peer-reviewed journals — Journals containing scholarly articles are approved through a peer-review process of multiple reviewers who hold advanced degrees within the discipline, teach within the field, are experts in the profession, and are very knowledgeable about the topic.

Person — Individuals, families, communities, and the integrated aspects of the biophysical, psychological, sociological, and spiritual person/family/community.

Persuasive research utilization — Using research to influence others.

Phenomenon of interest — The part of a patient's experience that you want to understand.

PICO question — A question about the effectiveness of interventions in which *P* represents population, *I* equals intervention, *C* stands for comparison intervention, and *O* is outcome.

PICo question — A question in which *P* represents population, *I* stands for phenomena of interest, and *Co* stands for context.

Pluralistic approach — In evidence-based practice, accepting evidence from quantitative and qualitative research as well as discourse as legitimate sources of evidence.

Population — The group of people that are of concern in the question. This group may be related by a disease, a health condition, risk profile, the environment in which they exist, age, or any combination of these factors.

Potential adopters — Practitioners, policy makers, patients, and other stakeholders who may accept or play a role in change guided by evidence.

Practice environment — Setting and social factors in which a change will occur; includes governing rules and cultural and social factors such as local politics, power structures, resource availability, leadership approaches, and peer groups.

Pre-appraised, digested evidence — Evidence sources where someone else has already done the hard work of searching, appraising, and summarizing the evidence.

Pre-appraised evidence — Evidence that has already been appraised and ranked for its quality and/or strength.

Predictive framework or model — Forecast of how phenomena will behave and how they relate to each other and tend to generate propositions and hypotheses.

Pressure ulcer — Localized injury to the skin and/or underlying tissue, usually over a bony prominence, as a result of pressure or pressure in combination with shear.

Printed information sheets — Printed patient information sheets prior to discharge that describe medications.

Prevalence — The ratio (for a given time period) of the number of occurrences of a disease or event to the number of units at risk in the population.

Primary source or primary study — An article or report in which researchers publish data they collected first hand.

Problem-solving — Defining problem and cause, generating alternative solutions, selecting alternative solutions, carrying out solutions, and evaluating effects.

Professional standards — Appropriate standards of care based on the Nursing Scope and Standards of Practice developed by professional organizations.

Process measures — Metrics for assessing what is being done.

Prompts — Cues in the clinical setting to enhance attention to an intervention.

Prospective data — Observations or data collected going forward in time.

Public Health Resource Unit (PHRU) — A division of the United Kingdom's National Health Service that provides Critical Appraisal Skills Program (CASP) tools.

Public policy — Whatever governments choose to do, or choose not to do.

PubMed — 30 million citations for biomedical literature from MEDLINE, life science journals, and online books. Citations may include links to full-text content from PubMed Central and publisher Web sites.

PubMed Central — A free Internet resource made available by the U.S. National Institutes of Health (NIH) and managed by the National Center for Biotechnology Information (NCBI) at the National Library of Medicine. It provides access to MEDLINE's 18 million abstracts and limited full-text articles from participating journals, publisher Web sites, and other Internet sites.

PubMed Central's Clinical Queries — A place to search for free, full-text systematic reviews within the National Library of Medicine's database, PubMed.

Qualifications — A quality/accomplishment that fits a person for some function.

Qualitative research — Methods of inquiry that include an array of methodologies that attempt to explore the meaning and experience of phenomena.

Questions of appropriateness — Clinical questions that address how appropriate a given activity or intervention is related to the context in which the care is given.

Questions of effectiveness — Clinical questions that relate to the efficacy of interventions on patient outcomes.

Questions of feasibility — Clinical questions that relate to the extent a particular activity would be practical or practicable.

Questions of meaningfulness — Clinical questions that address how people experience a particular phenomenon.

Randomized controlled trial (RCT) — An experimental research design in which the investigator randomly assigns participants in a trial to either a treatment or control (no treatment) group.

Randomized controlled trial (RCT) with concealed randomization — RCT in which participants are blindly assigned to a treatment or control group and the researcher manipulates whether or not the group receives the treatment or control.

RAPid — Formerly a program from JBI used to perform rapid appraisals of primary research. JBI no longer maintains the software but offers the rapid appraisal tools on their Web site.

Rapid critical appraisal — A method allowing clinicians to quickly appraise evidence to determine its validity and applicability to practice, and a user-friendly critical appraisal approach.

Readability — How easy it is to read and understand written material.

Regression equation — A statistical technique that is used to predict the behavior of a dependent variable.

Reliability — A quality of measurement that refers to consistency or reproducibility including two observers measuring consistent results (inter-rater reliability), within an instrument (internal reliability) or over time with the same instrument (test-retest reliability)

Relative data — a way of measuring rates where the numerator represents the number of cases and denominator is the number in the population of interest.

Reminders — An embedded memory aid.

Research — A diligent and systematic inquiry or investigation into a subject to discover or revise facts, theories, applications, etc.

Research knowledge — Knowledge gained through investigation.

Research process — A formal, systematic process of identifying and developing an area of inquiry and a research question, and using a methodology to generate data to answer the question.

Research utilization — A complex process in which knowledge, in this case in the form of research, is transformed from the findings of one or more studies into possible nursing interventions, the ultimate goal of which is use in practice.

Respect for patients' values — To give particular attention or regard to what patients deem important.

Retrospective data — data gathered after whatever is being assessed has already happened.

Review of the literature (ROL) — Encompasses a strategic search for current knowledge on a given subject. A person searches literature on a specific topic to find out what has been published on the subject. Depending on the focus, the search may include multiple databases within multiple disciplines. The results of the search may include informational articles, research findings, and theoretical papers.

Rigor — In the context of research, the degree that the researchers ensure high-quality methods are used that lead to valid or credible results or findings.

Safe sleep — Providing a sleeping environment for infants that lowers the risk of accidental suffocation or strangulations that includes a firm, flat sleeping surface free from loose blankets, sheets, crib bumpers, toys and placement of the infant on his/her back.

Safety huddle — Brief, regular meetings of those involved in patient care to address new or existing threats to safety.

School health nurse — A professional nurse who provides health services in schools.

School health provider — A broader term for people who provide health services in schools.

School health services — Services provided to children and sometimes families through the school.

Scale — Relates to how much of the scope of the issue you wish to address.

Scope — Relates to the breadth of the question. You might define scope in terms of setting, population, age, group, or other category.

Search strategy — The plan to find evidence in various databases that includes the keywords, how to link keywords together and filter sources by their type, year of publication, language, etc.

Secondary sources — Report on the work of others, not on the author's own original research findings.

Shared decision making — A decision-making process jointly shared by patients and their health-care provider; it is a key part of evidence-based practice because it brings together clinical expertise and patient preference.

Shared governance — A structural configuration of councils and committees that provides formal mechanisms that ensures nurses' responsibility, right, and power to make decisions and to control nursing practice.

Single-payer system — A system in which only a single entity pays the bill.

Skill set — A set of basic techniques that you need to carry out a task.

Social contract — The explicit or implicit obligations nurses meet in their relationship with patients and their families.

Special cause variation — non-random variation or irregularities in a process that are not inherent to the process.

Social policy — Policies that address things such as welfare, crime, education, and health care.

Standards of nursing practice — Authoritative statement by which the nursing profession describes the responsibilities for which its practitioners are accountable; the outcomes for which registered nurses are responsible; and by which the quality of practice, service, or education can be evaluated.

Standardized subject headings — Specific subject terms developed by the Library of Congress to organize large subjects logically into categories.

State Children's Health Insurance Program (SCHIP) — Funded by both the federal government and the states to provide health care to children whose families earn too much income to qualify for Medicaid but do not have enough money to pay for private insurance.

Strength (of evidence) — Relates to the quality or believability of the evidence.

Structure measures — Ways of assessing elements in a particular context such as characteristics of the physical facility, equipment, human resources, and organizational characteristics like training, payment, etc.

Structural supports — Supports that help nurses achieve expected performance levels and externalize the internal cultural value for evidence-based nursing practice.

Sudden infant death syndrome (SIDS) — One subgroup of SUID that is the sudden death of an infant less than one year of age that remains unexplained even after a thorough investigation including an autopsy, examination of the death scene and review of the clinical history.

Sudden unexpected infant death (SUID) — A broad term for any unexpected death of an infant less than 1 year of age in which the cause of death is not obvious before investigation, often occurring during sleep.

Synopses — Short, abridged summaries of a longer source of evidence.

Syntheses — Systematic reviews of quantitative or qualitative evidence that follow explicit methods of search, appraisal, and analysis of the evidence.

Systematic reviews — A rigorous secondary research method that incorporates a comprehensive search, critical appraisal, and synthesis of either quantitative or qualitative research; it addresses a focused clinical question using methods designed to reduce the likelihood of bias.

Tacit knowledge — Implicit or unspoken knowledge largely associated with expertise, experience, and tradition.

Theory-guided practice — The use of theory to describe, predict, and explain the phenomena important to nursing for the purpose of improving practice.

Tradition — An inherited pattern of thought or action that leads to a specific, long-standing practice.

Transferability — The degree to which the results of the study can be applied to other contexts.

Transparent — When an evidence source is transparent, the authors provide a great deal of details about purpose and methods so that someone else might reproduce the study or systematic review.

TRICARE — A program that provides health coverage to all military retirees, their spouses, survivors, and other qualified dependents.

Truncation — A symbol, typically an asterisk (*) in bibliographic databases, that can be applied to the end of a keyword to retrieve all the words beginning with the letters before the truncation symbol.

Unit practice councils — A formal venue to allow nurses to voice their concerns and be involved in making practice changes. They allow for the exploration of practice issues and create opportunities for supporting evidence-based practice.

U.S. Department of Health and Human Services (HHS) — The federal agency with primary responsibility of protecting the health of Americans and providing essential human services, especially for the most needy.

Validity — The quality of a measurement that represents how well the assessment truly represents the phenomenon.

Veterans Health Administration (VHA) — A federally funded and administered program for veterans. Health care is delivered in government-run health-care facilities.

Western Interstate Commission on Higher Education (WICHE) Project — Like the Conduct and Utilization of Research in Nursing (CURN) Project, a national project aimed at increasing nurses' utilization of research.

Wildcards — A symbol, typically a question mark in bibliographic databases, that can be inserted within a word to retrieve all the words with alternate spellings of the same word.

Workplace violence — Violence or the threat of violence against workers.

World Health Organization (WHO) — WHO is the directing and coordinating authority for health within the United Nations system. It is responsible for providing leadership on global health matters, shaping the health research agenda, setting norms and standards, articulating evidence-based policy options, providing technical support to countries, and monitoring and assessing health trends.

Worldview — Frame of reference and how we fit our experiences into our representation of the world

Index